Early Life Stage Mortality Syndrome in Fishes of the Great Lakes and Baltic Sea

Support for the publication of this proceedings was provided by

Great Lakes Fishery Commission

Early Life Stage Mortality Syndrome in Fishes of the Great Lakes and Baltic Sea

Edited by

Gordon McDonald
McMaster University

John D. Fitzsimons
Department of Fisheries and Oceans

Dale C. Honeyfield
U.S. Geological Survey

American Fisheries Society Symposium 21

Proceedings of the Symposium
Early Mortality Syndrome: Reproductive Disruptions in Fish of the Great Lakes, New York Finger Lakes, and the Baltic Region

Held at Dearborn, Michigan, USA
28 August 1996

American Fisheries Society
Bethesda, Maryland
1998

The American Fisheries Society Symposium series is a registered serial. Suggested citation formats follow.

Entire book

McDonald, G., J. D. Fitzsimons, and D. C. Honeyfield, editors. 1998. Early life stage mortality syndrome in fishes of the Great Lakes and Baltic Sea. American Fisheries Society, Symposium 21, Bethesda, Maryland.

Article within the book

Brown, S. B., D. C. Honeyfield, and L. Vandenbyllaardt. 1998. Thiamine analysis in fish tissues. Pages 73–81 *in* G. McDonald, J. D. Fitzsimons, and D. C. Honeyfield, editors. Early life stage mortality syndrome in fishes of the Great Lakes and Baltic Sea. American Fisheries Society, Symposium 21, Bethesda, Maryland.

The photograph of the larval salmonid on the cover was provided by Gun Åkerman, Institute of Applied Environmental Research, Laboratory for Aquatic Ecotoxicology, Stockholm University.

Library of Congress Catalog Card Number: 98-71305
ISBN 1-888569-08-5
ISSN 0892-2284

Printed in the United States of America on acid-free paper

American Fisheries Society
5410 Grosvenor Lane, Suite 110
Bethesda, Maryland 20814-2199, USA

Contents

Preface

Ever since the pioneering work of George Burdick in the 1960s on DDT-related mortality affecting early life stages of lake trout, there has been an increased awareness and appreciation of the sensitivity of embryonic stages to environmental stressors. In the 1970s and 1980s, John Gunn's seminal work on acid precipitation showed the extreme vulnerability of early life stages of lake trout to acidic runoff. In the 1990s still more evidence of the sensitivity of early life stages was provided in the elegant work of Mary Walker and Richard Peterson on the extreme susceptibility of larval lake trout to 2,3,7,8-tetrachlorodibenzo-*p*-dioxin and its establishment as a prototypical chlorinated organic toxicant. Given this history, we should not be surprised by the elevated occurrence of early mortality syndromes (EMS) now occurring in the progeny of various Great Lakes salmonids; however, it is unusual that these syndromes show so little relationship with anthropogenic toxicants. Indeed, the current mortality syndromes seem to have occurred during a period of reduced contaminant levels, with no direct human involvement, and in contrast seem to have been generated by the very food webs on which the affected species have depended for nourishment for many decades. It is noteworthy that EMS has been present for some time and while the causal factors that have generated the current epizootics of EMS remain to be clearly identified, a threshold has evidently been crossed in recent times. The consequences of this new set of conditions is evident in the high levels of EMS occurring in salmonids throughout the Great Lakes. Yet the problem extends beyond the Great Lakes: it affects salmonids in the New York Finger Lakes where it is called Cayuga Syndrome and the Baltic Sea where it is called M74.

Against this backdrop and with the increasing realization of the threat to hatchery-reared and wild salmonids posed by EMS, a special symposium was held at the 1996 Annual Meeting of the American Fisheries Society in Dearborn, Michigan. With the generous support of the Great Lakes Fishery Commission, 20 scientists from Canada, the United States, and Sweden were brought together for a one-day symposium to present their work on various aspects of early mortality syndromes. This book, which contains 18 of those papers, represents the end result of the presentations made at that symposium. Our intent is to provide the reader with comprehensive information on EMS in all its forms, its etiology, and recommendations for future research.

The completion of this book has involved an enormous effort by all of the authors, who were aided by the thoughtful and constructive reviews of many others. We gratefully acknowledge and thank the AFS Editorial Office staff, especially Stephen Kilduff and Janet Harry for their editing and typesetting, Bob Rand for the cover layout design, and Beth Staehle for her leadership. We are grateful to all of these individuals for the diligence and patience they have shown in bringing this project to fruition. Finally, we are indebted to Randy Eshenroder who has been a catalyst for the symposium, the book, and the continued dedication of many to improving the future of freshwater fisheries.

Gordon McDonald
John Fitzsimons
Dale Honeyfield

Reviewers

The editors thank the following people who contributed technical reviews of the manuscripts.

Ira Adelman	*University of Minnesota*
Patric Amcoff	*Swedish University of Agricultural Sciences*
Paul Brown	*Purdue University*
Scott Brown	*Environment Canada*
Paul Bowser	*Cornell University*
Bengt-Erik Bengtsson	*Stockholm University*
Douglas Conklin	*University of California-Davis*
Randy Eshenroder	*Great Lakes Fishery Commission*
Samuel Felton	*University of Washington*
Jeff Fisher	*Pacific Environmental Technologies*
John Fryer	*Oregon State University*
Ronald Hardy	*University of Idaho-Hagerman*
John Hnath	*Michigan Department of Natural Resources*
Christer Hogstrand	*University of Kentucky*
Mike Hornung	*University of Wisconsin-Madison*
Chris Kennedy	*Simon Fraser University*
Jenny Lundström	*Swedish University of Agricultural Sciences*
Susan Marcquenski	*Wisconsin Department of Natural Resources*
Douglas McFarland	*South Dakota State University*
Scott McKinley	*University of Waterloo*
Ken Minns	*Department of Fisheries and Oceans*
Arthur Niimi	*Department of Fisheries and Oceans*
Leif Norrgren	*Swedish University of Agricultural Sciences*
Vince Palace	*University of Manitoba*
Peter Pärt	*University of Uppsala*
Annette Pettersson	*University of Uppsala*
Annika Salama	*University of Helsinki*
Roy Stein	*Ohio State University*
Don Tillitt	*Biological Research Division, U.S. Geological Survey*
Glen Van der Kraak	*University of Guelph*

Symbols and Abbreviations

The following symbols and abbreviations may be found in this book without definition. Also undefined are standard mathematical and statistical symbols given in most dictionaries.

A	ampere
AC	alternating current
Bq	becquerel
C	coulomb
°C	Celsius
cd	candela
cm	centimeter
Co.	Company
Corp.	Corporation
cov	covariance
DC	direct current; District of Columbia
D	dextro configuration
d	day
d	dextrorotary
df	degrees of freedom
dL	deciliter
E	east
E	expected value
e	base of natural logarithm
e.g.,	for example
eq	equivalent
et al.	(et alii) and others
etc.	et cetera
eV	electron volt
F	filial generation; Farad
°F	degrees Fahrenheit
fc	footcandle (0.0929 lx)
ft	foot (30.5 cm)
ft^3/s	cubic feet per second ($0.0283\ m^3/s$)
g	gram
G	giga (10^9, as a prefix)
gal	gallon (3.79 L)
Gy	gray
h	hour
ha	hectare (2.47 acres)
hp	horsepower (746 W)
Hz	hertz
in	inch (2.54 cm)
Inc.	Incorporated
i.e.,	that is
IU	international unit
J	joule
K	Kelvin (degrees above absolute zero)
k	kilo (10^3, as a prefix)
kg	kilogram
km	kilometer
l	levorotary
L	levo configuration
L	liter (0.264 gal, 1.06 qt)
lb	pound (0.454 kg, 454g)
lm	lumen
log	logarithm (specify base)
Ltd.	Limited
lx	lux (10.8 fc)
M	mega (10^6, as a prefix); molar (as a suffix or by itself)
m	meter (as a suffix or by itself); milli (10^{-3}, as a prefix)
mi	mile (1.61 km)
min	minute
mol	mole
N	newton; normal; north
N	sample size
NS	not significant
n	ploidy; nanno (10^{-9}, as a prefix)
o	ortho (as a chemical prefix)
oz	ounce (28.4 g)
P	probability
p	para (as a chemical prefix)
p	pico (10^{-12}, as a prefix)
Pa	pascal
pH	negative log of hydrogen ion activity

ppm	parts per million (in the metric system, use mg/L, mg/kg, etc.)
ppt	parts per thousand
qt	quart (0.946 L)
R	multiple correlation or regression coefficient
r	simple correlation or regression coefficient
rad	radian
S	siemens (= mho, Ω^{-1}); south (for geography)
s	second
SD	standard deviation
SE	standard error
sr	steradian
T	tesla
tris	tris(hydroxymethyl)-aminomethane (a buffer)
UK	United Kingdom
U.S.	United States (adjective)
USA	United States of America (noun)
V	volt
V, Var	variance (population)
var	variance (sample)
W	watt (for power); west (for geography)
Wb	weber
yd	yard (0.914 m, 91.4 cm)
α or P_α	probability of type I error (false rejection of null hypothesis)
β	probability of type II error (false acceptance of null hypothesis)
Ω	ohm
μ	micro (10^{-6}, as a prefix)
$'$	minute (angular)
$''$	second (angular)
$^\circ$	degree (temperature as a prefix, angular as a suffix)
%	per cent (per hundred)
‰	per mille (per thousand)

American Fisheries Society Symposium 21:1–7, 1998

Introduction and Overview of Early Life Stage Mortality

DALE C. HONEYFIELD
Biological Resources Division, U.S. Geological Survey
Research and Development Laboratory, RR #4 Box 63
Wellsboro, Pennsylvania 16901, USA

JOHN D. FITZSIMONS
Bayfield Institute, Department of Fisheries and Oceans
867 Lakeshore Road, Box 5050, Burlington, Ontario L7R 4A6, Canada

SCOTT B. BROWN
Environment Canada, Canadian Centre for Inland Waters
867 Lakeshore Road, Box 5050, Burlington, Ontario L7R 4A6, Canada

SUSAN V. MARCQUENSKI
Wisconsin Department of Natural Resources, Box 7921, Madison, Wisconsin 53707, USA

GORDON MCDONALD
Department of Biology, McMaster University
1280 Main Street West, Hamilton, Ontario L8S 4K1, Canada

Early mortality syndrome (EMS) is the term now widely used to describe mortality affecting early life stages of various salmonid species in the Laurentian Great Lakes, particularly in Lakes Michigan and Ontario and, to a lesser extent, in Lakes Huron and Erie. The species affected include coho salmon *Oncorhynchus kisutch*, chinook salmon *O. tshawytscha*, steelhead or rainbow trout *O. mykiss*, brown trout *Salmo trutta*, and lake trout *Salvelinus namaycush*. The mortality rates are in excess of those attributable to poor fertilization, overripening of eggs, rearing environment, husbandry, or infectious disease. The clinical signs of EMS include loss of equilibrium, swimming in a spiral pattern, lethargy, hyperexcitability, and hemorrhage before death. For the most part, the symptoms develop just before and at first feeding. Early mortality syndrome in coho salmon and other salmonids was present in hatcheries in the 1960s, with mortality rates around 20% or less, and was compensated for by increasing the egg take at spawning (Marcquenski and Brown 1997). However, beginning in the early 1990s, mortality rates attributable to EMS in feral coho salmon rose dramatically in Lake Michigan hatcheries, to 60–90% (Figure 1; J. Hnath and M. Wolgamood, Michigan Department of Natural Resources, Fish Health Laboratory, personal communication). Similar syndromes have been reported for Atlantic salmon *Salmo salar* from the Finger Lakes in New York State (termed Cayuga syndrome; Fisher et al. 1995) and for Atlantic salmon in the Baltic Sea (termed M74 for the year in which it was first reported; Johansson et al. 1995). In recent years, mounting losses of Baltic salmon offspring to M74 (Figure 2; H. Börjeson, Swedish Salmon Research Institute, personal communication) have paralleled those for coho salmon (Figure 1). These mortality syndromes are entirely confined to eggs collected from feral broodstock in all affected regions. Eggs derived from broodstock maintained on commercial feeds do not exhibit these mortalities.

A common connection among the mortality syndromes (EMS, Cayuga syndrome, and M74) is that eggs of affected stocks have very low thiamine levels and that sac fry mortality can be dramatically reduced by therapeutic thiamine treatments of eggs or sac fry. Until new information is forthcoming, we consider these three early life stage mortality syndromes to be synonymous in that they result from a thiamine deficiency. Nevertheless, there may be aspects of early life stage mortality that are specific to a species, and there may be more than one possible mechanism by which the thiamine deficiency develops.

The link between early life stage mortality and thiamine was first demonstrated by Fitzsimons (1995), who found that immersing affected sac fry in thiamine increased survivability in the 1992 year-class of Lake Ontario lake trout. Subsequently, Fisher et al. (1996b) established the effectiveness of thiamine treatments for the 1993 year-class of Atlantic salmon from Cayuga Lake, and Bylund and

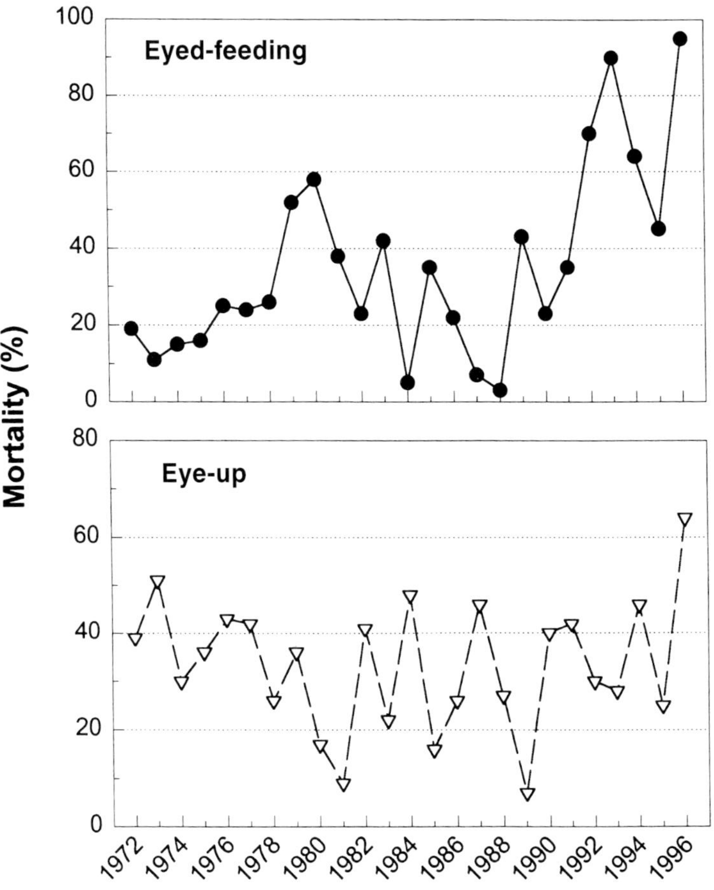

FIGURE 1.—Early life stage mortality in coho salmon family groups from Lake Michigan, 1972–1996. The top panel shows the mortality between eyed egg and feeding fry (**Eyed–feeding**), and the bottom panel shows mortality occurring from fertilization to eye-up (**Eye-up**). Data supplied by J. Hnath and M. Wolgamood, Michigan Department of Natural Resources, Fish Health Laboratory.

Lerche (1995) demonstrated it for the 1994 year-class of Baltic salmon. More recently, Hornung et al. (1996) reduced mortality from EMS in Great Lakes coho salmon and steelhead with thiamine treatments. Immersion of eggs and presymptomatic and postsymptomatic fry in thiamine has proven to be a highly effective treatment for progeny reared in hatcheries, and it is now routine practice at hatcheries that use feral broodstock to stock salmon into Lake Michigan and the Baltic Sea. Without these treatments, mortality rates for the progeny of feral broodstock could be as high as 100% for some species (Atlantic salmon in the Finger Lakes) and more than 60–90% for others (Marcquenski and Brown 1997), which would seriously compromise the sport and commercial fisheries that are dependent on this stocking.

Symposium Results

We gathered together investigators from both North America and Scandinavia for a 1-day symposium at the 1996 American Fisheries Society annual meeting in Dearborn. The purpose of this symposium was to review current research on present day early life stage mortality with a focus on thiamine deficiency: its symptoms, its treatment, and, most importantly, its causes. The papers presented in McDonald et al. (1998, this volume) describe EMS and M74 (chapters 2–7); thiamine analysis methods for biological tissues (chapters 8 and 9); thiamine levels in the food chain (chapters 10 and 17), in adults (chapters 8, 9, 11, and 12), and in early life stages (chapters 3, 9, 12, and 13); thiamine dynamics in individuals

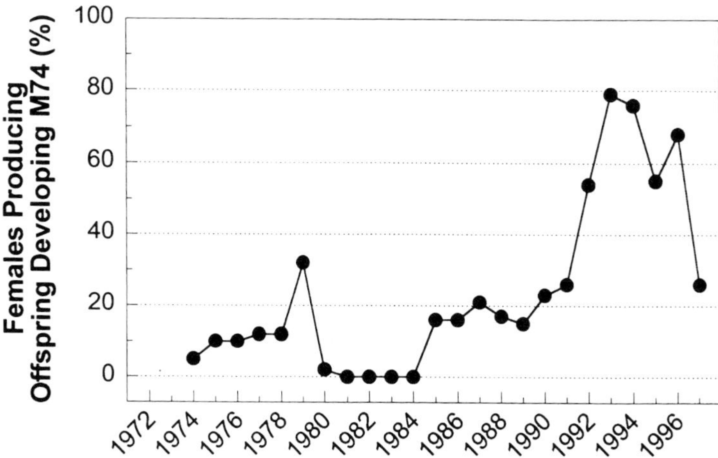

FIGURE 2.—Percentage of M74 among family groups of three different Baltic salmon populations representative of those inhabiting the Swedish part of the Baltic region. From 1974 to 1986, data are based on 100–200 family groups yearly, and from 1987 to 1996, data are based on 300–400 family groups yearly. Data supplied by H. Börjeson, Swedish Salmon Research Institute.

(chapter 11); potential causal agents of early life stage mortality, including interactions with contaminants (chapters 14 and 15) and thiaminase activity in forage fish species (chapters 15 and 16); development of treatment protocols for EMS based on thiamine immersion (chapters 5 and 13); and progress toward development of a laboratory model of EMS based on a thiamine antagonist, amprolium (chapter 18).

Based on the symposium presentations and other recent studies, we can now make the following generalizations:

1. Early life stage mortality will occur when egg thiamine levels are below certain thresholds (Fisher et al. 1996a; Amcoff et al. 1998b; Brown et al. 1998; Honeyfield et al. 1998a, all this volume).
2. Thiamine treatment of fry and eggs has proven therapeutically effective for a wide range of salmonids (Fitzsimons 1995; Fisher et al. 1996a; Amcoff et al. 1998a; Hornung et al. 1998, both this volume).
3. Other B vitamins (Fitzsimons 1995), ascorbic acid, and minerals (Fisher et al. 1996a; Honeyfield et al. 1998a) do not appear to be involved in the syndrome and are not therapeutically effective.
4. Carotenoids and other antioxidants are correlated to the presence of M74 in the Baltic (Börjeson and Norrgren 1997; Pettersson and Lignell 1998, this volume), but similar relationships have yet to be established for North American salmonids exhibiting EMS (Fisher et al. 1996a; Hornung et al. 1998; Palace et al. 1998, this volume).
5. Direct connections between EMS and hatchery practices, genetics, or pathogens have proven difficult to substantiate, despite repeated attempts (Fisher et al. 1995; Fitzsimons et al. 1995; Marcquenski and Brown 1997).

Future Research Needs

The symposium clearly reinforced the idea that EMS is a problem related to nutrition in the wild, the effects of which can only partially be offset by hatchery rearing practices. Not only does EMS jeopardize the stability of stocking programs based on feral broodstocks, but, more importantly, it undoubtedly impairs recruitment of lake resident populations (C. Edsall, U.S. Geological Survey, Great Lakes Science Center, personal communication), many of which in the Great Lakes are already experiencing low reproductive success. The extent of the effect of EMS in limiting reproduction relative to other factors is unknown because key indicators of effects in wild populations have not yet been developed. Conceivably, EMS is a major impediment to the restoration of self-sustaining natural populations in at least three systems: the Great Lakes, the Finger Lakes, and the Baltic Sea. Furthermore, the precise cause of the thiamine deficiency is unknown. It is clear, however, that the deficiency is not the result of low dietary thiamine per se (Fitzsimons et al. 1998, this volume); rather, it appears to be caused by the presence in the diet of some factor(s) such as thiaminase that acts to reduce the bioavailability of thiamine, either by destroying it or by converting it to an inactive analog or thiamine antagonist.

Does Forage Fish Thiaminase Prevent Sustainable Reproduction in Salmonid Populations?

In the Great Lakes, there is mounting evidence implicating alewife *Alosa pseudoharengus* and possibly smelt *Osmerus mordax* in the adult diet as a factor in the production of thiamine-deficient broodstock and eggs. Alewife and smelt as well as the Baltic sprat *Sprattus sprattus* are known to contain a thiamine-degrading enzyme, thiaminase (Gnaedinger 1964; Gnaedinger and Krzeczkowski 1966; Anglesea and Jackson 1985; Ji and Adelman 1998, this volume). Alewife and smelt represent a major dietary component for salmon and trout in the Finger Lakes and the Great Lakes (Miller and Holey 1992; Jones et al. 1993; Fisher et al. 1995). Recent surveys of lake trout and Atlantic salmon from several locations encompassing a variety of prey species support the hypothesis that low thiamine levels in the eggs are correlated with a diet rich in alewife (Fisher et al. 1996a; Fisher et al. 1998; Fitzsimons and Brown 1998, both this volume). This is particularly apparent in the Finger Lakes, where an exclusive diet of alewife appears to be the sole factor responsible for Cayuga syndrome in Atlantic salmon (Fisher et al. 1998). Although alewife have long been known to possess thiaminase activity (see Ji and Adelman 1998), the presence of this activity in this species is without a good biological explanation. One possibility is production from gut bacteria (D. Honeyfield, unpublished data), which would mean that thiaminase levels could vary independently of other changes in the fish species, including abundance, and its relative importance as a forage source. This type of mechanism offers a plausible explanation for the recent surge in early life stage mortality despite declining alewife abundance in some lake systems.

Unfortunately, although Ji and Adelman (1998) identified thiaminase activity in alewife and smelt samples collected in the spring and fall of 1987 from Lakes Superior, Michigan, and Huron, no measurements have been made during the recent surge in EMS. Thus, there is a critical need to examine thiaminase and thiamine levels in prey fish and how they may change temporally, spatially, seasonally, or with other factors.

Can a Thiamine Deficiency Be Produced in the Laboratory and Does it Result in EMS?

Feral salmonids in the Great Lakes have thiamine-deficient eggs that develop EMS, but the two may not be related. The most direct way to test whether low thiamine is causing EMS is to reproduce a thiamine deficiency under laboratory conditions. Ji et al. (1998, this volume) were unable to reduce blood thiamine pyrophosphate concentrations in parental lake trout using a diet lacking thiamine but could lower blood levels if frozen alewife were included in the diet. Honeyfield et al. (1998b, this volume) and Fynn-Aikins et al. (in press) reported a significant reduction in egg thiamine concentrations in lake trout and Atlantic salmon, respectively, by including the thiamine antagonist amprolium in the diet. In the Atlantic salmon study, fry mortality exceeded control mortality and appeared to represent a low level of EMS. Although these laboratory studies have been very useful in guiding the development of a thiamine deficiency model, so far neither the extremely low levels of thiamine reported for wild fish (see, for example, Amcoff et al. 1998b) nor the overt clinical symptoms and pathological characteristics (see, for example, Lundstrom et al. 1998, this volume) of EMS, Cayuga syndrome, or M74 have been unequivocally reproduced in the laboratory.

Thus, there is a critical need for a laboratory model for thiamine deficiency and EMS. Such a model will facilitate studies of thiamine dynamics and transport by a postulated carrier protein, the role of endocrine disruptors in EMS, and the effects of thiamine deficiency on natural spawning behavior.

Are There Thiamine–Contaminant Interactions?

Thiamine may have functions other than as an essential cofactor for thiamine-containing enzymes. For example, thiamine may participate in the metabolism of xenobiotics. Although it is not the case with Cayuga syndrome in Finger Lakes Atlantic salmon, EMS and M74 are more prevalent in contaminated systems, which implies possible contaminant–thiamine interactions (e.g., contaminants may increase the thiamine requirement of early life stages). Consequently, contaminant effects may be expressed only when bioavailability of thiamine is low. For example, D. E. Tillett (U.S. Geological Survey, Midwest Science Center, personal communication) found that thiamine treatments could reduce dioxin-induced embryo toxicity. Elevated hepatic mixed function oxidase (Norrgren et al. 1993) and lower concentrations of antioxidants in sac fry that develop M74 (Börjeson and Norrgren 1997) also suggest the possible involvement of dioxin-like contaminants. Moreover, between 1988 and 1992, Finnish researchers showed a correlation between increases in some dioxin-like contaminants and M74 (Paasivirta et al. 1995). In the Great Lakes, direct relationships between EMS or Cayuga syndrome and contaminants (Mac et al. 1993; Fitzsimons et al. 1995; Fisher et al. 1996b; Cook et al. 1997; Marcquenski and Brown 1997; Honeyfield et al. 1998a) or antioxidants (Palace et al. 1998) have been difficult to substantiate. However, there are insufficient data to exclude sublethal effects of contaminants or possible interaction with thiamine deficits. Contaminants such as PCBs and DDT, which accumulate in top predator species such as the salmonids, are known to reduce thiamine levels in laboratory rats (Yagi et al. 1979; Stacpoole et al. 1990). Despite the fact that the levels of chlorinated compounds have declined (P. Cook, U.S. Environmental Protection Agency, personal communication), they may still be an important factor when thiamine concentrations are very low.

Other Research Questions

The as yet unexplained nature of EMS prompts a whole host of questions, which are briefly enumerated below:

What are the sublethal effects of thiamine deficiency in adults and progeny? Aside from behavioral abnormalities ("wiggling") observed in parental Baltic salmon (Amcoff et al.1998b) and coho salmon from Lake Michigan (J. Hnath, Michigan Department of Natural Resources, Fish Health Laboratory, personal communication), the potential long-term consequences to swim-up fry surviving EMS are completely unknown.

Are other species that consume alewife experiencing reproductive difficulties that might be associated with thiamine deficits? Preliminary studies by George Ketola (U.S. Geological Survey, Tunison Laboratory, personal communication) have found relatively low egg thiamine levels in walleye *Stizostedion vitreum* from Lake Erie, which may be linked to reduced reproductive success in this species (D. Busch, U.S. Fish and Wildlife Service, personal communication).

What is the mechanism of thiamine transport within the adult female? What is the role of a putative thiamine carrier protein in that transport?

What link might there be between thiamine deficiency and environmental change? Do environmental factors such as starvation stress and changes in available algal species affect the thiamine and thiaminase content of prey species? What role might blue-green algae play as a source of thiaminase?

Are antioxidant compounds reduced or deficient when thiamine is low and mortality is high? What are the concentrations of individual vitamins that can be considered normal in wild fish reproducing naturally or thought to be unaffected by contaminants and other factors?

How does contaminant-induced oxidative stress factor into the pathogenesis of early life stage mortality?

Conclusion

Finally, one is left with the overall impression that EMS represents a new paradigm in environmental problems. In place of overt toxicity, we now may be seeing combinations of sublethal assaults that alone are relatively innocuous but that in concert severely affect a species. We are thus led to wonder what has happened in the last decade that has brought about an increase in early life stage mortality while contaminant levels are either stable or declining, and what could explain the apparent similarity between the Baltic Sea and the Great Lakes.

References

Amcoff, P., H. Börjeson, R. Eriksson, and L. Norrgren. 1998a. Effects of thiamine treatments on survival of M74-affected feral Baltic salmon. Pages 31–40 *in* McDonald et al. (1998).

Amcoff, P., H. Börjeson, J. Lindeberg, and L. Norrgren. 1998b. Thiamine concentrations in feral Baltic salmon exhibiting the M74 syndrome. Pages 82–89 *in* McDonald et al. (1998).

Anglesea, J. D., and A. J. Jackson. 1985. Thiaminase activity in fish silage and moist fish feed. Animal Feed Science and Technology 13:39–46.

Börjeson, H., and L. Norrgren. 1997. M74 syndrome: a review of potential etiological factors. Pages 153–166 *in* R. M. Rolland, M. Gilbertson, and R. E. Peterson, editors. Chemically induced alterations in functional development and reproduction of fishes. SETAC (Society of Environmental Toxicology and Chemistry), Pensacola, Florida.

Brown, S. B., J. D. Fitzsimons, V. P. Palace, and L. Vandenbyllaardt. 1998. Thiamine and early mortality syndrome in lake trout. Pages 18–25 *in* McDonald et al. (1998).

Bylund, G., and O. Lerche. 1995. Thiamine therapy of M 74 affected fry of Atlantic salmon *Salmo salar*. Bulletin of the European Association of Fish Pathologists 15:93–97.

Cook, P. M., E. Zabel, and R. Peterson. 1997. The TCDD toxicity equivalence approach for characterization of early life stage mortality risks associated with exposures of trout to TCDD and related chemicals. Pages 9–27 *in* R. M. Rolland, M. Gilbertson, and R. E. Peterson, editors. Chemically induced alterations in functional development and reproduction of fishes. SETAC (Society of Environmental Toxicology and Chemistry), Pensacola, Florida.

Fisher, J. P., S. Brown, P. R. Bowser, G. A. Wooster, and T. Chiotti. 1996a. Continued investigations into the role of thiamine and thiaminase-rich forage in the Cayuga syndrome of New York's landlocked Atlantic salmon. Pages 79–81 *in* B.-E. Bengtsson, C. Hill, and S. Nellbring, editors. Report from the second workshop on reproduction disturbances in fish. Swedish Environmental Protection Agency Report 4534, Stockholm.

Fisher, J. P., S. B. Brown, S. Connelly, T. Chiotti, and C. C. Krueger. 1998. Interspecies comparisons of blood thiamine in salmonids from the Finger Lakes, and effect of maternal size on blood and egg thiamine in Atlantic salmon with and without Cayuga syndrome. Pages 112–123 *in* McDonald et al. (1998).

Fisher, J. P., J. Fitzsimons, G. F. Combs, Jr., and J. M. Spitsbergen. 1996b. Naturally occurring thiamine deficiency causing reproductive failure in Finger Lakes Atlantic salmon and Great Lakes lake trout. Transactions of the American Fisheries Society 125:167–178.

Fisher, J. P., and six coauthors. 1995. Reproductive failure of landlocked Atlantic salmon from New York's Finger Lakes: investigations into the etiology and epidemiology of the "Cayuga syndrome." Journal of Aquatic Animal Health 7:81–94.

Fitzsimons, J. D. 1995. The effect of B-vitamins on a swim-up syndrome in Lake Ontario lake trout. Journal of Great Lakes Research 21(Supplement 1):286–289.

Fitzsimons, J. D., and S. B. Brown. 1998. Reduced egg thiamine levels in inland and Great Lakes lake trout and their relationship with diet. Pages 160–171 *in* McDonald et al. (1998).

Fitzsimons, J. D., S. B. Brown, and L. Vandenbyllaardt. 1998. Thiamine levels in food chains of the Great Lakes. Pages 90–98 *in* McDonald et al. (1998).

Fitzsimons, J. D., S. Huestis, and B. Williston. 1995. Occurrence of a swim-up syndrome in Lake Ontario lake trout in relation to contaminants and cultural practices. Journal of Great Lakes Research 21(Supplement 1):277–285.

Fynn-Aikins, K., P. R. Bowser, D. C. Honeyfield, J. D. Fitzsimons, and H. G. Ketola. In press. Effect of dietary amprolium on tissue thiamin and Cayuga Syndrome in Atlantic salmon. Transactions of American Fisheries Society.

Gnaedinger, R. H. 1964. Thiaminase activity in fish: an improved assay method. Fishery Industrial Research 2:55–59.

Gnaedinger, R. H., and R. A. Krzeczkowski. 1966. Heat inactivation of thiaminase in whole fish. Commercial Fisheries Review 28(8):11–14.

Honeyfield, D. C., J. G. Hnath, J. Copeland, K. Dabrowski, and J. H. Blom. 1998a. Correlation of nutrients and environmental contaminants in Lake Michigan coho salmon with incidence of early mortality syndrome. Pages 135–145 *in* McDonald et al. (1998).

Honeyfield, D. C., K. Fynn-Aikins, J. D. Fitzsimons, and J. A. Mota. 1998b. Effect of dietary amprolium on egg and tissue thiamine concentrations in lake trout. Pages 172–177 *in* McDonald et al. (1998).

Hornung, M. W., L. Miller, R. E. Peterson, S. V. Marcquenski, and S. Brown. 1996. Evaluation of nutritional and pathogenic factors in early mortality syndrome in Lake Michigan salmonids. Pages 82–83 *in* B.-E. Bengtsson, C. Hill, and S. Nellbring, editors. Report from the second workshop on reproduction disturbances in fish. Swedish Environmental Protection Agency Report 4534, Stockholm.

Hornung, M. W., L. Miller, R. E. Peterson, S. Marcquenski, and S. B. Brown. 1998. Efficacy of thiamine, astaxanthin, β-carotene, and thyroxine treatments in reducing early mortality syndrome in Lake Michigan salmonid embryos. Pages 124–134 *in* McDonald et al. (1998).

Ji, Y. Q., and I. R. Adelman. 1998. Thiaminase activity in alewives and smelt in Lakes Huron, Michigan, and Superior. Pages 154–159 *in* McDonald et al. (1998).

Ji, Y. Q., J. J. Warthesen, and I. R. Adelman. 1998. Thiamine nutrition, synthesis, and retention in relation to lake trout reproduction in the Great Lakes. Pages 99–111 *in* McDonald et al. (1998).

Johansson, N., P. Jonsson, O. Svanberg, A. Sodergren, and J. Thulin. 1995. Reproduction disorders in Baltic fish. Swedish Environmental Protection Agency Report 4347, Solna.

Jones, M. L., J. F. Koonce, and R. O'Gorman. 1993. Sustainability of hatchery-dependent salmonine fisheries in Lake Ontario: conflicts between predator demand and supply. Transactions of the American Fisheries Society 122:1008–1018.

Lundström, J., H. Börjeson, and L. Norrgren. 1998. Clinical and pathological studies of Baltic salmon suffering from yolk sac fry mortality. Pages 62–72 *in* McDonald et al. (1998).

Mac, M. J., T. R. Schwartz, C. C. Edsall, and A. M. Frank. 1993. Polychlorinated biphenyls in Great Lakes trout and their eggs: relations to survival and congener composition 1979–1988. Journal of Great Lakes Research 19:752–756.

Marcquenski, S. V., and S. B. Brown. 1997. Early mortality syndrome (EMS) in salmonid fishes from the Great Lakes. Pages 135–152 *in* R. M. Rolland, M. Gilbertson, and R. E. Peterson, editors. Chemically induced alterations in functional development and reproduction of fishes. SETAC (Society of Environmental Toxicology and Chemistry), Pensacola, Florida.

McDonald, G., J. D. Fitzsimons, and D. C. Honeyfield, editors. 1998. Early life stage mortality syndrome in fishes of the Great Lakes and Baltic Sea. American Fisheries Society, Symposium 21, Bethesda, Maryland.

Miller, M. A., and M. E. Holey. 1992. Diets of lake trout inhabiting nearshore and offshore Lake Michigan environments. Journal of Great Lakes Research 18:51–60.

Norrgren, L., T. Andersson, P. A. Bergqvist, and I. Bjorklund. 1993. Chemical, physiological and morphological studies of feral Baltic salmon (*Salmo salar*) suffering from abnormal fry mortality. Environmental Toxicology and Chemistry 12:2065–2076.

Paasivirta, J., and six coauthors. 1995. TCDD-toxicity and M74 syndrome of Baltic salmon (*Salmo salar L.*). Organohalogen Compounds 25:355–359.

Palace, V. P., S. B. Brown, C. L. Baron, J. D. Fitzsimons, and J. F. Klaverkamp. 1998. Relationships between induction of the phase I enzyme system and oxidative stress: relevance for lake trout from Lake Ontario and early mortality syndrome of their offspring. Pages 146–153 *in* McDonald et al. (1998).

Pettersson, A., and Å. Lignell. 1998. Low astaxanthin levels in Baltic salmon exhibiting the M74 syndrome. Pages 26–30 *in* McDonald et al. (1998).

Stacpoole, P. W., and six coauthors. 1990. Chronic toxicity of dichloroacetate: possible relation to thiamine deficiency in rats. Fundamental and Applied Toxicology 14:327–337.

Yagi, N., K. Kamohara, and Y. Itokawa. 1979. Thiamin deficiency induced by polychlorinated biphenyls (PCB) and dichlorodiphenyltrichloroethane (DDT) administration to rats. Journal of Pathology and Toxicology 2:1119–1125.

American Fisheries Society Symposium 21:8–17, 1998

Reproductive Disturbances in Baltic Fish: A Review

LEIF NORRGREN[1] AND PATRIC AMCOFF
Department of Pathology, Faculty of Veterinary Medicine, Swedish University of Agricultural Sciences, Box 7028, S-750 07 Uppsala, Sweden

HANS BÖRJESON
Swedish Salmon Research Institute, S-814 94 Älvkarleby, Sweden

PER-OLOV LARSSON
Institute of Marine Research, S-453 21 Lysekil, Sweden

Abstract.—Populations of Baltic salmon *Salmo salar* and cod *Gadus morhua* are facing acute threats because of poor reproduction. The salmon is afflicted with high yolk sac fry mortality, and the incidence of cod larvae mortality is high. There are also indications that anadromous Baltic brown trout *Salmo trutta* populations are affected by reproductive disorders. These top predators have significant ecological, economic, and socioeconomic importance. Other species are also suffering from poor reproductive success and declining populations. Burbot *Lota lota* populations are locally affected by inadequate sexual maturation, resulting in a failure to spawn; gonad anomalies have also been described in roach *Rutilus rutilus*. High egg mortality has been recorded for whiting *Merlangius merlangus*, flounder *Platichtys flesus*, and herring *Clupea harengus*. Attempts have been made to discover the cause of reproductive disorders in Baltic fish species, but the available data suggest several possible causes, both abiotic and biotic. Species with pelagic eggs such as cod and flatfish are dependent on salinity and oxygen concentrations, factors that often limit the volume of reproduction in the Baltic Sea. A variety of biotic causes (i.e., infectious diseases, parasitism, and toxic algae) have been shown to affect species such as roach and herring. There are indications that nutritional factors (i.e., thiamine and astaxanthin) are involved in the cause of the yolk sac fry mortality syndrome affecting the Baltic salmon. Furthermore, anthropogenic activities causing both local point sources (i.e., metals and persistent organic pollutants) and long-range transport and deposition of acidic rain and pesticides must also be considered as potential threats to Baltic fish species.

The Baltic Sea, one of the largest brackish seas in the world, is under severe ecological pressure as a result of industrialization, urbanization, agriculture, forestry, and hydrologic and climatic conditions. The drainage area, which is four times the area of the Baltic Sea, is inhabited by more than 100 million people. The Baltic Sea is divided into a few major basins, with the deepest parts in the Baltic proper. It is connected to the North Sea by the Kattegat and the Danish straits, both of which have constituting shelves restricting the inflow of salt water from the North Sea (Figure 1). Salinity decreases from 10–20‰ in the Kattegat Strait to 3–5‰ in the northern Gulf of Bothnia, forming a salinity gradient that affects the distribution of several species. Well-defined haloclines and thermoclines stratify the water mass. The biological diversity is low, with few but relatively abundant species forming simple food chains. The Baltic cod *Gadus morhua* is the most important species for Swedish commercial fisheries, contributing about 50% of the total value of commercial fishing, which was estimated at US$60 million in 1991. Anadromous Baltic salmon *Salmo salar* and brown trout *S. trutta* are also valuable species; their commercial value in sea and coastal fisheries is estimated at $3 million. The socioeconomic value of these species in coastal and river fisheries, however, is more important; it is estimated at between $3 and $30 million annually.

The capacity of the Baltic Sea ecosystem to withstand environmental disturbances is poor. Many species are living at the edge of their range, and there are numerous alarming signs concerning the health of the ecosystem. The Baltic Sea is directly and indirectly affected by many different environmental problems. Eutrophication (Rosenberg et al. 1990), acidification of spawning areas for several species of anadromous fish, halogenated hydrocarbons (Jansson et al. 1993), and heavy metal contamination are among the best known threats to aquatic life. Furthermore, other potential environmental threats such as leaking canisters of war gases dumped after

[1] To whom reprint requests should be addressed.

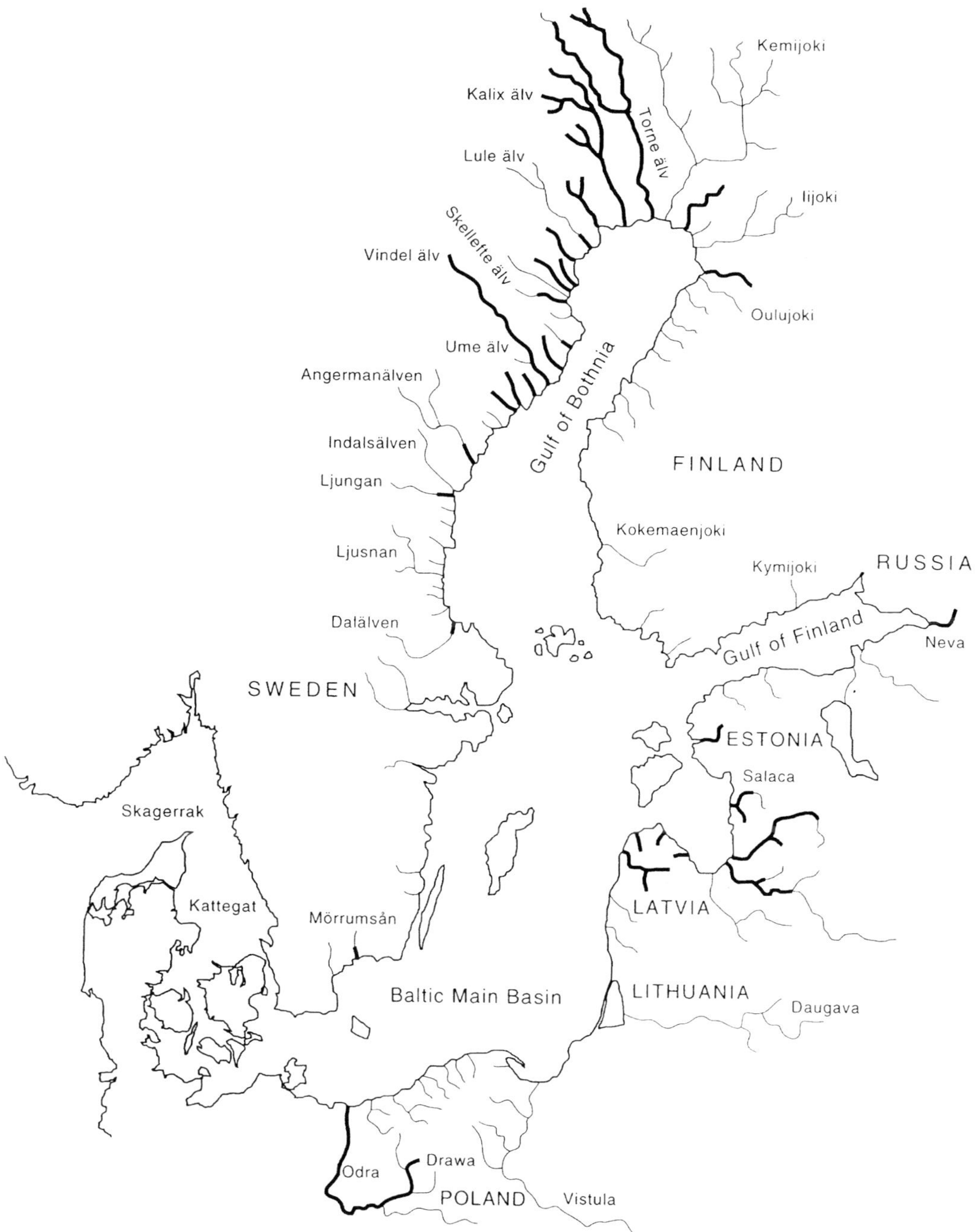

FIGURE 1.—The Baltic Sea. The rivers with naturally reproducing salmon populations are indicated by dark lines. (From Ackefors et al. 1991.)

the First World War (Henriksson et al. 1996), recently introduced industrial chemicals (brominated flame retardants, plasticizers, antifouling agents), and altered nutritional food webs attributable to the algal blooms caused by eutrophication also must be considered.

Vertebrates at higher trophic levels in the Baltic Sea have suffered from different types of environmentally induced diseases in recent decades. The number of grey seals *Halicoerus grypus* decreased dramatically during the 1960s, and the white-tailed sea eagle *Haliaeetus albicilla* was affected by poor reproduction (Helander et al. 1982). Reproductive failure in both seals and eagles has been correlated to a high body burden of persistent chloroorganic pollutants, including PCBs and DDT (Jensen et al. 1969; Helle et al. 1976). During the 1990s, stabilization of populations of both seals and sea eagles has been recorded. However, a variety of Baltic fish species have been shown to be affected by different types of environmental distress, especially reproductive disorders affecting both individuals and population levels. The Baltic Sea is inhabited by typical freshwater species (e.g., burbot *Lota lota*, perch *Perca fluviatilis*, and roach *Rutilus rutilus*). These species live in the same regions as marine species such as turbot *Scophthalmus maximus* and cod. In addition, anadromous species including salmon and brown trout inhabit these regions. During the period 1970–1997, different types of reproductive disorders, including inadequate gonad maturation, low fecundity, and early life stage mortality, were documented for a number of fish species in the Baltic Sea and in some major tributaries that constitute important spawning areas for anadromous species. The purpose of this paper is to summarize the situation for Baltic fish species with regard to reproductive disorders and early life stage mortality during the period 1970–1997.

Affected Baltic Fish Species

Baltic Cod

The two Baltic cod stocks, the eastern and the western (Bagge et al. 1994), have adapted to the low salinity in the Baltic Sea, but only to a certain extent. The eastern stock can reproduce in a salinity from 11‰ and upward (Nissling and Vallin 1996a). Higher salinities than that normally occur below the halocline (60–80 m) in the deeper basins of the Baltic proper, the Gdansk Basin, and the Gotland Basin (Figure 1). In the deeper waters of the Baltic Sea, however, low oxygen concentrations often limit reproductive success. Therefore, the term "reproduction volume" has been established (Larsson 1990); this is defined as the volume of water with conditions amenable to cod reproduction, that is, a sufficient salinity and oxygen concentration (>2.5 mg/L) for fertilization and embryo and larvae development. Reproduction volume varies between years and within spawning seasons. Salinity is normally increased by inflows of North Sea water via the Kattegat every 1–3 years (Matthäus and Lass 1995). In 1976–1977, very large inflows occurred, resulting in a number of large cod year-classes. The stocks increased to a maximum during the early 1980s, with a peak catch of 450,000 tons in 1984. However, after 1977 no major inflows of Atlantic water occurred until 1993. Since 1981, recruitment has decreased continuously, and this, together with overfishing, has led to a dramatic decline of the cod stocks (B. Sjöstrand, Institute of Marine Research, unpublished data, 1995). In 1993, the catch was only about 10% of the 1984 level. In 1991–1993, recruitment was far less than what was expected from the extent of the reproduction volumes. In 1979, Grauman and Sukhorukova (1982) found abnormal embryos of cod, and the frequency of abnormal embryos has increased steadily since then. In a comparison between cod from the Baltic and the Skagerrak, Pickova (1997) found that asymmetry was much more common in the early cleavage stages of eggs of Baltic cod. Asymmetric eggs from Skagerrak and Baltic cod raised for 24 months in Skagerrak water had a significantly lower hatching rate, and no difference in hatching rate was found for eggs from Baltic cod that spent <7 months in Skagerrak water. The numbers of symmetric eggs found in these groups, however, were so small that a reliable statistical evaluation was impossible. In rearing experiments, hatching rates have consistently been lower for eggs of Baltic cod than for those of Skagerrak cod (Pickova and Larsson 1992; Nissling et al. 1994; Pickova et al. 1996) and Barents Sea cod (Åkerman et al. 1996a, 1996b), indicating that spawn from the Baltic is of lower quality. On the whole, the indications of reproductive disturbances in Baltic cod are so strong that such an effect must be considered in assessment work and in management of the stocks.

Baltic Salmon

The Baltic salmon belongs to the Atlantic salmon species but is genetically isolated from the populations living in the North Atlantic (Ståhl 1987). At the beginning of this century, more than 60 rivers draining into the Baltic Sea had naturally reproducing salmon stocks. Damming in connection with construction of hydroelectric power plants has reduced the number of rivers available for natural salmon reproduction to about 20. The reduction of spawning areas, together with intensive sea fishing, has decreased recruitment of naturally reproduced smolts from 5 million to less than 0.5 million per year (Ackefors et al. 1991). In Sweden, a technique to rear smolt in hatcheries was developed during the 1950s, and smolts have been released to compensate for the losses of river production resulting from damming (Karlsson and Karlström 1994). In the mid-1980s, about 5.5 million hatchery-reared smolts were released annually from Swedish and Finnish salmon hatcheries to the Baltic Sea (Ackefors et al. 1991).

In 1974, a high incidence of yolk sac fry mortality was reported for the first time in Swedish compensatory fish farms (Börjeson et al. 1994). This phenomenon was designated the M74 syndrome and increased dramatically during the early 1990s. A peak in mortality was recorded in 1993, when 72% of the progeny from Swedish hatcheries died from M74. During the period 1994–1996, the mortality decreased slowly to 60%, and in 1997, it decreased further to 30%. Similar figures have been reported from Finnish salmon hatcheries (Soivio 1996). Electrofishing surveys in rivers with naturally reproducing salmon populations show low abundance of parr, indicating that these populations may be affected by the M74 syndrome (Karlsson and Karlström 1994). The M74 syndrome is linked to the progeny of certain females and develops during the yolk sac resorption process (Norrgren et al. 1993; Börjeson et al. 1994; Lundström et al. 1996). During this period, the yolk sac fry pass through a preclinical stage and enter the clinical stage, characterized by aggravating neurological symptoms. A few weeks after the first symptoms have been observed, the entire family group is dead. In addition to M74, since 1990–1991 feral spawning salmon caught for compensatory rearing programs have displayed wiggling and uncoordinated behavior. The behavior in the brood fish is strongly correlated to the development of M74 in their offspring (Börjeson et al. 1994; Amcoff et al. 1998, this volume). There are no indications that the M74 syndrome is caused by rearing conditions or infectious agents. An elevated activity in the cytochrome P450-dependent enzyme ethoxyresorufin-*O*-deethylase has been shown in yolk sac fry that develop M74 (Norrgren et al. 1993), which may indicate a possible role of toxic substances in the cause of this syndrome. Furthermore, yolk sac fry that develop M74 have been shown to have a deficiency in thiamine (vitamin B_1; Amcoff et al. 1998). The deficiency is treatable by immersion of the eggs or newly hatched yolk sac fry of the affected family groups in thiamine-enriched water (Bylund and Lerche 1995; Amcoff et al. 1996). Today, some Swedish salmon hatcheries use this method as a means to produce smolts in sufficient quantities. At present, it is too early to evaluate the consequences of this strategy because the future effect of thiamine immersion on roe and yolk sac fry cannot be predicted. Furthermore, naturally reproducing salmon populations cannot be treated with thiamine in this way.

Brown Trout

Vallin (1996) reported variances in egg and yolk sac fry survival in anadromous brown trout from a natural habitat, and there are indications that brown trout suffer from symptoms resembling those of M74. This has been noted sporadically in a few hatcheries where brown trout are reared in compensatory programs similar to those for Baltic salmon. A disturbance of brown trout reproduction is supported by electrofishing surveys that indicate decreased numbers of parr in a few important natural reproduction habitats. The documentation is not as extensive, however, as that for salmon. Another disturbance affecting brown trout and the Baltic salmon is hybridization. A high frequency of hybrids (41.5%) has been found in a restored section of the Dalälven River (Jansson and Öst 1997), and similarly high frequencies have also been detected in rivers with naturally reproducing populations (H. Jansson, Salmon Research Institute, personal communication).

Other Fish Species

There are numerous reports concerning other Baltic fish species affected by reproductive disorders (Table 1). In the southern part of the Baltic Sea, species with pelagic eggs (e.g., flounder *Platichtys flesus*, plaice *Pleuronectes platessa*, and whiting *Merlangius merlangus*) suffer from high egg mortality, low hatching rates, and different types of abnormalities (Westernhagen et al. 1981, 1988, 1989). In 1979, Grauman and Sukhorukova (1982) found the first abnormal embryos of sprat *Sprattus sprattus*. High mortality in herring *Clupea harengus* has been attributed to toxic algae (Aneer 1987), emissions from metal industries (Oulasvirta 1990), and chlorinated hydrocarbons (Hansen et al. 1985). Sprat and herring constitute the two most important food items for salmon, brown trout, and cod. In fourhorn sculpin *Myoxocephalus quadricornis* living in

TABLE 1.—Reproductive disturbances in Baltic fish; UDN denotes ulcerative dermal necrosis and PAH denotes polyaromatic hydrocarbons.

Species	Disturbance	References
Baltic flounder *Platichtys flesus*	Reduced hatching success correlated to ΣPCBs, embryo malformations	Westernhagen et al. 1981, 1988
Brown trout *Salmo trutta*	Indications of poor recruitment, adult spawning fish affected by UDN, hybridization with Baltic salmon	Johansson et al. 1982; Vallin 1996; Jansson and Ost 1997
Burbot *Lota lota*	Reduced spawning success, immature gonad maturation; acidification, elevated levels of PAHs and heavy metals as probable cause	Wit et al. 1990; Pulliainen et al. 1992; Kjellman et al. 1994
Cod *Gadus morhua*	Prolonged spawning period, poor recruitment, delayed hatching, abnormal embryos with spinal deformities, parasitic infestations, DNA adducts	Grauman and Sukhorukova 1982; Westernhagen et al. 1988; Larsson 1990; Pickova and Larsson 1992; Buchmann et al. 1993; Pedersen et al. 1993; Bagge et al. 1994; Nissling et al. 1994; Wieland et al. 1994; Akerman et al. 1996a, 1996b; Ericson et al. 1996; Nissling and Vallin 1996a, 1996b; Pickova et al. 1996, 1997; Vallin and Nissling 1996
Eelpout *Zoarces viviparus*	Abnormal progeny; high levels of PAHs as probable cause	Jacobsson et al. 1993; Ojaveer and Tanner 1996
Fourhorn sculpin *Myoxocephalus quadricornis*	Vertebral deformities related to pulp mill effluents	Hardig et al. 1988; Bengtsson 1991
Herring *Clupea harengus*	Reduced spawning period, egg mortality resulting from PAHs and heavy metals	Hansen et al. 1985; Aneer 1987; Oulasvirta 1990
Northern pike *Esox lucius*	Skeletal jaw deformities	Lindesjoo and Thulin 1992
Perch *Perca fluviatilis*	Poor recruitment, larval and skeletal deformities, larval mortality	Andersson et al. 1988; Sandstrom et al. 1988, 1991; Sandstrom 1994; Karas et al. 1991
Plaice *Pleuronectes platessa*	Embryo mortality and malformation	Westernhagen et al. 1988
Roach *Rutilus rutilus*	Immature gonad maturation, reduced gonadal growth, hermaphrodism, oocyte degeneration	Sandstrom et al. 1988; Luksiene and Sandstrom 1994; Wiklund and Bylund 1994
Salmon *Salmo salar*	M74 syndrome, high yolk-sac fry mortality; deficiency in vitamins B_1 and A, adult spawning fish displaying wiggling behavior correlated (99%) to M74, hybridization with brown trout, UDN	Norrgren et al. 1993; Borjeson et al. 1994, 1996; Karlsson and Karlstrom 1994; Bylund and Lerche 1995; Amcoff et al. 1996, 1998, this volume; Lundstrom et al. 1996, 1998, this volume; Soivio 1996; Jansson and Ost 1997; Vourinen et al. 1997
Sprat *Sprattus sprattus*	Larval abnormalities	Grauman and Sukhorukova 1982
Turbot *Scophthalmus maximus*	Endoparasite infestations causing larval mortality	Pedersen 1993
Whiting *Merlangius merlangus*	Reduced hatching success correlated to ΣDDT, dieldrin, and ΣPCBs	Westernhagen et al. 1989

pulp mill effluent areas, severe curving of the vertebral column was common (Härdig et al. 1988; Bengtsson 1991). Jacobsson et al. (1993) and Ojaveer and Tanner (1996) showed that eelpout *Zoarces viviparus* with high body burdens of polyaromatic hydrocarbons gave rise to deformed progeny. Local populations of burbot in the Bothnian Bay failed to spawn in the years 1987–1990 because of incomplete gonad maturation (Pulliainen et al. 1992). In some estuaries, the percentage of nonmaturing burbot was as high as 93–100%. The only location in the investigated region with a high degree of mature fish (100%) was the Tornio River at Pajala, 150 km from the river mouth in the Gulf of Bothnia, a location that is relatively uninfluenced by anthropogenic activities; this finding suggests the involvement of contaminants in the decreased maturation rates elsewhere in the region. Reduced spawning success of burbot as a result of acidification has also been described (Kjellman et al. 1994). Local populations of perch living close to pulp and paper mill effluents have been shown to be affected by poor recruitment (Karås et al. 1991), larval deformities, and mortality (Sandström et al. 1988, 1991; Sandström 1994). Reduced gonadal development, acute fin erosion, and indications of ovarian atresia have also been recorded (Sandström et al. 1988). The abnormalities decreased with increased distance from the source of the emissions. Serious gonadal anomalies with oocyte atresia and tissue degeneration have been recorded in roach stocks of Finnish coastal waters. In some cases, the gonads display hermaphrodism, with both male and female genital products being found in different parts of the same ovary (Wiklund and Bylund 1994). Reduced gonad growth in roach is also documented in areas with pulp mill effluents (Sandström et al. 1988). Oocyte degeneration, asynchronic gonad and oocyte growth, and an increased variation in gonad development affect local roach populations living in cooling water discharges (Luksiene and Sandström 1994).

Possible Causes and Explanations of Reproductive Disorders and Population Disturbances

Abiotic Factors

Reproductive disorders in Baltic fish species must be considered in light of the specific conditions that characterize the Baltic Sea ecosystem. The subarctic environment with long winters, ice cover and low water temperatures, low oxygen concentrations, and the reduced salinity gradient from south to north may have a negative effect on early development in certain species. During the 20th century, periods of oxygen depletion of some areas of the Baltic Sea have resulted in anoxia in benthic habitats and, thus, loss of biological productivity. In recent decades, the situation has worsened because of a combination of low saltwater inflow and increased eutrophication. For species with pelagic eggs, such as cod, low salinity has been shown to increase the vertical distribution of larvae (Nissling et al. 1994). The avoidance of stressful oxygen conditions by maintenance of egg buoyancy is an important factor for successful spawning in Baltic cod (Nissling and Vallin 1996b). In recent years, because of reduced salinity, cod eggs have been most abundant below the halocline (50–80 m), where oxygen levels are less suitable (Wieland et al. 1994; Nissling and Vallin 1996b). Consequently, the concentration of oxygen may play an important role in the survival of Baltic cod embryos (Wieland et al. 1994).

Biotic Factors

Important biotic factors that affect recruitment include parasitism, infectious diseases, malnutrition, and eutrophication resulting in altered primary production and, consequently, altered food webs. Parasitic infestations may cause larval mortality in Baltic cod (Buchmann et al. 1993; Pedersen et al. 1993) and turbot (Pedersen 1993). Brown trout and salmon are occasionally affected by ulcerative dermal necrosis, a fungal infection that causes high mortality during their migration in their native rivers for spawning (Johansson et al. 1982). In Baltic salmon afflicted with M74, lowered concentrations of carotenoids (Börjeson et al. 1994; Börjeson and Norrgren 1997; Pettersson and Lignell 1998, this volume), thiamine (Amcoff et al. 1998), tocopherol, and ubiquinone (Börjeson and Norrgren 1997) have been recorded. The causes of these sometimes severely lowered levels may be ecological, resulting from alterations in the community composition of algae and microorganisms of the Baltic Sea ecosystem. Baltic herring also are affected by high egg mortality, which has been suggested to be caused by algae exudates associated with eutrophication (Aneer 1987).

Chemical Contamination

Chloroorganic materials such as DDT, PCBs, tetrachlorodibenzodioxins/furans and other highly persistent bioaccumulative compounds are widespread in the Baltic Sea ecosystem and generally at higher levels than in adjacent saltwater areas (Koistinen et al. 1989). These pollutants come from atmospheric deposition (Falandysz 1994), pulp mill effluents, and other point sources. A variety of halogenated hydrocarbons accumulate in fish, particularly in fat-rich fish such as the Baltic salmon (Paasivirta et al. 1995; Larsson et al. 1996). Larval deformities and increased mortality in pelagic eggs of plaice, flounder, whiting, and herring have been suggested to be caused by these compounds (Westernhagen et al. 1981, 1988, 1989; Hansen et al. 1985). Baltic flounder eggs with total concentrations (Σ) of PCBs exceeding 120 ng/g (weight per weight, w/w) showed reduced survival, and at concentrations near or higher than 250 ng/g, the viable hatch was less than 15% (Westernhagen et al. 1981). In whiting, the ovarian threshold values for the major contaminants ΣDDT, dieldrin, and ΣPCBs were 20, 10, and 200 ng/g (w/w), respectively, giving rise to abnormal mortality (>90%) (Westernhagen et al. 1989). In Baltic herring, 18 ng of 1,1-dichloro-2,2-bis(*p*-chlorophenyl)ethane per gram of ovary (w/w) reduced reproductive success, and similar effects were recorded with ΣPCB values of 240 ng per gram of ovary (w/w; Hansen et al. 1985). High concentrations of polychlorinated dibenzodioxins/furans and heavy metals such as cadmium, copper, and lead were suggested to be responsible for inadequate maturation of burbot in the Gulf of Bothnia (Wit et al. 1990; Pulliainen et al. 1992). Pulp mill effluents contain many different environmentally active compounds, including chlorinated hydrocarbons, resin acids, dissolved nutrients, and dissolved and particulate organic matter (Karås et al. 1991). These substances may cause a variety of responses, including eutrophication and toxic stress (Karås et al. 1991; Sandström 1994). The debate regarding pulp mill effluents has mainly concerned chloroorganic compounds and their effects on biota. In the Baltic Sea, a number of abnormalities have been observed in fish living close to pulp mill effluents, including skeletal jaw deformities in northern pike *Esox lucius* (Lindesjöö and Thulin 1992) and vertebral curvature in perch (Sandström et al. 1991) and fourhorn sculpin (Härdig et al. 1988; Bengtsson 1991). Several studies have found induced activities of the cytochrome P450-dependent enzyme system in Baltic cod compared with Barents Sea cod (Åkerman et al. 1996a) and in fish exposed to pulp mill effluents, such as perch (Andersson et al. 1988; Karås et al. 1991), roach, and bream *Abramis brama* (Lindström-Seppä and Oikari 1990). There is also evidence of increased rates of larval mortality and malformed embryos in perch (Karås et al. 1991) and reduced gonad growth in roach and perch (Sandström et al. 1988). Sandström (1994) reported improved survival rates in perch, which he attributed to improved technical methods in the pulp and paper mills that resulted in decreased emissions of chloroorganic compounds. The concentrations of metals in the Baltic Sea are similar in magnitude to those in the North Atlantic. However, there are some reports of high concentrations of metals involved in reproductive disorders, such as in burbot in the Bothnian Bay (Wit et al. 1990; Pulliainen et al. 1992) and in high egg mortality in Baltic herring in the Gulf of Bothnia (Oulasvirta 1990).

Effect of Commercial Fishing

Two-thirds of the annual catch of Baltic salmon is taken in unselective offshore fisheries on a mixed stock of hatchery-reared and naturally reproducing salmon (Swedish Salmon Research Institute, Annual Report, 1995, unpublished data). The latter constitutes one-tenth of the total stock biomass. The pressure on naturally reproducing populations has been severe because of the high fishing pressure (Karlsson and Karlström 1994). The situation for the cod has also been worsened by commercial fishing, mainly for the large spawning cod (Bagge et al. 1994). Today, large Baltic cod are rare, and because there seems to be a relationship between the size of cod and success in spawning, high fishing pressure on large cod may have resulted in decreased recruitment (Vallin and Nissling 1996).

Conclusions and Future Perspectives

Human activities resulting in eutrophication and pollution of the Baltic Sea must be further evaluated. A search for the possible causes of fish reproductive disorders in major species, such as cod, salmon, and brown trout, and population declines in other species must be undertaken using a multidisciplinary approach. The complex interrelations between fluctuations in the fish ecosystem and other specific characteristics of the Baltic Sea also should be considered. The significance of various chloroorganic micropollutants and their metabolites must be evaluated in aquatic food chains, especially with regard to biomagnification, biotransformation, and interactions with different antioxidant systems. Fluctuations in primary production and variations in species composition of algae must also be considered because several species of algae that produce toxins such as cyanobacteria have been shown to affect fish (Aneer 1987). It must be understood that production of reactive metabolites is an integral part of both detoxification and normal biological processes and that it is highly controlled by antioxidant defenses, which normally cope with the free radicals generated. Only when there is an imbalance between free radical production and the protective antioxidant-dependent systems does damage occur, as seen in the relatively high occurrence of DNA adducts in Baltic cod eggs and larva, which indicates an uncontrolled production of free radicals (Ericson et al. 1996). The concentrations of many xenobiotics have decreased in Baltic fauna during recent decades since substances such as PCBs and DDT were banned (Olsson and Reutergårdh 1986; Bignert et al. 1995).

There are indications, however, that during this period other types of substances have also decreased in a similar or more extensive manner, as exemplified by reduced concentrations of vitamins in Baltic salmon affected by the M74 syndrome (Börjeson et al. 1994, 1996; Börjeson and Norrgren 1997; Amcoff et al. 1998; Pettersson and Lignell 1998). This relatively larger decrease in essential substances, which are of vital importance in detoxification systems, may explain the imbalance between reactive metabolites and antioxidants and, thus, the dramatic increase in reproductive disorders in Baltic fish species. The complex situation in the Baltic Sea is also indicated by recent investigations showing increased concentrations of coplanar PCBs (CB77, CB126, CB169) and two of the most toxic polychlorinated dibenzofurans in muscle tissue of Finnish salmon during the early 1990s (Paasivirta et al. 1995; Vourinen et al. 1997). This further complicates the assessment of the effect of chloroorganic pollutants and other toxic substances on biota in the Baltic Sea.

References

Ackefors, H., N. Johansson, and B. Wahlberg. 1991. The Swedish compensatory programme for salmon in the Baltic: an action plan with biological and economic implications. ICES Marine Science Symposium 192:109–119.

Åkerman, G., and six coauthors. 1996a. Studies of reproductive disorders in cod *(Gadus morhua)* and salmon (*Salmo salar*), using biomarkers, indicate environmental pollution as the common cause. Pages 63–64 *in* Bengtsson et al. (1996).

Åkerman, G., and five coauthors. 1996b. Comparison of reproductive success of cod, *Gadus morhua*, from the Barents Sea and Baltic Sea. Marine Environmental Research 42:139–144.

Amcoff, P., H. Börjeson, J. Lindeberg, and L. Norrgren. 1998. Thiamine concentrations in feral Baltic salmon exhibiting the M74 syndrome. Pages 82–89 *in* G. McDonald, J. D. Fitzsimons, and D. C. Honeyfield, editors. Early life stage mortality syndrome in fishes of the Great Lakes and Baltic Sea. American Fisheries Society, Symposium 21, Bethesda, Maryland.

Amcoff, P., L. Norrgren, H. Börjeson, and J. Lindeberg. 1996. Lowered concentrations of thiamine (vitamin B1) in M74-affected feral Baltic salmon (*Salmo salar*). Pages 38–39 *in* Bengtsson et al. (1996).

Andersson, T., L. Förlin, J. Härdig, and Å. Larsson. 1988. Physiological disturbances in fish living in coastal water polluted with bleached kraft pulp mill effluent. Canadian Journal of Fisheries and Aquatic Sciences 45:1525–1536.

Aneer, G. 1987. High natural mortality of Baltic herring (*Clupea harengus*) eggs caused by algal exudates. Marine Biology 94:163–169.

Bagge, O., F. Thurow, E. Steffensen, and J. Bay. 1994. The Baltic cod. Dana 10:1–28.

Bengtsson, Å. 1991. Effects of bleached pulp mill effluents on vertebral defects in fourhorn sculpin (*Myoxocephalus quadricornis* L.) in the Gulf of Bothnia. Archiv fuer Hydrobiologie 121:373–384.

Bengtsson, B.-E., C. Hill, and S. Nellbring, editors. 1996. Report from the second workshop on reproduction disturbances in fish. Swedish Environmental Protection Agency Report 4534, Stockholm.

Bignert, A., and five coauthors. 1995. Time-related factors influence the concentrations of DDT, PCBs and shell parameters in eggs of Baltic guillemot (*Uria aalge*), 1861–1989. Environmental Pollution 89:27–36.

Buchmann, K., J. L. Larsen, and I. Dalsgaard. 1993. Diseases and injuries associated with mortality of hatchery-reared Baltic cod (*Gadus morhua*) larvae. Acta Veterinaria Scandinavica 3:385–390.

Bylund, G., and O. Lerche. 1995. Thiamine therapy of M74 affected fry of Atlantic salmon *Salmo salar*. Bulletin of the European Association of Fish Pathologists 15(3):93–97.

Börjeson, H., L. Förlin, and L. Norrgren. 1996. Investigation of antioxidants in salmon affected by the M74 syndrome. Pages 95–96 *in* Bengtsson et al. (1996).

Börjeson, H., and L. Norrgren. 1997. The M74 syndrome: a review of etiological factors. Pages 153–166 *in* R. M. Rolland, M. Gilbertson, and R. E. Peterson, editors. Chemically induced alterations in functional development and reproduction of fishes. SETAC (Society of Environmental Toxicology and Chemistry), Pensacola, Florida.

Börjeson, H., L. Norrgren, T. Andersson, and P.-A. Bergqvist. 1994. The Baltic salmon-situation in the past and today. Pages 14–25 *in* L. Norrgren, editor. Reproduction disturbances in fish. Swedish Environmental Protection Agency Report 4346, Uppsala.

Ericson, G., G. Åkerman, B. Liewenborg, and L. Balk. 1996. Comparison of DNA damage in the early life stages of cod *Gadus morhua*, originating from the Barents Sea and Baltic Sea. Marine Environmental Research 42:119–123.

Falandysz, J. 1994. Polychlorinated biphenyl concentrations in cod-liver oil: evidence of a steady-state condition of these compounds in the Baltic area oils and levels noted in Atlantic oils. Archives of Environmental Contamination and Toxicology 27:266–271.

Grauman, G., and L. Sukhorukova. 1982. On the emergence of sprat and cod abnormal embryos in the open Baltic. ICES (International Council for the Exploration of the Sea) C.M. 1982/J:7, Copenhagen.

Hansen, P.-D., H. von Westernhagen, and H. Rosenthal. 1985. Chlorinated hydrocarbons and hatching success in Baltic herring spring spawners. Marine Environmental Research 15:59–76.

Härdig, J., T. Andersson, B.-E. Bengtsson, L. Förlin, and Å. Larsson. 1988. Long-term effects of bleached kraft mill effluents on red and white blood cell status, ion balance, and vertebral structure in fish. Ecotoxicology and Environmental Safety 15:96–106.

Helander, B., M. Olsson, and L. Reutergårdh. 1982. Residue levels of organochlorine and mercury compounds in unhatched eggs and the relationships to breeding success in white-tailed eagles *Haliaeetus albicilla* in Sweden. Holarctic Ecology 5:349–366.

Helle, E., M. Olsson, and S. Jensen. 1976. DDT and PCB levels and reproduction in ringed seals from the Bothnian Bay. Ambio 5:188–189.

Henriksson, J., A. Johannisson, P.-A. Bergqvist, and L. Norrgren. 1996. The toxicity of organoarsenic-based warfare agents: in vitro and in vivo studies. Archives of Environmental Contamination and Toxicology 30:213–219.

Jacobsson, A., E. Neumann, and M. Olsson. 1993. Tånglaken som indikator på effekter av giftiga ämnen. Naturvårdsverket, Kustrapport 1992:2. (In Swedish.)

Jansson, B., and eight coauthors. 1993. Chlorinated and brominated persistent organic compounds in biological samples from the environment. Environmental Toxicology and Chemistry 12:1163–1174.

Jansson, H., and T. Öst. 1997. Hybridization between Atlantic salmon (*Salmo salar*) and brown trout (*S. trutta*) in a restored section of the River Dalälven, Sweden. Canadian Journal of Fisheries and Aquatic Sciences 54:2033–2039.

Jensen, S., A. G. Johnels, M. Olsson, and G. Otterlind. 1969. DDT and PCB in marine animals from Swedish waters. Nature 224:247–250.

Johansson, N., K. M. Svensson, and G. Fridberg. 1982. Studies on the pathology of ulcerative dermal necrosis (UDN) in Swedish salmon, *Salmo salar*, and sea trout, *Salmo trutta* populations. Journal of Fish Diseases 5:293–308.

Karås, P., E. Neuman, and O. Sandström. 1991. Effects of pulp mill effluent on the population dynamics of perch, *Perca fluviatilis*. Canadian Journal of Fisheries and Aquatic Sciences 48:28–34.

Karlsson, L., and Ö. Karlström. 1994. The Baltic salmon (*Salmo salar* L.): its history, present situation and future. Dana 10:61–85.

Kjellman, J., R. Hudd, A. Leskela, J. Salmi, and H. Lehtonen. 1994. Estimations and prognosis of recruitment failures due to episodic acidifications on burbot (*Lota lota* L.) of the River Kyronjoki. Aqua Fennica 24:51–57.

Koistinen, J., J. Paasivirta, and P. J. Vuorinen. 1989. Dioxins and other planar polychloroaromatic compounds in Baltic, Finnish and Arctic fish samples. Chemosphere 19:527–530.

Larsson, P., C. Backe, G. Bremle, A. Eklöv, and L. Okla. 1996. Persistent pollutants in a salmon population (*Salmo salar*) of the southern Baltic Sea. Canadian Journal of Fisheries and Aquatic Sciences 53:62–69.

Larsson, P.-O. 1990. Baltic Sea cod. Pages 171–189 *in* Report of the ICES (International Council for the Exploration of the Sea) study group on cod stock fluctuations. App. III. Syntheses of Atlantic cod stocks. ICES C.M. 1990/G:50, Copenhagen.

Lindesjöö, E., and J. Thulin. 1992. A skeletal deformity of northern pike (*Esox lucius*) related to pulp mill effluents. Canadian Journal of Fisheries and Aquatic Sciences 49:166–172.

Lindström-Seppä, P., and A. Oikari. 1990. Biotransformation activities of feral fish in water receiving bleached pulp mill effluents. Environmental Toxicology and Chemistry 9:1415–1424.

Luksiene, D., and O. Sandström. 1994. Reproductive disturbance in a roach (*Rutilus rutilus*) population affected by cooling water discharge. Journal of Fish Biology 45:613–625.

Lundström, J., H. Börjeson, and L. Norrgren. 1998. Clinical and pathological studies of Baltic salmon suffering from yolk sac fry mortality. Pages 62–72 *in* G. McDonald, J. D. Fitzsimons, and D. C. Honeyfield, editors. Early life stage mortality syndrome in fishes of the Great Lakes and Baltic Sea. American Fisheries Society, Symposium 21, Bethesda, Maryland.

Lundström, J., L. Norrgren, and H. Börjeson. 1996. Clinical and morphological studies of Baltic salmon yolk-sac fry suffering from the M74 syndrome. Pages 26–27 *in* Bengtsson et al. (1996).

Matthäus, W., and H. U. Lass. 1995. The recent salt inflow into the Baltic Sea. Journal of Physical Oceanography 25:280–286.

Nissling, A., P. Solemdal, M. Svensson, and L. Westin. 1994. Survival, activity and feeding ability of Baltic cod (*Gadus morhua*) yolk-sac larvae at different salinities. Journal of Fish Biology 45:435–445.

Nissling, A., and L. Vallin. 1996a. The potential for successful spawning of Baltic cod—a question of interactions between spawning stocks and environmental conditions. Pages 68–69 *in* Bengtsson et al. (1996).

Nissling, A., and L. Vallin. 1996b. The ability of Baltic cod to maintain neutral buoyancy and the opportunity for survival in fluctuating conditions in the Baltic Sea. Journal of Fish Biology 48:217–227.

Norrgren L., T. Andersson, P.-A. Bergqvist, and I. Björklund. 1993. Studies of adult feral Baltic salmon (*Salmo salar*) and yolk-sac fry suffering from abnormal mortality. Environmental Toxicology and Chemistry 12:2065–2075.

Ojaveer, H., and R. Tanner. 1996. Polycyclic aromatic hydrocarbons in eelpout (*Zoarces viviparus*) from Estonian waters of the Baltic Sea. Pages 53–54 *in* Bengtsson et al. (1996).

Olsson, M., and L. Reutergårdh. 1986. DDT and PCB pollution trends in the Swedish aquatic environment. Ambio 15:103–109.

Oulasvirta, P. 1990. Effects of acid–iron effluent from a titanium dioxide factory on herring eggs in the Gulf of Bothnia (Finland). Finnish Fisheries Research 11:7–16.

Paasivirta, J., and six coauthors. 1995. TCDD-toxicity and M74 syndrome of Baltic salmon (*Salmo salar*, L.). Organohalogen Compounds 25:355–359.

Pedersen, B. H. 1993. Embryos and yolk-sac larva of turbot *Scophthalmus maximus* are infested with an endoparasite from the gastrula stage onwards. Diseases of Aquatic Organisms 17:57–59.

Pedersen, B. H., K. Buchmann, and M. Køie. 1993. Baltic larval cod *Gadus morhua* are infested with a protistan endoparasite in the yolk sac. Diseases of Aquatic Organisms 16:29–33.

Pettersson, A., and Å. Lignell. 1998. Low astaxanthin levels in Baltic salmon exhibiting the M74 syndrome. Pages 26–30 *in* G. McDonald, J. D. Fitzsimons, and D. C. Honeyfield, editors. Early life stage mortality syndrome in fishes of the Great Lakes and Baltic Sea. American Fisheries Society, Symposium 21, Bethesda, Maryland.

Pickova, J. 1997. Lipids in eggs and somatic tissues in cod and salmoides. Importance of individual fatty acids and antioxidants. Swedish University of Agricultural Sciences, Report 18, Uppsala.

Pickova, J., P. C. Dutra, A. Castling, and P.-O. Larsson. 1996. Fatty acid composition in fertilized eggs of cod (*Gadus morhua*) originating from the Baltic Sea and the Skagerrak. Pages 71–72 *in* Bengtsson et al. (1996).

Pickova, J., and P.-O. Larsson. 1992. Rearing experiments with cod. Comparison between Baltic cod and Skagerrak coastal cod. ICES (International Council for the Exploration of the Sea) C.M. 1992/F:12, Copenhagen.

Pulliainen, E., K. Korhonen, L. Kankaauranta, and K. Mäki. 1992. Non-spawning burbot on the northern coast of the Bothnian Bay. Ambio 21:170–175.

Rosenberg, R., and five coauthors. 1990. Marine euthrophication case studies in Sweden. Ambio 19:102–108.

Sandström. O., E. Neuman, and P. Karås. 1988. Effects of a bleached pulp mill effluent on growth and gonad function in Baltic coastal fish. Water Science and Technology 20:107–118.

Sandström. O., P. Karås, and E. Neuman. 1991. Pulp mill effluent effects on species distribution and recruitment in Baltic coastal fish. Finnish Fisheries Research 12:101–110.

Sandström, O. 1994. Incomplete recovery in a coastal fish community exposed to effluent from a modernized Swedish bleached kraft mill. Canadian Journal of Fisheries and Aquatic Sciences 51:2195–2205.

Soivio, A. 1996. M74 in Finland. Pages 42–43 *in* Bengtsson et al. (1996).

Ståhl, G. 1987. Genetic population structure of Atlantic salmon. Pages 121–140 *in* N. Ryman and F. Utter, editors. Population genetics and fishery management. University of Washington Press, Seattle.

Vallin, L. 1996. Reproductive success of anadromous brown trout (*Salmo trutta*) from three small streams in Got land, Sweden—an experimental study. Pages 91–92 *in* Bengtsson et al. (1996).

Vallin, L., and A. Nissling. 1996. Experimental studies of viability of eggs and larvae of cod, *Gadus morhua*, of different origin, with particular consideration to the stock in the Baltic. Pages 65–67 *in* Bengtsson et al. (1996).

Vourinen, P. J., and six coauthors. 1997. The M74 syndrome of Baltic salmon (*Salmo salar*) and organochlorine concentrations in the muscle of female salmon. Chemosphere 34:1151–1166.

Westernhagen, H. von, P. Cameron, V. Dethlefsen, and D. Jansson. 1989. Chlorinated hydrocarbons in North Sea whiting (*merlangus*, L.) and effects on reproduction. I. Tissue burden and hatching success. Helgolaender Meeresuntersuchungen 43:45–60.

Westernhagen, H. von, V. Dethlefsen, P. Cameron, J. Berg, and G. Furstenberg. 1988. Developmental defects in pelagic fish embryos from the western Baltic. Helgoländer Meeresuntersuchungen 42:13–36.

Westernhagen, H. von, and five coauthors. 1981. Bioaccumulating substances and reproductive success in Baltic flounder (*Platichthys flesus*). Aquatic Toxicology 1:85–99.

Wieland, K., U. Waller, and D. Schnack. 1994. Development of Baltic cod eggs at different levels of temperature and oxygen content. Dana 10:163–177.

Wiklund, T., and G. Bylund. 1994. Reproductive disorder in roach (*rutilus*) in the northern Baltic Sea. Bulletin of the European Association of Fish Pathologists 14:159–162.

Wit, C. de, and nine coauthors. 1990. Results from the first year of the Swedish dioxin survey. Chemosphere 20:1473–1480.

American Fisheries Society Symposium 21:18–25, 1998

Thiamine and Early Mortality Syndrome in Lake Trout[1]

Scott B. Brown[2]
Department of Fisheries and Oceans, Freshwater Institute
Winnipeg, Manitoba R3T 2N6, Canada

John D. Fitzsimons
Department of Fisheries and Oceans, Bayfield Institute
Burlington, Ontario L7R 4A6, Canada

Vince P. Palace[3]
University of Manitoba, Department of Zoology, Winnipeg, Manitoba R3T 2N6, Canada

Lenore Vandenbyllaardt
Nore-Tech Laboratory Services, Box 20 Group 70 RR # 1
Anola, Manitoba R0E 0A0, Canada

Abstract.—Reproductive success and vitamin B_1 (thiamine pyrophosphate, thiamine monophosphate, and free thiamine) concentrations were assessed in feral female lake trout *Salvelinus namaycush* from Lake Ontario and Lake Manitou. We monitored fertilization success, survival to hatch, incidence of blue-sac disease, other anomalies, and lake trout early mortality syndrome (EMS). Fertilization and hatching success were high, whereas mortality from blue-sac disease and other anomalies was low in egg batches from both lakes. There was no mortality from EMS in families from Lake Manitou. However, EMS occurred after hatching in the offspring of 48% of the females collected from Lake Ontario. We measured thiamine in liver, red blood cells, eggs, and developing embryos. Relative to fish collected in reference lakes, females in Lake Ontario had depressed hepatic, red blood cell, and egg thiamine concentrations. Although more extensive investigation of thiamine balance is required, it may be possible to use red blood cell thiamine pyrophosphate as a predictive index for EMS susceptibility in offspring. Total thiamine concentrations in developing embryos declined by 50% between fertilization and swim-up. Free thiamine reserves declined most rapidly, whereas levels of thiamine pyrophosphate increased between the eyed embryo and hatch stages. A high proportion (67%) of lake trout families in which the initial egg free thiamine reserves or embryonic concentrations of thiamine pyrophosphate levels were <0.8 nmol/g exhibited EMS. Below this threshold (0.8 nmol/g), the occurrence of EMS was variable (0–100%) and only weakly related to free thiamine concentrations ($r^2 = 0.32$, $P = 0.014$). This observation implies the possibility of additional interactions with other factors.

The presence of maternally transmitted noninfectious ailments that cause yolk sac embryo and swim-up stage mortality has at least partly compromised the sustainability of naturally reproducing populations of salmonids in the lower Great Lakes (Fitzsimons et al. 1995; Marcquenski 1996), the New York Finger Lakes (Fisher et al. 1995), and the Baltic Sea (Johansson et al. 1995). The ailments have been referred to as early mortality syndrome (EMS) in the salmonids from the lower Great Lakes (Marcquenski 1996), Cayuga syndrome in Atlantic salmon *Salmo salar* from the Finger Lakes region (Fisher et al. 1995), and M74 in Baltic Sea salmon (Johansson et al. 1995). One common characteristic of these embryonic mortality syndromes is that treatment of eggs or offspring with prophylactic doses of thiamine alleviates the clinical symptoms (Bylund and Lerche 1995; Fitzsimons 1995). Moreover, analysis of total thiamine levels suggests that low concentrations in eggs are also associated with the ailments (Amcoff et al.1996; Fisher et al.1996).

To enhance understanding of thiamine-related ailments in salmonids, it is essential to determine the cause of the low levels of thiamine and how they relate to developmental processes. Adequate levels of thiamine (particularly the phosphorylated forms) are essential for normal carbohydrate metabolism and neurological function. The diphosphate ester (thiamine pyrophosphate) acts as a cofactor for key enzymatic steps in carbohydrate metabolism (e.g.,

[1] Portions of this publication were presented at the Second Workshop on Reproductive Disturbances in Fish, Stockholm, Sweden (1995).

[2] Present address: Environment Canada, Canada Centre for Inland Waters, 867 Lakeshore Road, Box 5050, Burlington, Ontario L7R 4A6, Canada.

[3] Present address: Institute of Cardiovascular Science, 352 Tache Avenue, Winnipeg, Manitoba R2H 2A6, Canada.

decarboxylation of α-ketoacids and transketolase reactions), and the phosphorylated forms also play a critical role in nerve function (Combs 1992). Although studies by Fisher et al. (1996) and Amcoff et al. (1996) associate low thiamine concentrations with the observed embryonic mortality in EMS, Cayuga syndrome, and M74, they do not provide sufficient data to assess the roles of the different thiamine forms or to evaluate dose response relationships.

To obtain more information about the role of thiamine in embryonic development, we collected feral female lake trout *Salvelinus namaycush* tissues and gametes from a stock with a history of EMS (Lake Ontario) and an EMS-free stock (Lake Manitou). After fertilization, reproductive competence was assessed by monitoring developmental defects and survival of embryos until swim-up. We analyzed different thiamine forms (thiamine monophosphate, thiamine pyrophosphate, and free thiamine) using high-performance liquid chromatography (HPLC) technology (Brown et al. 1998, this volume). Study objectives were to characterize (1) the prevalence and extent of EMS in lake trout egg batches from Lake Ontario and Lake Manitou; (2) the relationship between thiamine content in females, eggs, and developing embryos; and (3) the association between thiamine content and EMS.

Materials and Methods

Fish and Gamete Collection

Lake trout were captured in Lake Ontario ($N = 30$) near Port Weller and in Lake Manitou ($N = 6$) on Manitoulin Island in Lake Huron by small-mesh trap nets set over spawning beds between 20 October and 14 November 1994. Fish were anesthetized in 3-aminobenzoic acid ethyl ester (1:5,000, volume per volume), rinsed in freshwater, and dried. Eggs from ripe fish were expressed into a dry measuring flask and egg volume was recorded. Only females whose eggs showed no evidence of overripening were used. An egg sample (10 g) from each female was placed in a Whirl-Pac® bag and immediately frozen between slabs of dry ice and stored at less than −90°C until analyzed. The remaining eggs were transferred to dry glass jars and placed on ice for transport to the Bayfield Institute laboratory. Semen (1–2 mL), collected from male fish by inserting a glass pipette into the urogenital opening, was placed into dry glass jars and held on ice during transport to the laboratory. After egg collection, blood was removed from the caudal vessels using heparinized 10-mL syringes with 18-gauge needles. Plasma and blood cells were separated by centrifugation and plasma was immediately frozen on dry ice in polyethylene vials. To remove plasma from the red blood cells, they were washed twice by resuspension in isotonic sodium chloride (approximately 300 mosmol/L) and recentrifugation. Fish were killed by a blow to the head and liver tissue was quickly dissected, weighed, and packaged in Whirl-Pac bags. Tissues were immediately frozen between slabs of dry ice and stored at less than −90°C until analyzed. The ages of fish from Lake Ontario were determined using implanted coded wire tags that indicated the date of stocking.

Egg Fertilization and Incubation

Three replicate batches of eggs (20 mL, ≈200 eggs) from each female were fertilized with composite milt (100 μL per 20 mL of eggs) of males ($N = 6$) from the same lake. Fertilized eggs were water-hardened and reared at 7°C in an incubation facility as described previously (Fitzsimons et al. 1995). A photoperiod of 12 h of light and 12 h of dark was maintained throughout development. Fertilized eggs were examined for developmental anomalies or mortality, and dead eggs or embryos were removed daily. The success of fertilization, hatching deformities, blue-sac disease (Wolf 1957), lake trout EMS, and overall survival were monitored in the offspring of each female. Samples of developing embryos (5–10 individuals) for thiamine analysis were taken at six times after fertilization and placed in sterile vials, quick frozen on dry ice, and stored at less than −90°C until analyzed. To standardize sampling among egg batches collected and fertilized on different dates, sampling occurred at the same cumulative temperature units (CTU; calculated as the incubation temperature in degrees Celsius times the number of days after fertilization) for each egg batch: fertilization (0 CTU), eyed embryo (247 CTU), prehatch embryo (524 CTU), posthatch embryo (686 CTU), pre-swim-up embryo (836 CTU), and post-swim-up embryo (964 CTU).

Thiamine Analysis

Thiamine pyrophosphate, thiamine monophosphate, and thiamine were extracted and quantified by reversed phase HPLC in tissues, eggs, and embryos from each female as described by Brown et al. (1998). Mean assay sensitivity for thiamine and its phosphates was 0.012 pmol. Average recoveries of low and high doses of thiamine compounds added to tissue samples ranged from 91.4 to 104.5%. Average coefficients of variation for between assay reproducibility ranged from 4.8 to 12.8%.

Statistics

To compare variables based on the presence of EMS in offspring from Lake Ontario females, the measurements were grouped. The first group (LON) represented families (N = 14) displaying a low occurrence of EMS (range, 0–4%). The second group (LON-EMS) represented families (N = 13) displaying a higher occurrence of EMS (range, 30–97%). Egg batches from three females (two from the LON group and one from the LON-EMS group) exhibited poor fertilization success (<25%). These families had too few survivors to provide accurate estimates for subsequent measurements and were eliminated from the analysis. The Systat statistical package (Wilkinson et al. 1992) was used to analyze the data. Bartlett's test was applied to test for homogeneity of variance and, where necessary, data were log-transformed. Significance was determined by one-way analysis of variance (ANOVA) on means of replicate measures of variables from each female. Because offspring from the same family were sampled at successive times during development, repeated-measures ANOVA (Wilkinson et al. 1992) was used to determine the significance of measured variables in developing offspring. Comparisons of egg diameter were made using analysis of covariance with total body weight adjusted for expressed egg volume (total weight minus expressed egg weight) as the covariate. Comparisons of body weight were made using analysis of covariance with age as the covariate. Pairwise comparisons were conducted by applying the least-significant-difference test to the least-squares means produced by the ANOVAs. Linear relationships between variables were examined by Pearson's product-moment correlation. For all tests, a P-value < 0.05 was considered significant. For clarity of presentation, arithmetic means with standard errors have been used in the tables and figures. A Fulton-type condition factor (Bagenal and Tesch 1978) was calculated as:

$$CF = \frac{100 \times (\text{total fish weight} - \text{expressed egg weight})}{\text{length}^3},$$

where CF = condition factor.

TABLE 1.—Number of fish, size (weight and length), condition, age, and egg size in female lake trout from Lake Manitou (LM), Lake Ontario with a low (<10%) offspring incidence of early mortality syndrome (LON), and Lake Ontario with high (>10%) offspring incidence of EMS (LON-EMS). Values represent mean (SE). Significant differences are indicated (P < 0.05) by different letters after the mean. Under Lake Manitou, NA = not analyzed.

Variable	LM	LON	LON-EMS
N	6	14	13
Weight (kg)	2.58 (0.14)	3.63 (0.31)	3.13 (0.21)
Length (cm)	64.0 (0.4)	69.2 (1.6)	67.1 (1.5)
Condition factor	0.99 (0.14)	1.06 (0.15)	1.02 (0.12)
Age (years)	NA	9.9 z (0.8)	7.6 y (0.5)
Egg diameter (mm)	5.53 z (0.05)	5.38 y (0.06)	5.23 y (0.08)

Results and Discussion

Fish Characteristics

Fish from Lake Ontario spanned a range of sizes (1.75–5.55 kg) that did not differ between groups when tested with age as a covariate (Table 1). The fish from Lake Manitou fell within the size range of the Lake Ontario fish, but their sizes could not be compared directly with those of the Lake Ontario groups because aging structures were unavailable. Fish condition was similar among all groups. In Lake Ontario fish, females that produced offspring exhibiting high occurrence of EMS were approximately 2 years younger than those that produced offspring exhibiting low occurrence of EMS. The fish from Lake Manitou produced larger eggs than those from Lake Ontario (Table 1). Egg diameter was related to fish size (r^2 = 0.251, P = 0.013) in fish from Lake Ontario. However, similar to the observations of Fitzsimons et al. (1995), egg size was unrelated to the presence of EMS in the offspring.

Fertilization and Reproductive Success

Fertilization and survival to hatch did not differ between egg batches, whereas mortality from bluesac disease and other anomalies was low in egg batches from both lakes (Table 2). There was no mortality attributable to EMS in offspring of Lake Manitou females. Posthatch mortality (>10%) attributable to EMS occurred between 800 and 1,000 CTU

TABLE 2.—Percentage of fertilization, hatching success, blue-sac disease relative to hatch, other anomalies (e.g., bent backs), EMS relative to hatch, and overall survival through 0–1,138 cumulative temperature units in embryos of female lake trout from Lake Manitou (LM), Lake Ontario with a low EMS incidence (LON), and Lake Ontario with a high EMS incidence (LON-EMS). Values represent mean (SE). Significant differences ($P < 0.05$) are indicated by different letters after the mean.

Variable	LM	LON	LON-EMS
Fertilization	86.6 (3.3)	90.2 (2.3)	88.6 (3.2)
Hatching success	73.5 (6.0)	76.2 (6.2)	83.3 (5.3)
Blue-sac disease relative to hatch	4.6 (1.9)	10.9 (4.0)	3.0 (0.8)
Other anomalies	1.4 (0.6)	1.9 (0.9)	0.5 (0.1)
EMS relative to hatch	0	0.9 z (0.8)	71.1 y (6.2)
Overall survival	69.1 z (6.9)	68.6 z (7.9)	20.8 y (5.2)

(Figure 1) and affected offspring from 48% of the females collected from Lake Ontario. The prevalence and clinical signs of EMS (e.g., loss of equilibrium, fish lying on their sides at the bottom of the tank, erratic swimming behavior, hyperexcitability) were similar to those previously reported in lake trout (Fitzsimons et al. 1995). Families suffering significant levels of EMS had low overall survival (Table 2).

Thiamine Levels

In fish from Lake Manitou, thiamine in liver and red blood cells occurred mostly as the metabolically functional enzyme cofactor (thiamine pyrophosphate; Table 3). The hepatic and egg thiamine concentrations of Lake Manitou fish were comparable with those found in lake trout collected at the Experimental Lake Area in northwestern Ontario (Brown et al. 1998), where offspring survival is high (Delorme 1995). Similar concentrations of thiamine pyrophosphate (Table 3) were also observed in juvenile rainbow trout *Oncorhynchus mykiss* fed a commercial diet supplemented with exogenous thiamine (Masumoto et al. 1987). In contrast to the forms found in other tissues, free thiamine was the predominant vitamin form (86%) in eggs of lake trout from Lake Manitou. Significant egg reserves of free

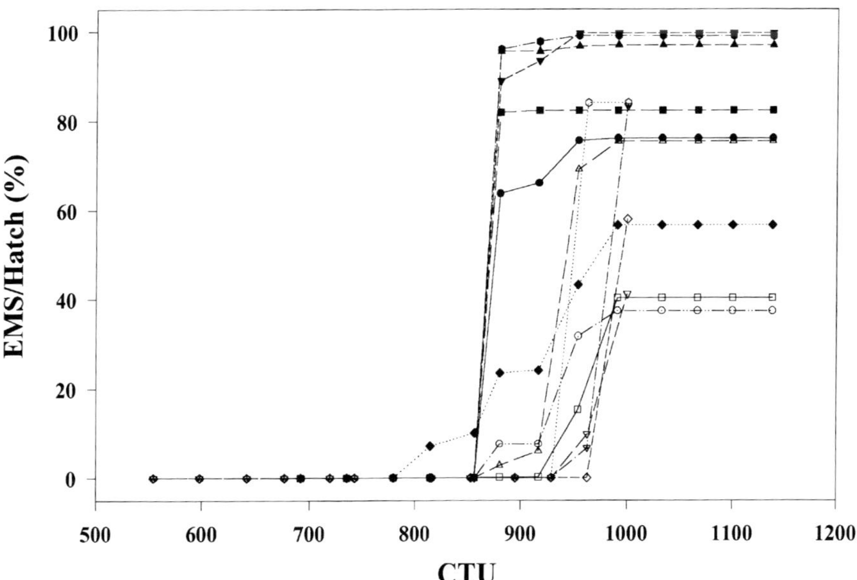

FIGURE 1.—Relationship between mortality as a percentage of the number of progeny hatched from Lake Ontario females ($N = 13$) with high incidence (>10%) of early mortality syndrome (EMS) and cumulative temperature units (CTU) after fertilization. Posthatch mortality attributable to EMS occurred between 800 and 1,000 CTU. Values represent the mean of three replicates of 200 progeny per female.

TABLE 3.—Thiamine pyrophosphate, thiamine monophosphate, and free thiamine levels (nmol/g) in liver and red blood cells of female lake trout from Lake Manitou (LM), Lake Ontario with a low EMS incidence (LON), and Lake Ontario with a high EMS incidence (LON-EMS). Values represent mean (SE) of duplicate measures from 6 (LM), 14 (LON), or 13 (LON-EMS) fish. Significant differences are indicated ($P < 0.05$) by different letters after the mean. For Lake Manitou, NA = not analyzed.

	Thiamine pyrophosphate			Thiamine monophosphate			Free thiamine		
Tissue	LM	LON	LON-EMS	LM	LON	LON-EMS	LM	LON	LON-EMS
Liver	10.19 z (0.91)	7.00 y (0.58)	5.98 y (0.66)	0.34 (0.07)	0.22 (0.05)	0.13 (0.05)	0.31 (0.10)	0.17 (0.06)	0.24 (0.07)
Red blood cells	NA	0.34 z (0.03)	0.24 y (0.02)	NA	0.06 (0.02)	0.07 (0.02)	NA	0.12 (0.01)	0.16 (0.04)

thiamine are common among lake trout reared on vitamin-fortified hatchery diets or collected from locations where EMS does not occur (Fitzsimons and Brown 1996; Honeyfield et al. 1998, this volume).

Relative to female lake trout collected from Lake Manitou, fish from Lake Ontario had depressed tissue levels of thiamine (Table 3). Hepatic reserves of thiamine pyrophosphate in Lake Ontario females were about 60–70% of those found in fish from Lake Manitou. Red blood cell thiamine pyrophosphate in Lake Ontario fish was 30% that of female fish collected from the Experimental Lake Area (Brown et al. 1998). Moreover, the depressed levels of thiamine found in the lake trout collected from Lake Ontario (Table 3) were comparable with those found in juvenile rainbow trout exhibiting overt signs of thiamine deficiency after consuming a thiamine-deficient diet (Masumoto et al. 1987).

Hepatic concentrations of thiamine pyrophosphate in the Lake Ontario females were unrelated to either the presence of lower egg levels of thiamine or the presence of EMS. However, maternal concentrations of thiamine pyrophosphate in washed red blood cells correlated to the amount of free thiamine ($r^2 = 0.518$, $P < 0.001$) in eggs and to the presence of EMS ($r^2 = 0.252$, $P = 0.009$; Figure 2). When red blood cell thiamine pyrophosphate concentrations were less than 0.33 nmol/g, 63% of females produced offspring exhibiting EMS. Honeyfield et al. (1998) found that different tissue concentrations are not depleted at the same rate when inhibitors of thiamine uptake are fed to fish to produce deficient broodstock and eggs. Although more extensive investigation of thiamine balance is required, it may be possible

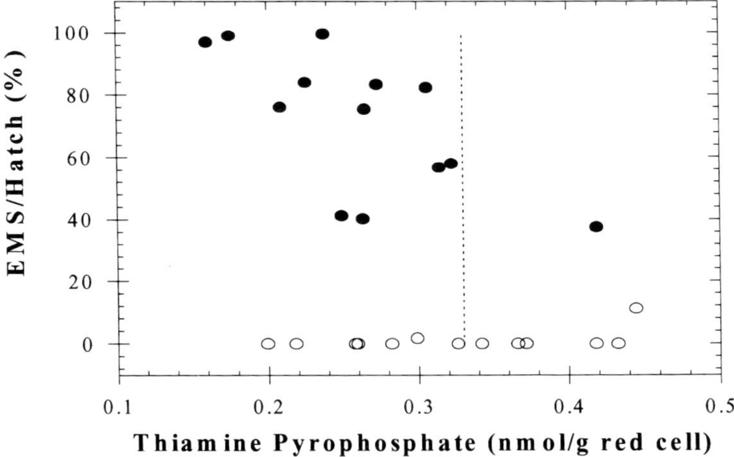

FIGURE 2.—Relationship between thiamine pyrophosphate levels in red blood cells of mothers and incidence of EMS as a percentage of the number of embryos hatched from Lake Ontario females. Symbols indicate values for eggs from Lake Ontario with a low incidence of EMS (○) and with a high incidence of EMS (●). At red blood cell thiamine levels less than 0.33 nmol/g (dotted line), there is an high occurrence of EMS (63%).

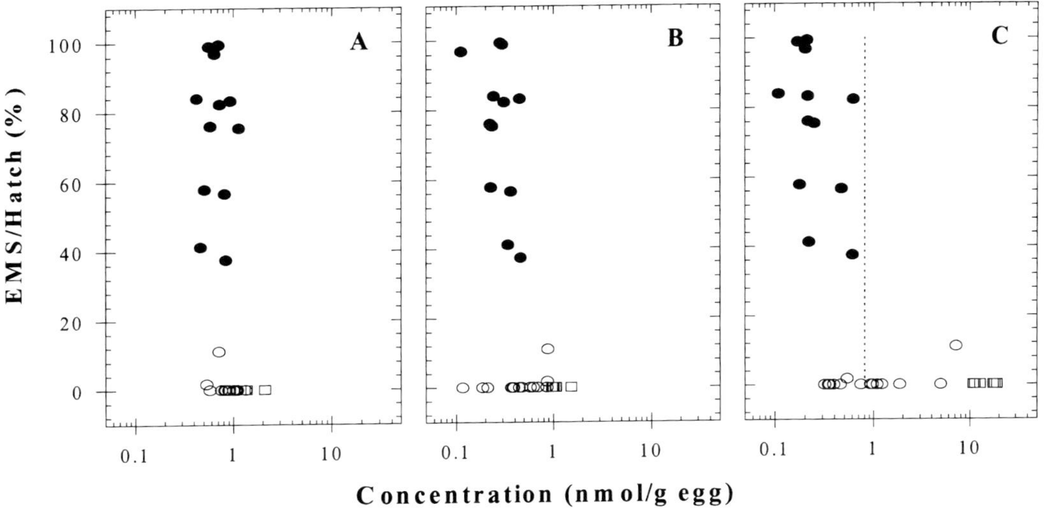

FIGURE 3.—Relationship between incidence of EMS as a percentage of the number of embryos hatched from Lake Ontario females and egg levels of thiamine pyrophosphate (**A**), thiamine monophosphate (**B**), and free thiamine (**C**). Symbols indicate values for eggs from Lake Manitou (□), Lake Ontario with a low incidence of EMS (○), and Lake Ontario with a high incidence of EMS (●). At egg free thiamine levels less than 0.8 nmol/g (dotted line), there is a high occurrence of EMS (67%).

to use red blood cell thiamine pyrophosphate as a predictive index for EMS susceptibility in offspring.

Although all forms of thiamine were lower in eggs of lake trout from Lake Ontario, the levels of free thiamine showed the greatest difference (Table 3). The Lake Ontario fish that produced offspring with a low incidence of EMS had free thiamine levels that were 10% of those of the Lake Manitou fish. Free thiamine levels in eggs produced by females from Lake Ontario whose offspring developed EMS were still lower, 3% of the thiamine levels found in eggs from Lake Manitou females. There was also a shift in thiamine forms: phosphorylated thiamine made up a larger portion of the total thiamine in eggs from Lake Ontario. A high proportion (67%) of lake trout families in which the initial egg free thiamine reserves were <0.8 nmol/g developed EMS (Figure 3A). Below this threshold, the amount of EMS was variable (0–100%) and loosely but significantly related to free thiamine concentrations ($r^2 = 0.32$, $P < 0.05$). Egg concentrations of phosphorylated thiamine forms were unrelated to the amount of EMS (Figure 3, B and C). A similar relationship between egg free thiamine and EMS in developing offspring was observed in coho salmon *Oncorhynchus kisutch* from Lake Michigan (Hornung et al. 1998, this volume). In coho salmon, the threshold egg free thiamine concentration for greater prevalence of EMS was 0.3 nmol/g. Similar to our findings in lake trout, the extent of EMS-related mortality below this threshold concentration in coho salmon eggs was variable and unrelated to further changes in thiamine level (Hornung et al. 1998). The high variability of EMS mortality below a critical threshold level raises the possibility that interactions by factors other than thiamine could also contribute to the development of EMS.

Total thiamine concentrations in developing offspring from all groups declined by 50% between fertilization and swim-up (Table 4). In the only other study of thiamine dynamics in the developing embryo, thiamine concentrations measured by microbial assay in eggs and embryos of hatchery-reared rainbow trout (Sato et al. 1987) were comparable with our findings for total thiamine in the Lake Manitou families. In lake trout, free thiamine reserves declined most extensively in developing embryos (Table 4), whereas levels of thiamine pyrophosphate (active enzyme cofactor) initially declined and then between 247 and 684 CTU (eyed and posthatch embryos; Table 4) increased. It appears that egg free thiamine may serve as a reservoir to supply substrate for production of thiamine pyrophosphate. Thiamine monophosphate levels remained constant during development in the Lake Manitou families (Table 4). In the families from Lake Ontario, thiamine monophosphate declined after hatching but returned to levels found in the freshly fertilized eggs by swim-up.

TABLE 4.—Thiamine pyrophosphate, thiamine monophosphate, and free thiamine levels (nmol/g) in eggs and developing offspring of female lake trout from Lake Manitou (LM), Lake Ontario with a low EMS incidence (LON), and Lake Ontario with a high EMS incidence (LON-EMS) at various stages of development. Values represent mean (SE) of duplicate measures from 6 (LM), 14 (LON), or 13 (LON-EMS) fish. Significant differences between groups are indicated ($P < 0.05$) by different letters after the mean.

	Thiamine pyrophosphate			Thiamine monophosphate			Free thiamine		
Embryonic stage	LM	LON	LON-EMS	LM	LON	LON-EMS	LM	LON	LON-EMS
Fertilized egg	1.29 z	0.90 y	0.70 y	1.10 z	0.51 y	0.30 x	14.85 z	1.53 y	0.39 x
	(0.18)	(0.06)	(0.06)	(0.09)	(0.07)	(0.03)	(1.51)	(0.54)	(0.05)
Eyed embryo	0.80 z	0.27 y	0.24 y	0.98 z	0.39 y	0.41 y	13.73 z	1.31 y	0.39 x
	(0.06)	(0.03)	(0.03)	(0.05)	(0.06)	(0.05)	(0.72)	(0.59)	(0.05)
Prehatch embryo	1.28 z	0.83 y	0.59 y	1.49 z	0.35 y	0.22 x	9.93 z	0.95 y	0.37 x
	(0.12)	(0.07)	(0.03)	(0.01)	(0.04)	(0.02)	(1.06)	(0.25)	(0.05)
Posthatch embryo	5.09 z	1.17 y	0.59 x	1.37 z	0.30 y	0.15 x	5.34 z	0.47 y	0.28 y
	(0.44)	(0.12)	(0.05)	(0.04)	(0.04)	(0.02)	(1.23)	(0.12)	(0.05)
Pre-swim-up embryo	5.63 z	1.05 y	0.56 x	0.73 z	0.25 y	0.02 x	1.40 z	0.17 y	0.07 x
	(0.32)	(0.17)	(0.05)	(0.05)	(0.03)	(0.01)	(0.10)	(0.05)	(0.02)
Post-swim-up embryo	6.63 z	1.10 y	0.47 x	0.91 z	0.29 y	0.08 y	1.30 z	0.12 y	0.05 x
	(0.24)	(0.25)	(0.15)	(0.09)	(0.16)	(0.01)	(0.22)	(0.03)	(0.02)

Posthatch levels of thiamine pyrophosphate less than 0.8 nmol/g corresponded to a high incidence (80%) of EMS in embryos. Further study is required to substantiate the finding that the formation of phosphorylated thiamine in embryos represents a critical step in the development of EMS. However, we note that the elevations in embryonic levels of thiamine pyrophosphate (eyed stage to first feeding) were coincident with the occurrence of rearing losses attributable to early mortality syndrome in the various salmonid species that have been examined (Marcquenski 1996).

Although these results do not explicitly demonstrate cause and effect, it is clear that fish capable of producing eggs and embryos with higher thiamine levels are less likely to exhibit EMS. The high variability in the occurrence of EMS when thiamine concentrations are low implies that other factors may also contribute to the development of EMS. In a companion study (Palace 1996), it was determined that the presence of EMS in offspring of female lake trout from Lake Ontario was unrelated to maternal, egg, or embryo levels of vitamin E, vitamin C, or the carotinoid astaxanthin.

Acknowledgments

This work was partially supported by the Fish Health Monitoring project in the Department of Fisheries and Oceans Toxic Chemicals Program. We thank J. Klaverkamp, K. Mills, R. Evans, and P. Amcoff for their comments on a previous draft. P. Mettner and J. Radford aided in the capture of fish and the collection of samples. The assistance of B. Williston is gratefully acknowledged.

References

Amcoff, P., L. Norrgren, H. Borjeson, and J. Lindeberg. 1996. Lowered concentrations of thiamine (vitamin B_1) in M74-affected feral Baltic salmon (*Salmo salar*). Pages 38–39 *in* B.-E. Bengtsson, C. Hill, and S. Nellbring, editors. Report from the second workshop on reproduction disturbances in fish. Swedish Environmental Protection Agency Report 4534, Stockholm.

Bagenal, T. B., and F. W. Tesch. 1978. Age and growth. Pages 101–136 *in* T. Bagenal, editor. Methods for assessment of fish production in fresh waters, 3rd edition. Blackwell Scientific Publications, Oxford, UK.

Brown, S. B., D. C. Honeyfield, and L. Vandenbyllaardt. 1998. Thiamine analysis in fish tissues. Pages 73–81 *in* G. McDonald, J. D. Fitzsimons, and D. C. Honeyfield, editors. Early life stage mortality syndrome in fishes of the Great Lakes and Baltic Sea. American Fisheries Society, Symposium 21, Bethesda, Maryland.

Bylund, G., and O. Lerche. 1995. Thiamine therapy of M74 affected fry of Atlantic salmon, *Salmo salar*. Bulletin of the European Association of Fish Pathologists 15(3):93–97.

Combs, G. F. 1992. The vitamins. Academic Press, San Diego, California.

Delorme, P. D. 1995. The effect of toxaphene, chlordane and 2,3,4,7,8-pentachlorodibenzofuran on lake trout and white sucker in an ecosystem experiment and the distribution and effects of 2,3,4,7,8-pentachlorodibenzofuran on white suckers and broodstock rainbow trout in laboratory experiments. Doctoral dissertation. University of Manitoba, Winnipeg.

Fisher, J. P., J. D. Fitzsimons, G. F. Combs, and J. M. Spitzbergan. 1996. Naturally occurring thiamine deficiency causing reproductive failure in Finger Lakes Atlantic salmon and Great Lakes lake trout. Transactions of the American Fisheries Society 125:167–178.

Fisher, J. P., and six coauthors. 1995. Reproductive failure of landlocked Atlantic salmon from New York's Finger Lakes: investigation into etiology and epidemiology of the "Cayuga syndrome." Journal of Aquatic Animal Health 7:81–95.

Fitzsimons, J. D. 1995. The effect of B-vitamins on a swim-up syndrome in Lake Ontario lake trout. Journal of Great Lakes Research 21 (Supplement 1):286–289.

Fitzsimons, J. D., and S. B. Brown. 1996. Effect of diet on thiamine levels in Great Lakes lake trout and relationship with early mortality syndrome. Pages 76–78 *in* B.-E. Bengtsson, C. Hill, and S. Nellbring, editors. Report from the second workshop on reproduction disturbances in fish. Swedish Environmental Protection Agency Report 4534.

Fitzsimons, J. D., S. Huestis, and B. Williston. 1995. Occurrence of a swim-up syndrome in Lake Ontario lake trout in relation to contaminants and cultural practices. Journal of Great Lakes Research 21 (Supplement 1):277–285.

Honeyfield, D. C., K. Fynn-Aikins, J. D. Fitzsimons, and J. A. Mota. 1998. Effect of dietary amprolium on egg and tissue thiamine concentrations in lake trout. Pages 172–177 *in* G. McDonald, J. D. Fitzsimons, and D. C. Honeyfield, editors. Early life stage mortality syndrome in fishes of the Great Lakes and Baltic Sea. American Fisheries Society, Symposium 21, Bethesda, Maryland.

Hornung, M. W., L. Miller, R. E. Peterson, S. Marcquenski, and S. B. Brown. 1998. Efficacy of thiamine, astaxanthin, β-carotene, and thyroxine treatments in reducing early mortality syndrome in Lake Michigan salmonid embryos. Pages 124–134 *in* G. McDonald, J. D. Fitzsimons, and D. C. Honeyfield, editors. Early life stage mortality syndrome in fishes of the Great Lakes and Baltic Sea. American Fisheries Society, Symposium 21, Bethesda, Maryland.

Johansson, N., P. Jonsson, O. Svanberg, A. Sodergren, and J. Thulin. 1995. Reproduction disorders in Baltic fish. Swedish Environmental Protection Agency Report 4347, Stockholm.

Marcquenski, S. V. 1996. Characterization of early mortality syndrome (EMS) in salmonids from the Great Lakes. Pages 73–75 *in* B.-E. Bengtsson, C. Hill, and S. Nellbring, editors. Report from the second workshop on reproduction disturbances in fish. Swedish Environmental Protection Agency Report 4534, Stockholm.

Masumoto, T., R. W. Hardy, and E. Casillas. 1987. Comparison of transketolase activity and thiamine pyrophosphate levels in erythrocytes and liver of rainbow trout (*Salmo gairdneri*) as indicators of thiamine status. Journal of Nutrition 117:1422–1426.

Palace, V. P. 1996. Oxidative stress in lake trout (*Salvelinus namaycush*) exposed to organochlorine contaminants that induce phase I biotransformation enzyme system. Doctoral dissertation. University of Manitoba, Winnipeg.

Sato, M., R. Yoshinaka, R. Kuroshima, H. Morimoto, and S. Ikeda. 1987. Changes in water soluble vitamin contents and transaminase activity of rainbow trout egg during development. Nippon Suisan Gakkaishi 53:795–799.

Wilkinson, L., M. Hill, J. P. Welna, and G. K. Birkenbeuel. 1992. Systat for Windows: statistics version 5. Systat Inc. Evanston, Illinois.

Wolf, K. 1957. Blue-sac disease investigations: microbiology and laboratory induction. Progressive Fish-Culturist 19:14–18.

American Fisheries Society Symposium 21:26–30, 1998

Low Astaxanthin Levels in Baltic Salmon Exhibiting the M74 Syndrome

ANNETTE PETTERSSON[1]
Department of Limnology, Uppsala University, Norbyvägen 20, S-752 36 Uppsala, Sweden

ÅKE LIGNELL
AstaCarotene AB, Idrottsvägen 4, S-134 40 Gustavsberg, Sweden

Abstract.—The carotenoid levels in Baltic salmon *Salmo salar* appear to have decreased as the incidence of the M74 syndrome has increased during the last 20 years. Our preliminary investigations suggested a relationship between a low level of the carotenoid astaxanthin in yolk sac fry of Baltic salmon and elevated mortality attributable to M74. The objective of this study was to further detail this relationship during the spawning seasons of 1994 and 1995 in salmon taken from hatcheries on the Baltic Sea, the Swedish west coast, and Lake Vänern. Total carotenoids and astaxanthin were measured in female muscle tissue and eggs. The carotenoid concentration and the ratio of astaxanthin to total carotenoids were significantly lower in the muscle of Baltic salmon females than in the muscle of feral females from salmon stocks on the Swedish west coast and in Lake Vänern. A relationship between low muscle levels of astaxanthin in Baltic salmon females and M74 in the progeny was observed, and yolk sac fry from eggs with low astaxanthin content tended to exhibit M74 more often than fry from eggs with high astaxanthin concentration. The low levels of astaxanthin observed in Baltic salmon eggs and yolk sac fry may be part of a general astaxanthin deficiency in the feral Baltic salmon.

In 1974 an abnormally high mortality of yolk sac fry of Baltic salmon *Salmo salar* was discovered at Swedish hatcheries. The incidence of the syndrome, designated M74, increased successively from 1974 and peaked in the early 1990s, when up to 95% of the produced fry were lost in some hatcheries (Norrgren et al. 1994). No known diseases and causes of mortality have been associated with the clinical signs seen in this syndrome. Fry suffering from M74 lack normal motor activity and show discoloration of the skin and exophthalmia ("popeye"). Morphological changes include ruptures of blood vessels in the form of hemorrhages close to the heart, white precipitates in the yolk sac, and more vacuoles and lower glycogen content in the liver (Börjeson et al. 1994; Lundström et al. 1996). Death usually occurs within 3 weeks after hatching, before the fry begin to feed, although high mortality has also been registered in later stages of development (Lundström et al. 1996). The M74 syndrome is strongly linked to individual females, and a correlation has been found between a "wiggling" behavior in females and M74 in their progeny (Börjeson et al. 1994). Thiamine deficiency appears to be an important biochemical marker of M74. It is possible to cure the wiggling of adult salmon and reduce mortality rates by thiamine treatment, and thiamine bathing of eggs and newly hatched fry is now used in the hatcheries to improve fry recruitment (Amcoff et al. 1996; Bengtsson and Hill 1996).

Baltic salmon tend to have pale flesh color. According to anglers and hatchery personnel, flesh pigmentation has decreased during the last 20 years. The usual pink color of salmon flesh is caused by high concentrations of carotenoids, especially astaxanthin (diketo-dihydroxy-β-carotene). During egg formation, astaxanthin is mobilized from the female muscle and liver and laid down in the growing ovary; it is found in unesterified form in the mature egg (Torrissen et al. 1989).

Low levels of astaxanthin in yolk sac fry of Baltic salmon are related to elevated mortality from M74 (Lignell 1994). The objective of this study was to further document the dynamics of astaxanthin in the M74 syndrome. In this paper, we present and discuss data showing a relationship between low levels of astaxanthin in female muscle tissue and eggs and high mortality rates of Baltic salmon yolk sac fry.

Methods

Sampling and Storage

The Swedish compensatory program for salmon is described elsewhere (Larsson 1980; Ackefors et al. 1991). In short, wild salmon are caught while migrating up their home rivers in the autumn. Females are stripped and their eggs are fertilized artifi-

[1]To whom correspondence should be addressed.

cially. In the hatchery, the fertilized eggs from each female are kept separate from those of other females and are incubated at ambient river temperature.

Unfertilized eggs and dorsal muscle samples from stripped females were collected from five different Baltic salmon hatcheries located at River Luleälv, River Umeälv, River Ångermanälven, River Dalälven, and River Mörrumsån during the spawning seasons in 1994 and 1995. For comparison, eggs and female muscle from salmon stocks not displaying M74 were also sampled from two Swedish west coast hatcheries (North Atlantic salmon) at River Lagan and River Götaälv and from one hatchery reproducing the landlocked Lake Vänern salmon at River Klarälven. In addition, dorsal muscle samples from ten juvenile salmon caught in the main basin of the Baltic Sea in June 1995 were analyzed.

When analyses could not be conducted immediately after sampling, samples were stored at −20°C for no more than 2 weeks and at −70°C when a longer storage period was needed. Reference material was also kept at this lower temperature to prevent degradation of carotenoids.

Carotenoid and Astaxanthin Analyses

Weighted samples, consisting of 3–6 eggs and 1.5–2.5 g of muscle tissue, were homogenized in glass vials using Ultra-Turrax homogenizer (Janke & Kunkel GmbH & Co., Ltd., Ika-Werke, Staufen, Germany) and extracted in 4–5 mL of 100% acetone. After centrifugation at 1,500 g and recovery of the acetone extract, the pelleted material was resuspended and, if necessary, extracted a second time in acetone. The acetone extracts were pooled, and the carotenoid content was determined by measuring the absorbance in a spectrophotometer at 474 nm. An extinction coefficient of 193 cm^{-2} mg^{-1} was used for calculations. The acetone extract was thereafter mixed vigorously with cyclohexane (1:1), and the carotenoids were collected in the hexane phase.

Carotenoid composition was determined by high-pressure liquid chromatography (HPLC) after evaporation of the cyclohexane extract to dryness with nitrogen and dissolution of the carotenoids in chloroform:methanol (2:1). Samples (20 μL) were filtered through a 0.45-μm hydrophobic membrane filter to remove particulate residues before injection. The HPLC system (E. Merck, Darmstadt, Germany) consisted of a L6200A Intelligent pump, a D-2000 injector, and a L4200 visible–ultraviolet detector set at 474 nm with 0.1 absorbance units at full scale. A linear elution gradient with methanol:water:ethyl acetate was adopted, from 82:8:10 at the start to 29:1:70 after 16 min. External and internal carotenoid standards (astaxanthin and canthaxanthin, 99% pure, F. Hoffman-La Roche & Co., Ltd., Basle, Switzerland) were used to determine the recovery of carotenoids during extraction and the reproducibility of the analysis methods applied. The recovery of the carotenoids in the acetone extracts, after concentration and transfer to chloroform:methanol, was generally >90% for both muscle tissue and egg extracts. However, in the acetone extracts of muscle tissue, unidentified yellow substances that were not transferred to the cyclohexane phase were found. All of the solvents and chemicals used were of analytical grade and were purchased from Merck & Co. (Darmstadt, Germany).

Results

Carotenoid levels and astaxanthin:carotenoid ratios found in feral female muscle after stripping in 1994 and 1995 in Baltic Sea, North Atlantic, and Lake Vänern salmon hatcheries are summarized in Table 1. The three groups of salmon represented three significantly different (P = 0.001) carotenoid lev-

TABLE 1.—Total carotenoid levels and astaxanthin:carotenoid ratios found in dorsal muscle of feral female salmon from the Baltic Sea, North Atlantic, and Lake Vänern during spawning in 1994 and 1995 and in juvenile salmon caught in the main basin of the Baltic Sea in June 1995. Parenthetical values are SDs.

Origin	N	Total carotenoids (mg/kg)	Range (mg/kg)	Astaxanthin:total carotenoids	Range
Baltic Sea	137	0.4 (0.2)[a]	0.1–1.0	0.47 (0.20)	0.13–0.78
North Atlantic	75	2.6 (1.3)	0.6–4.6	0.92 (0.03)	0.89–0.98
Lake Vänern	35	0.7 (0.3)	0.3–1.5	0.71[b]	0.65–0.78
Juvenile	10	0.8 (0.5)	0.5–1.6	0.57 (0.10)	0.38–0.61

[a] Significantly different from North Atlantic and Lake Vänern salmon (P = 0.001, z-test).

[b] Determined only in pooled samples (N = 5) in 1995.

TABLE 2.—Ratio of astaxanthin to total carotenoids in muscle of seven feral female salmon from the River Umeälv, stripped in November 1994, and egg and yolk sac fry mortality in the offspring.

Female number	Astaxanthin:total carotenoid ratio	Egg mortality (%)	Yolk sac fry mortality (%)	Surviving yolk sac fry (%)
1	0.37	100		0
2	0.20		100	0
3	0.47		100	0
4	0.58		40	60
5	0.58		0	100
6	0.68		0	100
7	0.78		0	100

els, with the highest found in North Atlantic salmon and the lowest in Baltic salmon. The Lake Vänern salmon displayed an intermediate carotenoid level. Astaxanthin was the dominant carotenoid in Lake Vänern (>65% of total carotenoids) and North Atlantic (>89% of total carotenoids) feral salmon muscle tissue. In Baltic Sea salmon, astaxanthin levels in muscle tissue showed substantial variation in different females (13–78%), and the mean value of astaxanthin was less than 50% of total carotenoids. Moreover, astaxanthin constituted only 50–60% of total carotenoids in the flesh of juvenile salmon caught in the main basin of the Baltic Sea in June 1995 (Table 1). It is important to note that an internal carotenoid standard was not added to these samples. Therefore, astaxanthin levels are presented only as ratios of total carotenoids; otherwise, they could be overestimated because of the presence of the unidentified yellow substances in the acetone extract (see "Methods"). Results from the River Umeälv hatchery indicate that fry (and egg) mortality attributable to M74 increases when the astaxanthin ratio is less than 0.5–0.6 of total carotenoids in the female muscle (Table 2).

Approximately 65% of the Baltic salmon egg batches analyzed during the spawning season in 1994 contained astaxanthin concentrations of less than 2 mg/kg, whereas astaxanthin levels in salmon eggs from Lake Vänern (2.8–4.7 mg/kg) and the North Atlantic (5.5–9.0 mg/kg) were generally higher (Table 3). Yolk sac fry mortality attributable to M74 was 100% from eggs with astaxanthin levels ≤1.0 mg/kg, and M74 was not recorded in batches with egg astaxanthin concentrations ≥3.0 mg/kg. In Baltic salmon egg batches with astaxanthin concentrations between 1 and 3 mg/kg, the frequency of M74 tended to be higher at the lower egg astaxanthin concentrations: 62% of the batches with <2 mg/kg and 42% of the batches with >2 mg/kg exhibited M74 in the yolk sac stage (Table 3). The frequency of M74 varied between 50 and 60% in the Baltic salmon hatcheries in 1994 (data not shown).

Discussion

A relationship between low muscle levels of astaxanthin in feral Baltic salmon females and M74 in their progeny was observed in this study (Table 2), and yolk sac fry from egg batches with low astaxanthin concentrations tended to exhibit M74 more often than fry from egg batches with high astaxanthin concentrations (Table 3). Moreover, the flesh of juvenile salmon caught in the Baltic main basin showed low concentrations of astaxanthin and astaxanthin to total carotenoid ratios of only 0.5–0.6 (Table 1). These results indicate that the low levels of astaxanthin observed in Baltic salmon eggs and yolk sac fry (Lignell 1994) may be part of a general astaxanthin deficiency in the feral salmon.

The cause of the low astaxanthin levels in Baltic salmon is unknown. Salmon are unable to synthesize astaxanthin and therefore are dependent on a dietary supply of this carotenoid. Our working hypothesis is that a change in the food web during the last 20–25 years has resulted in a decline in the availability of astaxanthin in the salmon diet. The ecosystem of the Baltic Sea is extremely vulnerable to environmental disturbances because of the low number of species and is strongly affected by anthropogenic effects such as eutrophication and emissions of inorganic and organic pollutants. Herring *Clupea harengus* is considered to be the main prey species of Baltic salmon. Preliminary results indicate that herring is a very poor source of astaxanthin, but the carotenoid levels found in Baltic herring are not significantly lower than in sprat *Sprattus sprattus*, the

TABLE 3.—Distribution of egg batches of Baltic Sea, North Atlantic, and Lake Vänern salmon with different levels of astaxanthin during the spawning season in 1994. Parenthetical values are the number of Baltic Sea salmon egg batches exhibiting M74.

		Astaxanthin (mg/kg egg)				
Origin	*N*	<1	1–2	2–3	3–4	>4
Baltic Sea	44	6 (6)	23 (14)	13 (5)	2 (0)	0
North Atlantic	30	0	0	0	0	30
Lake Vänern	30	0	0	5	19	6

second most important prey species, or in Swedish west coast herring. However, considering the great variation in carotenoid content found, more analyses are needed before any conclusion can be drawn.

Astaxanthin has been proven to be one of the most potent antioxidative agents known, protecting polyunsaturated lipids from lipid peroxidation in studies of animals both in vitro and in vivo (Kurashige et al. 1990; Nishigaki et al. 1994). Oxidative damage may be prevented by astaxanthin acting as a singlet oxygen ($^1O_2$) quencher and trapping chain-propagating lipid-peroxyl radicals (Krinsky 1989). In a study by Christiansen et al. (1995), astaxanthin supplementation in the diet promoted muscle pigmentation and growth of Atlantic salmon parr. Moreover, a relationship was found between dietary astaxanthin concentration and antioxidant status (retinol, α-tocopherol, and ascorbic acid) in both liver and muscle, suggesting "antioxidant-sparing" effects of astaxanthin. Juvenile rainbow trout *Oncorhynchus mykiss* were reported to show improved muscle pigmentation and liver function and greater defensive potential level against oxidative stress when fed astaxanthin. However, growth was not significantly different from that of the control fish without astaxanthin supplementation in the diet (Nakano et al. 1995). Börjeson et al. (1996) reported decreased levels of the antioxidants α-tocopherol and ubiquinone in the liver of fry that exhibited M74. Concentrations of both α-tocopherol and ubiquinone increased after thiamine therapy, indicating an antioxidant-sparing effect of thiamine (Börjeson et al. 1996). Using the thiobarbituric acid test (Uchiyama and Mihara 1978), an elevated level of malondialdehyde was found in fry afflicted with M74 (Pettersson and Lignell 1996). Thus, increased lipid peroxidation is evident in the later stages of the M74 syndrome. The M74 syndrome-affected eggs also had a higher content of the polyunsaturated fatty acid docosahexanoic acid than eggs not affected by M74 (Pickova et al., in press), which could suggest that individuals with a higher demand for oxidative protection are more susceptible to M74.

The M74 syndrome shows several similarities with the early mortality syndrome found in salmonids of the Great Lakes (Fitzsimons 1996) and with the Cayuga syndrome in landlocked Atlantic salmon of New York State's Finger Lakes (Fisher et al. 1995). In all three of these syndromes, thiamine deficiency in the female flesh, eggs, and fry is evidently correlated to the high mortality of the salmonid fry. However, whether the reduced levels of thiamine have similar causes, such as dietary deficiencies or increased breakdown of thiamine attributable to some inactivating factors (Larsson and Haux 1996), is still an open question. In this context, the antioxidative properties of astaxanthin are interesting because thiamine is a substance susceptible to oxidation.

Acknowledgments

This project was funded by the Swedish Environmental Protection Agency within the FiRe research program. We are deeply grateful to the staffs at the Swedish salmon hatcheries for their help with sample collection and transport. We especially thank Elisabeth Elfving for valuable assistance in the laboratory.

References

Ackefors, H., N. Johansson, and B. Wahlberg. 1991. The Swedish compensatory program for salmon in the Baltic—an action plan with biological and economical implications. ICES Marine Science Symposium 192:109–119.

Amcoff, P., L. Norrgren, H. Börjeson, and J. Lindeberg. 1996. Lowered concentrations of thiamine (vitamin B1) in M74-affected feral Baltic salmon (*Salmo salar*). Pages 38–39 *in* Bengtsson et al. (1996).

Bengtsson, B.-E., and C. Hill. 1996. Review of recent research efforts on reproductive disturbances in Baltic fish. Pages 21–22 *in* Bengtsson et al. (1996).

Bengtsson, B.-E., C. Hill, and S. Nellbring, editors. 1996. Report from the second workshop on reproduction disturbances in fish. Swedish Environmental Protection Agency Report 4534, Stockholm.

Börjeson, H., L. Förlin, and L. Norrgren. 1996. Investigation of oxidants and prooxidants in salmon affected by the M74 syndrome. Pages 95–96 *in* Bengtsson et al. (1996).

Börjeson, H., L. Norrgren, T. Andersson, and P.-A. Bergqvist. 1994. The Baltic salmon-situation in the past and today. Pages 14–25 *in* L. Norrgren, editor. Report from the Uppsala workshop on reproduction disturbances in fish. Swedish Environmental Protection Agency Report 4346, Uppsala.

Christiansen, R., J. Glette, Ø. Lie, O. J. Torrissen, and R. Waagbo. 1995. Antioxidant status and immunity in Atlantic salmon, *Salmo salar* L., fed semi-purified diets with and without astaxanthin supplementation. Journal of Fish Diseases 18:317–328.

Fisher, J. P., J. M. Spitsbergen, T. Iamonte, E. E. Little, and A. DeLonay. 1995. Pathological and behavioral manifestations of the "Cayuga syndrome," a thiamine deficiency in larval landlocked Atlantic salmon. Journal of Aquatic Animal Health 7:269–283.

Fitzsimons, J. 1996. Overview of M74/early mortality syndrome research in the Great Lakes. Pages 23–24 *in* Bengtsson et al. (1996).

Krinsky, N. I. 1989. Antioxidant functions of carotenoids. Free Radical Biology and Medicine 7:617–635.

Kurashige, M., E., Okimasu, M. Inoue, and K. Utsumi. 1990. Inhibition of oxidative injury of biological membranes by astaxanthin. Physiological Chemistry and Physics and Medical NMR 22:27–38.

Larsson, D. G., and C. Haux. 1996. Possible roles of thiamine, thiaminases and other thiamine inactivating factors in the EMS/M74 syndrome. Pages 40–41 *in* Bengtsson et al. (1996).

Larsson, P.-O. 1980. Smolt rearing and the Baltic salmon fishery. Pages 157–186 *in* J. Thorpe, editor. Salmon ranching. Academic Press, London.

Lignell, Å. 1994. Astaxanthin in yolk-sac fry from feral Baltic salmon. Pages 94–96 *in* L. Norrgren, editor. Report from the Uppsala workshop on reproduction disturbances in fish. Swedish Environmental Protection Agency Report 4346, Uppsala.

Lundström J., L. Norrgren, and H. Börjeson. 1996. Clinical and morphological studies of Baltic salmon yolk-sac fry suffering from the M74 syndrome. Pages 26–27 *in* Bengtsson et al. (1996).

Nakano T., M. Tosa, and M. Takeuchi. 1995. Improvement of biochemical features in fish health by red yeast and synthetic astaxanthin. Journal of Agricultural and Food Chemistry 43:1570–1573.

Nishigaki, I., A. A. Dmitrovskii, W. Miki, and K. Yagi. 1994. Suppressive effect of astaxanthin on lipid peroxidation induced in rats. Journal of Clinical Biochemistry and Nutrition 16:161–166.

Norrgren, L., B.-E. Bengtsson, and H. Börjeson. 1994. Summary of the workshop "reproduction disturbances in fish." Pages 7–11 *in* L. Norrgren, editor. Report from the Uppsala workshop on reproduction disturbances in fish. Swedish Environmental Protection Agency Report 4346, Uppsala.

Pettersson, A. and Å. Lignell. 1996. Decreased astaxanthin levels in the Baltic salmon and the M74 syndrome. Pages 28–29 *in* Bengtsson et al. (1996).

Pickova, J., A. Kiessling, A. Pettersson, and P. Dutta. In press. Comparison of fatty acid composition and astaxanthin content in health and by M74 affected salmon eggs from three Swedish river stocks. Comparative Biochemistry and Physiology.

Torrissen, O. J., W. Hardy, and K. D. Shearer. 1989. Pigment composition of salmonids—carotenoid deposition and metabolism. CRC Critical Reviews in Aquatic Sciences 1(2):209–225.

Uchiyama, M., and M. Mihara. 1978. Determination of malonaldehyde precursor in tissues by thiobarbituric acid test. Analytical Biochemistry 86:271–278.

American Fisheries Society Symposium 21:31–40, 1998

Effects of Thiamine Treatments on Survival of M74-Affected Feral Baltic Salmon

PATRIC AMCOFF[1]
Department of Pathology, Faculty of Veterinary Medicine
Swedish University of Agricultural Sciences, Box 7028, S-750 07 Uppsala, Sweden

HANS BÖRJESON
Swedish Salmon Research Institute, S-814 94 Älvkarleby, Sweden

ROLAND ERIKSSON
Heden Salmon Hatchery, Hedenforsvägen 24, S-961 46 Boden, Sweden

LEIF NORRGREN
Department of Pathology, Faculty of Veterinary Medicine
Swedish University of Agricultural Sciences

Abstract.—Since 1974, feral salmon *Salmo salar* populations of the Baltic Sea have suffered from a yolk sac fry mortality known as the M74 syndrome. Mortality rates of 40–95% have been recorded during the 1990s in compensatory rearing stations along the east coast of Sweden. The M74 syndrome has been linked to the offspring of specific females and associated with low thiamine (vitamin B_1) concentrations in both female tissues and their progeny. This study evaluated the effect of thiamine treatments on mortality and thiamine concentrations in progeny with and without M74. Eggs and newly hatched yolk sac fry were immersed in water containing thiamine at concentrations of 100, 500, or 2,000 mg/L. Hardening of eggs in water containing thiamine at 500 or 2,000 mg/L completely eliminated M74-related mortality, whereas treatment with thiamine at 100 mg/L only partially reduced M74 mortality. The mean thiamine concentrations at the yolk sac fry stage (21–23 d after hatching) in untreated normal and M74-affected groups were between 0.70–1.0 and 0.19–0.26 nmol/g, respectively. At the same sampling, the mean thiamine concentrations in groups in which eggs were water-hardened in thiamine at 500 or 2,000 mg/L were between 0.8 and 9.4 times higher than the concentrations in the untreated groups. A thiamine threshold limit interval of 0.34–0.47 nmol/g was estimated for the development of M74 in yolk sac fry.

Feral anadromous salmon *Salmo salar* populations of the Baltic Sea have been severely constrained during the later part of the 20th century by commercial fishing and by reduced access to natural habitats and spawning grounds because of damming for construction of hydroelectric power plants (Karlsson and Karlström 1994). To compensate for losses of natural production, a rearing program was developed in Sweden in the 1950s. The strategy has been to catch ascending sexually maturing salmon and to maintain them in indoor pools until ovulation. Eggs are then stripped and fertilized, and the fry are reared until smoltification, when the smolts are released into their native river.

Since 1974, the feral Baltic salmon populations have suffered from yolk sac fry mortality caused by a condition known as the M74 syndrome. The M74 syndrome, which develops during the yolk sac resorption process, is female dependent, and the mortality rate in affected family groups is usually 100% (Norrgren et al. 1993; Lundström et al. 1998, this volume). In the early 1990s, an increased incidence of M74 was recorded at compensatory rearing stations along the entire east coast of Sweden, with mortality peaking at 85% in 1993 (Börjeson and Norrgren 1997). A number of factors have been hypothesized to be involved in the etiology of the M74 syndrome, including toxicants and reduced contents of essential antioxidants and nutrients (Norrgren et al. 1993; Börjeson and Norrgren 1997; Amcoff et al. 1998; Pettersson and Lignell 1998, both this volume). Amcoff et al. (1998) have shown that the development of M74 is related to the thiamine (vitamin B_1) status of the offspring. Thiamine deficiency in larval fish has been associated with early mortality syndrome (EMS) and the Cayuga syndrome (CS; Fisher et al. 1996; Brown et al. 1998, this volume). Early mortality syndrome affects several salmonid species in the Great Lakes basin, causing high yolk sac fry mortality at swim-up (Skea et al. 1985;

[1] To whom correspondence should be addressed.

Fitzsimons et al. 1995), whereas CS is associated with high Atlantic salmon yolk sac fry mortality in the Finger Lakes of New York State (Fisher et al. 1995a, 1995b). The pathogenesis of M74 resembles that of EMS and CS, and generally low thiamine concentrations in the affected offspring have been observed (Fisher et al. 1996; Amcoff et al. 1998; Lundström et al. 1998). Yolk sac fry affected by the syndromes have shown improved survival after immersion in thiamine-enriched water, indicating that thiamine is involved in the cause of all three syndromes (Bylund and Lerche 1995; Fitzsimons 1995; Fisher et al. 1996).

The objectives of this investigation were to evaluate the effects of prophylactic thiamine treatments on the survival of Baltic salmon and to measure thiamine concentrations in M74-afflicted offspring to determine appropriate dose levels and to examine the response to treatment at different developmental stages.

Methods

Fish Material

From July to September, 1994 and 1995, spawning migrating Baltic salmon of both sexes were caught in salmon traps at the Boden Brood Stock Fishery on the River Luleälven. The fish were maintained in indoor pools with flowing river water, mature individuals were weighed, and a condition factor was calculated [(body weight in grams) ÷ (length in cubic centimeters) × 100]. In late October 1994 and 1995, 414 and 370 females, respectively, were stripped. Of these, the spawn from 10 and 20 females were randomly selected in 1994 and 1995, respectively, for evaluation of the effects of different thiamine treatments on their thiamine content and mortality during egg and larval development. Each egg batch was rinsed twice in a 0.9% NaCl solution to remove remnants of ruptured eggs and to optimize fertilization (Scott and Baynes 1980). Milt from two males was added to each batch, together with 0.5 L of NaCl solution (0.9%), and left for 3 min for fertilization. The eggs were subsequently rinsed three times in a 0.9% NaCl solution to remove excess milt. Eggs were then water-hardened for 3 h with or without a supplement of thiamine hydrochloride, as described below, in 4°C river water. After water hardening, all egg batches were disinfected by immersion in an iodophor solution of Buffodine® (Evans Vanodine International Ltd., Preston, UK) (1%, volume per volume) for 10 min and then incubated in separate hatching trays with flowing river water at the Heden Salmon Hatchery on the River Luleälven and followed until swim-up. The mortality rates were monitored during prehatch development, as was the occurrence of M74 mortality from the posthatch period until swim-up. Dead offspring were removed regularly. The water temperature from the time of stripping until swim-up varied between 0.1–4°C from October to April and 4–15°C in May and June. To standardize the sampling of yolk sac fry that hatched on different dates, accumulated posthatch centigrade degree-days (d°C) were used. The date of hatching was defined as the date when 50% of the eggs had hatched. Each family group hatched over a period of 2–3 d. The first sampling (S1) was performed 1 week after fertilization. Yolk sac fry were sampled 5 d after hatching at 32–34d°C (S2) and again 21–23 d after hatching at 148–172d°C (S3). Eggs and yolk sac fry were killed by rapid freezing and stored in airtight plastic bags at −70°C until thiamine analysis, which was performed within 2 months. Absorption of thiamine in the differently treated groups was estimated as the actual increase of thiamine concentration in the treated groups compared with the untreated controls on the same sampling occasion.

Immersion Experiments

Solutions of 100, 500, and 2,000 mg of thiamine hydrochloride (T-4625, Sigma Chemical Co., St. Louis, Missouri) per liter of river water (4°C) were prepared and buffered with $NaHCO_3$ to pH < 6.9. Solutions were aerated for 30 min to remove excess CO_2 before immersions using 1 L of solution per 1,000 individuals. The untreated controls were handled identically except that they were immersed in river water.

Immersion experiment 1 (Ie1).—The egg batch (7,450–14,500 eggs) from each of the 10 females caught and stripped in 1994 was divided into three subgroups of equal size. One subgroup (Ie1-100E) was immersed in thiamine at 100 mg/L during water hardening. The remaining two subgroups were both hardened in river water: one was kept as an untreated control (Ie1-C) and the other (Ie1-500YSF) was immersed in thiamine at 500 mg/L for 1.5 h 2 d after hatching (13d°C). All subgroups were sampled twice (S2 and S3) for thiamine analysis.

Immersion experiment 2 (Ie2).—The egg batch (2,750–11,900 eggs) from each of the 20 females caught and stripped in 1995 was divided into four subgroups of equal size. Two of these subgroups were immersed in thiamine at 500 (Ie2-500E) or 2,000 (Ie2-2000E) mg/L during water hardening. The remaining two subgroups were hardened in river water: one was kept as an untreated control (Ie2-C) and the other (Ie2-2000YSF) was immersed in thiamine at 2,000 mg/L for 1.5 h 2 d after hatching (11d°C). To minimize the risk of interference from thiamine attached to the chorion, egg samples (S1) from all family groups were taken 1 week after treatment. Yolk sac fry were collected twice (S2 and S3) from all family groups.

Thiamine Assay

Total thiamine, in the form of unphosphorylated free thiamine, was extracted using acid and enzymatic hydrolysis (Amcoff et al. 1998). Thiamine was converted by derivation with alkaline $K_3Fe(CN)_6$ to the fluorescent compound thiochrome and was then analyzed by high-performance liquid chromatography. All samples were analyzed in duplicate, and all data are presented on a wet weight basis (ww).

Statistics

To test for differences in weight, condition factor, and fecundity between females producing normal or M74-affected offspring, and to test for differences in mortality, thiamine concentrations, and absorption of thiamine between normal and M74-affected groups, the two-tailed Student's unpaired t-test was used. To compare the absorption of thiamine in groups exposed to different concentrations of thiamine, simple regression analysis was used and P-values were calculated using analysis of variance. Absorbed thiamine concentrations (nanomoles per gram) were subjected to $\log_{10}$ transformation [$Y' = \log_{10}(\text{absorption} + 1)$] and plotted against the exposure concentrations (100, 500, and 2,000 mg/L). In all testing, the work of Zar (1984) was consulted, and the statistics were calculated using the StatView 4.5 data analysis system (Abacus Concepts, Inc., Berkeley, California). The significance levels are presented as $P \leq 0.05$, $P \leq 0.01$, or $P \leq 0.001$.

Results

The mean mortality attributable to M74 in the progeny of all stripped female salmon (414 and 370) from the River Luleälven was 62 and 50% in 1994 and 1995, respectively. Among the fish used in this investigation, 4 of 10 (40%) family groups evaluated in 1994 and 16 of 20 (80%) family groups evaluated in 1995 developed M74. In 1994, females that produced progeny affected by M74 were significantly larger ($P \leq 0.05$) than females that produced normal offspring, although this was not the case in 1995 (Tables 1 and 2).

TABLE 1.—Female weight, condition factor, and fecundity with prehatch and posthatch mortality in normal (N = 6) and M74 (N = 4) groups for immersion experiment 1 (Ie1) in 1994. Significant differences between groups are indicated by different letters after the means.

Variable or egg subgroup	Normal groups	M74 groups	Statistics
Weight (kg)	8.4 ± 2.5 z	12 ± 0.97 y	$P \leq 0.05$
Condition factor[a]	1.2 ± 0.13	1.2 ± 0.15	NS
Fecundity (eggs/kg)	1,300 ± 300	1,000 ±140	NS
	Prehatch mortality (%)[b]		
Ie1-C[c]	1.8 ± 1.7	2.1 ± 1.0	NS
Ie1-100E[d]	1.2 ± 1.3	2.1 ± 1.1	NS
Ie1-500YSF[e]	1.8 ± 1.7	2.1 ± 1.1	NS
	Posthatch mortality (%)[f]		
Ie1-C	1.5 ± 1.3 z	100 ± 0 y	$P \leq 0.001$
Ie1-100E	1.9 ± 1.6 z	82 ± 23 y	$P \leq 0.01$
Ie1-500YSF	1.4 ± 1.5 z	67 ± 40 y	$P \leq 0.01$

[a] (Body weight in grams) ÷ (Length in cubic centimeters) × 100.

[b] Total egg mortality from fertilization to hatching.

[c] Untreated controls.

[d] Eggs hardened in 100 mg of thiamine per liter per 1,000 individuals.

[e] Yolk sac fry immersed in 500 mg of thiamine per liter per 1,000 individuals at 13d°C posthatch.

[f] Total yolk sac fry mortality from hatching to swim-up.

TABLE 2.—Female weight, condition factor, and fecundity with prehatch and posthatch mortality in normal ($N = 4$) and M74 ($N = 16$) groups for immersion experiment 2 (Ie2) in 1995. Significant differences between groups are indicated by different letters after the means.

Variable or egg subgroup	Normal groups	M74 groups	Statistics
Weight (kg)	8.1 ± 1.7	7.7 ± 2.2	NS
Condition factor[a]	1.1 ± 0.10	1.2 ± 0.10	NS
Fecundity (eggs/kg)	1,100 ± 470	880 ± 260	NS
	Prehatch mortality (%)[b]		
Ie2-C[c]	8.5 ± 11	5.2 ± 9.0	NS
Ie2-500E[d]	6.6 ± 11	5.3 ± 6.5	NS
Ie2-2000E[e]	13 ± 17	13 ± 11	NS
Ie2-2000YSF[f]	8.5 ± 11	5.2 ± 9.0	NS
	Posthatch mortality (%)[g]		
Ie2-C	1.5 ± 1.2 z	100 ± 0 y	$P \leq 0.001$
Ie2-500E	1.8 ± 1.1	2.3 ± 0.9	NS
Ie2-2000E	4.0 ± 3.2	7.0 ± 6.1	NS
Ie2-2000YSF	1.5 ± 1.3	33 ± 36	NS

[a] (Body weight in grams)÷(Length in cubic centimeters) × 100.

[b] Total egg mortality from fertilization to hatching.

[c] Untreated controls.

[d] Eggs hardened in 500 mg of thiamine per liter per 1,000 individuals.

[e] Eggs hardened in 2,000 mg of thiamine per liter per 1,000 individuals.

[f] Yolk sac fry immersed in 2,000 mg of thiamine per liter per 1,000 individuals at 11d°C posthatch.

[g] Total yolk sac fry mortality from hatching to swim-up.

Mortality Rates

In 1994, prehatch mortality (1.2–2.1%) did not differ significantly between thiamine-treated and untreated groups or between the groups that developed into normal or M74-affected offspring (Table 1). Posthatch mortality was significantly higher in the M74 controls and the treated M74 groups ($P \leq 0.01$–0.001) than in normal groups. All fish in untreated M74 groups died, whereas the normal family groups displayed a posthatch mortality of 1.4–1.9%. The M74 groups of Ie1-100E and Ie1-500YSF showed mean posthatch mortality rates of 82 and 67%, respectively; 2 of 4 treated M74 family groups displayed partial M74 development averaging 30% (Ie1-500YSF) and 60% (Ie1-100E), and the other two family groups experienced 100% mortality.

In 1995, no differences were observed in prehatch mortality between normal (6.6–13%) and M74 groups (5.2–13%; Table 2). At swim-up, the normal control groups showed a mean posthatch mortality of 1.5%, compared with 100% for the M74 control groups ($P \leq 0.001$). Posthatch mortality in the treated normal groups ranged from 1.5 to 4%. An average M74 mortality of 33% was observed in the treated M74 groups for Ie2-2000YSF, whereas the mean posthatch mortality rates in Ie2-500E and Ie2-2000E were 2.3 and 7.0%, respectively.

Thiamine Concentrations

Untreated yolk sac fry (Ie1-C) that did not develop M74 had mean thiamine concentrations of 0.71 and 0.70 nmol/g (ww) at S2 and S3, respectively (Table 3). Their thiamine levels were significantly higher ($P \leq 0.01$) than those of fry in untreated groups that developed M74, which had mean thiamine concentrations at S2 and S3 of 0.21 and 0.19 nmol/g (ww). The M74 groups from Ie1-100E contained significantly lower ($P \leq 0.05$–0.01) concentrations of thiamine at S2 and S3, 0.29 and 0.27 nmol/g (ww), than normal groups for these treatments, which contained 0.88 (S2) and 0.69 (S3) nmol/g (ww). The results obtained after immersion of yolk sac fry in thiamine at 500 mg/L (Ie1-500YSF) were 0.91 and 0.70 nmol/g (ww) in the normal groups at S2 and S3 and 0.30 and 0.22 nmol/g (ww) in the M74 groups at S2 and S3.

TABLE 3.—Mean thiamine concentrations ± SD (nmol/g, wet weight) in normal ($N = 6$) and M74 ($N = 4$) groups for immersion experiment 1 (Ie1) in 1994. Significant differences between groups are indicated by different letters after the means. NA, not analyzed.

Sample	Normal groups	M74 groups	Statistics
	Ie1-C[a]		
S1[b]	NA	NA	
S2[c]	0.71 ± 0.29 z	0.21 ± 0.12 y	$P \leq 0.01$
S3[d]	0.70 ± 0.25 z	0.19 ± 0.08 y	$P \leq 0.01$
	Ie1-100E[e]		
S1	NA	NA	
S2	0.88 ± 0.35 z	0.29 ± 0.05 y	$P \leq 0.05$
S3	0.69 ± 0.18 z	0.27 ± 0.08 y	$P \leq 0.01$
	Ie1-500YSF[f]		
S1	NA	NA	
S2	0.91 ± 0.25 z	0.30 ± 0.11 y	$P \leq 0.01$
S3	0.70 ± 0.16 z	0.22 ± 0.10 y	$P \leq 0.001$

[a] Untreated controls.

[b] Eggs sampled 1 week after fertilization.

[c] Yolk sac fry sampled 7 d after hatching at 32–34d°C posthatch.

[d] Yolk sac fry sampled 21–23 d after hatching at 148–172d°C posthatch.

[e] Eggs hardened in 100 mg of thiamine per liter per 1,000 individuals.

[f] Yolk sac fry immersed in 500 mg of thiamine per liter per 1,000 individuals at 13d°C posthatch.

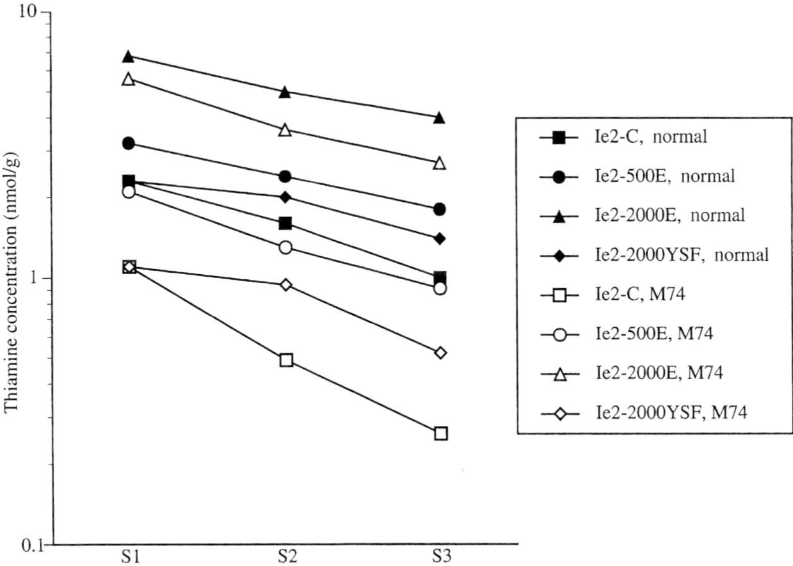

FIGURE 1.—Mean thiamine concentrations (nmol/g, wet weight) on sampling occasions S1–S3 in immersion experiment 2 (Ie2). The groups Ie2-C (100% M74) are controls; in Ie2-500E (0% M74) and Ie2-2000E (0% M74), eggs were hardened in 500 or 2,000 mg of thiamine per liter per 1,000 eggs; in Ie2-2000YSF (33% M74), yolk sac fry were immersed in 2,000 mg of thiamine per liter per 1,000 individuals at 11d°C posthatch. Normal and M74 indicate groups developing normally and groups developing M74.

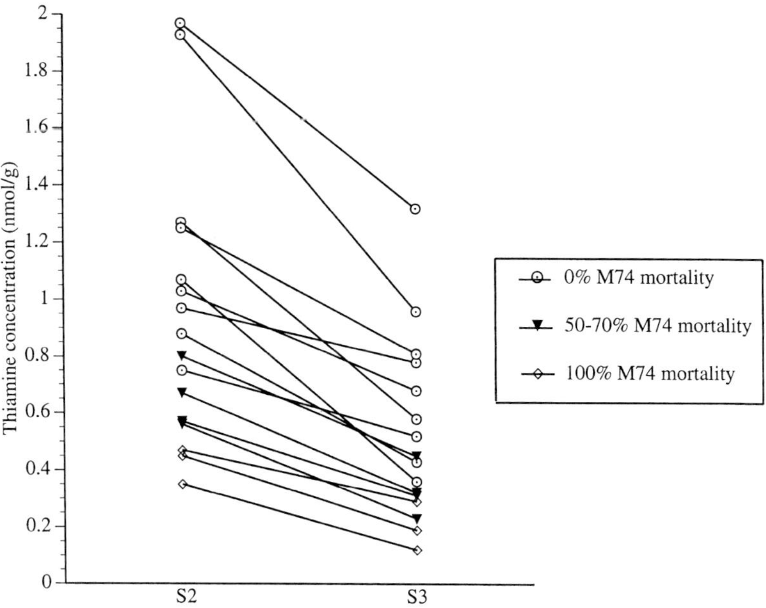

FIGURE 2.—Thiamine concentrations (nmol/g, wet weight) in M74 groups ($N = 16$), including those with partial M74 development ($N = 4$), after immersions of yolk sac fry in 2,000 mg of thiamine per liter per 1,000 individuals at 11d°C posthatch (Ie2-2000YSF). Yolk sac fry were sampled at S2 (5 d after hatching, 32–34d°C) and S3 (21–23 d after hatching, 148–172d°C).

Mean thiamine concentrations in normal groups from Ie2-C were 2.3 (S1), 1.6 (S2), and 1.0 (S3) nmol/g (ww), which were significantly higher ($P \leq 0.01$–0.001) than the corresponding concentrations in the groups that developed M74: 1.1 (S1), 0.49 (S2), and 0.26 (S3) nmol/g (ww; Table 4, Figure 1). Because of the rapid development of M74 in 10 of the 16 untreated M74 family groups (Ie2-C), it was possible to sample only 6 of the untreated M74 groups at the third sampling time (S3). Of the groups immersed at water hardening in 500 (Ie2-500E) or 2,000 (Ie2-2000E) mg/L, mean thiamine concentrations in all M74-affected groups were significantly ($P \leq 0.05$–0.001) lower than in the normal groups at all three (S1–S3) sampling times. Immersion of yolk sac fry in 2,000 mg/L (Ie2-2000YSF) resulted in mean thiamine concentrations for S2 and S3 of 2.0 and 1.4 nmol/g (ww), respectively, in normal groups, which were significantly ($P \leq 0.01$–0.001) greater than the mean thiamine concentrations of 0.94 (S2) and 0.52 (S3) nmol/g (ww) measured in the M74 groups. Two of three family groups from the Ie2-2000YSF treatment that developed 100% M74 at S3 had the lowest thiamine concentrations of all the treated family groups in this investigation, 0.12 and 0.19 nmol/g (ww; Figure 2). Only M74 controls had thiamine contents similar to these values. The M74 groups from Ie2-2000YSF that did not develop M74 at swim-up ($N = 9$) had a significantly higher ($P \leq 0.05$) mean thiamine concentration (0.72 ± 0.30 nmol/g, ww) than the groups ($N = 3$) that developed 100% M74 (0.20 ± 0.084 nmol/g, ww) at S3. The family groups from Ie2-2000YSF that showed partial (50–70%) M74 development ($N = 4$) had a mean thiamine concentration of 0.33 ± 0.090 nmol/g (ww) at S3. The lowest thiamine concentrations in yolk sac fry with no M74 development (S3) were 0.34 and 0.36 nmol/g (ww) in Ie1 and Ie2, respectively, and the highest detected concentrations in family groups with complete M74 development (S3) were 0.38 and 0.47 nmol/g (ww) in Ie1 and Ie2. These results suggest a threshold limit interval of thiamine concentrations between 0.34 and 0.47 nmol/g (ww) for development of M74.

Absorption of Thiamine

No significant differences were found between normal and M74 groups in absorption of thiamine in the treated groups. In Ie1, the mean thiamine absorption in Ie1-100E and Ie1-500YSF was between 0 and 0.17 nmol/g in both the normal and M74 groups at S2 and S3. In Ie2, the mean thiamine absorption in the

TABLE 4.—Mean thiamine concentrations ± SD (nmol/g, wet weight) in normal ($N = 4$) and M74 ($N = 16$) groups for immersion experiment 2 (Ie2) in 1995. The mean with the asterisk (*) is based on six samples. Significant differences between groups are indicated by different letters after the means.

Sample	Normal groups	M74 groups	Statistics
		Ie2-C[a]	
S1[b]	2.3 ± 0.85 z	1.1 ± 0.25 y	$P \leq 0.001$
S2[c]	1.6 ± 0.74 z	0.49 ± 0.20 y	$P \leq 0.001$
S3[d]	1.0 ± 0.51 z	0.26 ± 0.12 y*	$P \leq 0.01$
		Ie2-500E[e]	
S1	3.2 ± 0.36 z	2.1 ± 0.34 y	$P \leq 0.001$
S2	2.4 ± 0.46 z	1.3 ± 0.35 y	$P \leq 0.001$
S3	1.8 ± 0.39 z	0.91 ± 0.28 y	$P \leq 0.001$
		Ie2-2000E[f]	
S1	6.8 ± 0.99 z	5.6 ± 0.97 y	$P \leq 0.05$
S2	5.0 ± 0.59 z	3.6 ± 0.79 y	$P \leq 0.01$
S3	4.0 ± 0.52 z	2.7 ± 0.69 y	$P \leq 0.001$
		Ie2-2000YSF[g]	
S1	2.3 ± 0.85 z	1.1 ± 0.25 y	$P \leq 0.001$
S2	2.0 ± 0.68 z	0.94 ± 0.48 y	$P \leq 0.01$
S3	1.4 ± 0.55 z	0.52 ± 0.32 y	$P \leq 0.001$

[a] Untreated controls.
[b] Eggs sampled 1 week after fertilization.
[c] Yolk sac fry sampled 7 d after hatching at 32–34 d°C posthatch.
[d] Yolk sac fry sampled 21–23 d after hatching at 148–172 d°C posthatch.
[e] Eggs hardened in 500 mg of thiamine per liter per 1,000 individuals.
[f] Eggs hardened in 2,000 mg of thiamine per liter per 1,000 individuals.
[g] Yolk sac fry immersed in 2,000 mg of thiamine per liter per 1,000 individuals at 11 d°C posthatch.

normal and M74 groups was 0.26–0.45 nmol/g in Ie2-2000YSF (S2 and S3) and 0.65–1.0 and 2.4–4.5 nmol/g in Ie2-500E and Ie2-2000E (S1, S2, and S3), respectively. The absorption on sampling occasions S1–S3 in both the normal and M74 groups of Ie2-2000E was significantly ($P \leq 0.05$) higher than those in the normal and M74 groups of Ie2-500E. At S3, both the normal and M74 groups of Ie2-2000YSF had significantly ($P \leq 0.05$) less absorption of thiamine (0.26–0.40 nmol/g) than the normal and M74 groups of Ie2-500E (0.65–0.80 nmol/g).

A significant ($P \leq 0.001$) dose-dependent absorption of thiamine was found at sampling time S2 in groups exposed during water hardening (regression equation: $y = 0.064 + 2.79x \times 10^{-4}$; $R^2 = 0.904$; Figure 3A). Also, groups exposed to thiamine as newly hatched yolk sac fry showed a significant ($P \leq 0.032$) absorption of thiamine at S2 (regression equation: $y = 0.026 + 5.70x \times 10^{-5}$; $R^2 = 0.154$; Figure 3B).

Discussion

Treatment of Baltic salmon eggs with thiamine reduced M74 mortality; our data indicate that concentrations of at least 500 mg/L applied during water hardening are necessary to counteract the development of M74. Mean M74 mortality in family groups immersed as yolk sac fry in thiamine at 500 or 2,000 mg/L varied between 33 and 67%, suggesting that single immersions in 500 or 2,000 mg/L at the yolk sac fry stage may not be sufficient to completely reverse the development of M74. In the present investigation, several treated M74 family groups exhibited partial (30–70%) M74 development, whereas complete M74 development was observed in all untreated M74 groups. This partial M74 development may be attributable to individual variations in susceptibility to thiamine deficiency and to the initial thiamine concentrations within family groups.

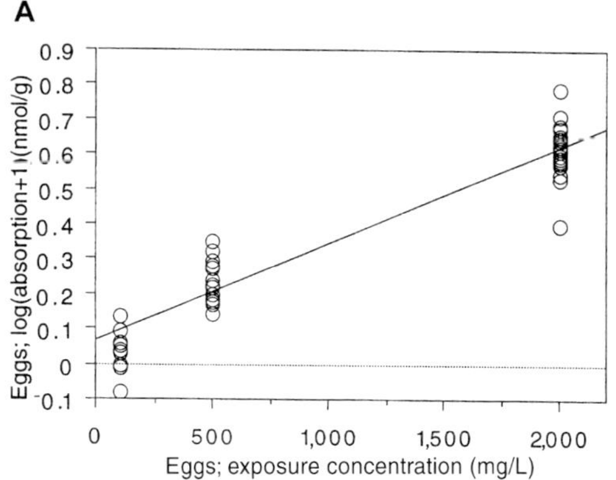

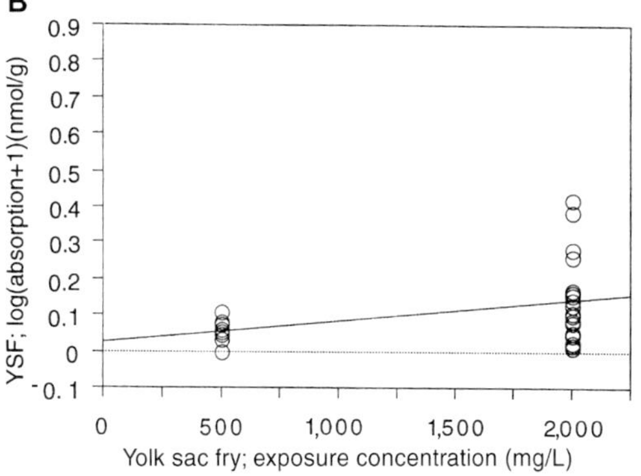

FIGURE 3.—Regression plots of thiamine absorption (nmol/g) and exposure concentrations at S2 in groups (N = 50) treated during water hardening in 100, 500, and 2,000 mg/L per 1,000 individuals (A) and in groups (N = 30) treated in 500 and 2,000 mg/L per 1,000 individuals as newly hatched yolk sac fry (YSF; B). The thiamine absorption was subjected to $\log_{10}$ transformation [$Y' = \log_{10}(\text{absorption} + 1)$].

To compare the absorption efficiency between groups treated at different times, the regression plots of absorbed thiamine and exposure concentrations may be used. The mean absorption at S2 in M74 groups treated in 500 mg/L during water hardening, the lowest exposure concentration resulting in a complete elimination of M74 mortality, was 0.81 nmol/g. By using the regression equation for groups exposed as newly hatched yolk sac fry, a rough estimation of the dosage required to achieve full survival may be calculated. This resulted in a suggested treatment concentration of at least 4,000 mg of thiamine per liter per 1,000 individuals. This is considerably higher than the 2,000 mg/L used, which might explain the M74 development in several groups from Ie2-2000YSF.

There are several possible methods of thiamine treatment, including thiamine injection into broodfish during oogenesis and absorption at water hardening, during the eyed egg stage, or during the posthatch period. Brown et al. (1998) have shown that the pool of thiamine phosphate esters varies during ontogenesis, with an increase of the coenzyme thiamine diphosphate during the yolk sac fry stage, so thiamine treatment should begin as early as possible. The survival data from this study suggest that with the thiamine concentrations used, treatment during the water-hardening process are more efficient than exposure after hatching to obtain a high survival. The dose-dependent absorption of thiamine in eggs treated during water hardening may indicate a passive absorption of thiamine, whereas in yolk sac fry treated after hatching, considerably less dose-related absorption was demonstrated. One possible explanation of why thiamine absorption is higher in treated eggs than in treated yolk sac fry is the incorporation of water into the egg perivitelline space during water hardening. This incorporation may account for as much as 25% of the total egg weight (Li et al. 1989). Consequently, thiamine taken up into the egg during water hardening may serve as a source of thiamine during progressive development of the embryo. Further research, however, is required to determine adequate dosages and to define the optimal timing and duration of treatment.

The findings of this and other studies (Bylund and Lerche 1995; Fitzsimons 1995; Fisher et al. 1996) clearly show that M74, EMS, and CS are syndromes that can be treated with thiamine. Bylund and Lerche (1995) immersed Baltic salmon yolk sac fry from one female producing progeny with partial M74 development in thiamine hydrochloride at 800 and 8,000 mg/L for 30–60 min. Both treatments resulted in reduction of M74 mortality from 60 to 15%. Atlantic salmon yolk sac fry affected by the CS also increased their survival at swim-up from 0 to 96% after immersion for 1 h in thiamine hydrochloride at 10,000 mg/L (Fisher et al. 1996). Fitzsimons (1995) showed that lake trout *Salvelinus namaycush* affected by EMS responded to thiamine treatment with a reduced total mortality of 22%, compared with 53% in untreated groups. This result was reached after 15 consecutive immersions of yolk sac fry in thiamine hydrochloride at 1,000 mg/L for a period of 2 min every second day.

Because of the high incidence of M74 in the 1990s, some Swedish compensatory rearing stations have had difficulties raising adequate numbers of smolts. Since it became known that it was possible to reduce M74 development by immersion in thiamine solutions, some rearing stations have used this treatment, but at different developmental stages. At some rearing stations, only yolk sac fry with clinical signs of M74 are immersed; this usually requires three or four treatments to obtain good survival. At other rearing stations, high survival rates are achieved by treating newly hatched yolk sac fry on five–seven consecutive occasions until swim-up. The results of this investigation emphasize the importance of the correct distribution of thiamine in therapeutic treatments to eliminate M74 with regard to time, concentration, and treatment method. Moreover, the potential for latent disturbances that may be manifested at later stages in treated M74-affected yolk sac fry should not be underestimated, and further studies with thiamine are necessary to demonstrate the reliability of thiamine treatments.

This work demonstrates that therapeutic thiamine treatments may limit M74 mortality, but effectiveness depends on when that treatment is applied. The highest survival was achieved when eggs were water-hardened in thiamine at concentrations of at least 500 mg/L. There were no differences in thiamine absorption between the M74 and the normally developing groups. The mean thiamine concentrations in eggs and yolk sac fry that developed M74 were significantly lower than in eggs and yolk sac that developed normally, and a thiamine threshold limit interval for the development of M74 in yolk sac fry was estimated at 0.34–0.47 nmol/g.

Acknowledgments

This investigation was financed by grants from the FiRe group at the Swedish Environmental Protection Agency and the National Board of Fisheries. The staff at the Boden Brood Stock Fishery and the Heden Salmon Hatchery, Vattenfall AB, are acknowledged for assisting in the sampling procedures.

References

Amcoff, P., H. Börjeson, J. Lindeberg, and L. Norrgren. 1998. Thiamine concentrations in feral Baltic salmon exhibiting the M74 syndrome. Pages 82–89 *in* McDonald et al. (1998).

Brown, S. B., J. D. Fitzsimons, V. P. Palace, and L. Vandenbyllaardt. 1998. Thiamine and early mortality syndrome in lake trout. Pages 18–25 *in* McDonald et al. (1998).

Bylund, G., and O. Lerche. 1995. Thiamine therapy of M74 affected fry of Atlantic salmon (*Salmo salar*). Bulletin of the European Association of Fish Pathologists 15:93–97.

Börjeson, H., and L. Norrgren. 1997. M74 syndrome: a review of potential etiological factors. Pages 153–166 *in* R. M. Rolland, M. Gilbertson, and R. E. Peterson, editors. Chemically induced alterations in functional development and reproduction of fishes. SETAC (Society of Environmental Toxicology and Chemistry), Pensacola, Florida.

Fisher, J. P., J. D. Fitzsimons, G. F. Combs, Jr., and J. M. Spitsbergen. 1996. Naturally occurring thiamine deficiency causing reproductive failure in Finger Lakes Atlantic salmon and Great Lakes lake trout. Transactions of the American Fisheries Society 125:167–178.

Fisher, J. P., and six coauthors. 1995a. Reproductive failure of landlocked Atlantic salmon from New York's Finger Lakes: investigations into the etiology and epidemiology of the "Cayuga syndrome." Journal of Aquatic Animal Health 7:81–94.

Fisher, J. P., J. M. Spitsbergen, T. Iamonte, E. E. Little, and A. DeLonay. 1995b. Pathological and behavioral manifestations of the "Cayuga syndrome," a thiamine deficiency in larval landlocked Atlantic salmon. Journal of Aquatic Animal Health 7:269–283.

Fitzsimons, J. D. 1995. The effect of B-vitamins on a swim-up syndrome in Lake Ontario lake trout. Journal of Great Lakes Research 21(Supplement 1):286–289.

Fitzsimons, J. D., S. Huestis, and B. Williston. 1995. Occurrence of a swim-up syndrome in Lake Ontario lake trout in relation to contaminants and cultural practices. Journal of Great Lakes Research 21(Supplement 1):277–285.

Karlsson, L., and Ö. Karlström. 1994. The Baltic salmon (*Salmo salar*, L.): its history, present situation and future. Dana 10:61–85.

Li, X., E. Jenssen, and H. J. Fyhn. 1989. Effects of salinity on egg swelling in Atlantic salmon (*Salmo salar*). Aquaculture 76:317–334.

Lundström, J., H. Börjeson, and L. Norrgren. 1998. Clinical and pathological studies of Baltic salmon suffering from yolk sac fry mortality. Pages 62–72 *in* McDonald et al. (1998).

McDonald, G., J. D. Fitzsimons, and D. C. Honeyfield, editors. 1998. Early life stage mortality syndrome in fishes of the Great Lakes and Baltic Sea. American Fisheries Society, Symposium 21, Bethesda, Maryland.

Norrgren, L., T. Andersson, P.-A. Bergqvist, and I. Björklund. 1993. Chemical, physiological and morphological studies of feral Baltic salmon (*Salmo *salar*) suffering from abnormal fry mortality. Environmental Toxicology and Chemistry 12:2065–2075.

Pettersson, A., and Å. Lignell. 1998. Low astaxanthin levels in Baltic salmon exhibiting the M74 syndrome. Pages 26–30 *in* McDonald et al. (1998).

Scott, A. P., and S. M. Baynes. 1980. A review of the biology, handling and storage of salmonid spermatozoa. Journal of Fish Biology 17:707–739.

Skea, J. C., J. Symula, and J. Miccoli. 1985. Separating starvation losses from other early feeding fry mortality in steelhead trout (*Salmo gairdneri*) chinook salmon (*Oncorhynchus tshawytscha*) and lake trout (*Salvelinus namaycush*). Bulletin of Environmental Contamination and Toxicology 35:82–91.

Zar, J. H., editor. 1984. Biostatistical analysis, second edition. Prentice-Hall, Inc., Englewood Cliffs, New Jersey.

American Fisheries Society Symposium 21:41–61, 1998

Descriptive Studies of Mortality and Morphological Disorders in Early Life Stages of Cod and Salmon Originating from the Baltic Sea

GUN ÅKERMAN AND LENNART BALK
Institute of Applied Environmental Research, Laboratory for Aquatic Ecotoxicology Stockholm University, S-611 82 Nyköping, Sweden

Abstract.—The reproductive success of cod *Gadus morhua* from the Baltic Sea and the Barents Sea was compared. The offspring of 17 family pairs from the Baltic Sea and 12 family pairs from the Barents Sea were investigated during the embryonic and larval development stages. Frequencies of mortality over time and frequencies of different disorders at hatch were analyzed. The results indicated that the reproductive success of cod from the Baltic Sea was seriously impaired. The Baltic cod showed high mortality before hatch. In newly hatched larvae, different kinds of disorders were seen, such as vertebrae deformity, disrupted yolk sac or subcutaneous edema in the yolk sac, and precipitate in the yolk. To compare mortality and early developmental abnormalities in Baltic cod and Baltic salmon *Salmo salar*, the offspring of 20 salmon family pairs, caught in the River Dalälven in Sweden, were investigated analogically. The results showed that the majority of the salmon offspring experienced a thiamine deficiency-dependent mortality at different stages of larval development and that five family pairs experienced high mortality before hatch. In salmon, different kinds of disorders were also seen at hatch, such as vertebrae deformity, blood disorders, subcutaneous edema in the yolk sac, and precipitate in the yolk. The disorders at hatch were not correlated to later thiamine deficiency-dependent mortality. Aliquots of newly fertilized salmon eggs were injected with thiamine by the nanoinjection method. This treatment had only a minor effect on the frequency of disorders at hatch, but it protected the salmon larvae almost completely from later thiamine deficiency-dependent mortality. This indicates that factors other than thiamine deficiency are involved in the developmental disorders. In both salmon and cod from the Baltic Sea, the mortality and disorders among the offspring were mainly correlated to the female, and in both species some females produced offspring that experienced high mortality before hatch. Both salmon and cod also showed disorders that might have similar biochemical mechanisms, because the formation of precipitates and edema in the yolk sac occurs in both species.

The Baltic Sea is a brackish-water sea that contains a young ecosystem compared with other marine ecosystems. The Baltic Sea consists of three main basins: the Bothnian Bay, the Bothnian Sea, and the Baltic proper. The Baltic proper opens into the North Sea via a narrow outlet, the Kattegat. The species that invaded after the last glacial period were marine species, with wide salinity tolerance from the North Sea, and limnic species, with salinity tolerance from the glacial lakes. Today, the Baltic Sea is inhabited by few but relatively abundant species, and several are living close to their osmotic tolerance limit. The salinity in the surface water decreases from about 20‰ in Kattegat, to 6–8‰ in the Baltic proper, to 2–4‰ in the northern part, the Bothnian Bay. The deep water has a higher salinity and is only partly mixed with the surface water. The exchange of surface water depends mainly on irregular inflows of marine water, which are dependent on factors such as low and high atmospheric pressure and heavy storms working in concert. Oxygen deficiency is common in some parts of the Baltic Sea below the halocline during stagnation periods.

Today, the Baltic Sea is surrounded by urban industrial countries, which results in anthropogenic effects such as eutrophication and discharges of inorganic and organic pollutants. The hydrographic characteristics of the Baltic Sea, notably its low water turnover rate (about 40 years), low water temperatures, and pronounced thermoclines and haloclines, contribute to an accumulation of persistent organic compounds and heavy metals in the sediments and biota. Certain compounds, such as DDT, 1,1-dichloro-2,2-bis(*p*-chlorophenyl)ethane, and PCBs, have decreased in some species, probably as a result of their being banned, but many "new" and "old" chemicals continue to enter the ecosystem with known and unknown toxicological effects (Bignert et al. 1993).

Several fish species in the Baltic Sea show signs of reproductive disorders. The most obvious occurs in the Atlantic salmon *Salmo salar* and is designated the M74 syndrome, but there are indications of reproductive failure also in sea trout *Salmo trutta* (Bengtsson et al. 1994), cod *Gadus morhua* (Westernhagen et al. 1988; Larsson 1994; Åkerman et al. 1996a), eel *Anguilla anguilla* (Moriarty 1990; Larsson et al. 1991), and perch *Perca fluviatilis*. The reproductive disorders in perch show a geographical connection to the pulp mill industry (Karås et al. 1991). In burbot *Lota lota*, a high frequency of individuals with retarded gonadal development has been reported in the Gulf of Bothnia (the northern part of the Bothnian Bay; Pulliainen et al. 1992).

The underlying reasons for the reproductive disturbances among all of these fish species in the Baltic Sea are not known. Because the Baltic Sea is characterized by low diversity and simple food chains, the observed reproductive disturbances represent a more serious threat here than in other ecosystems.

Cod is one of the most important species for Swedish fisheries. There are five separate cod populations in Swedish waters, but the largest and most important one is the eastern Baltic cod population. This population has adapted, to a certain degree, to the low salinity of brackish water. Salinity levels sufficient for reproduction are present in the deeper parts of the Baltic proper. However, because of the increased eutrophication, the oxygen concentration is often too low for developing offspring. Long stagnation periods, therefore, have led to serious declines in the population. Recently, during the years 1993–1994, large inflows of marine water, attributable to meteorological events, improved the salinity and oxygen conditions in the spawning areas. However, despite the favorable conditions for reproduction, no abundant year-classes of the cod have been found (Larsson 1994).

During the last 23 years, high mortality has occurred among salmon yolk sac larvae (M74 syndrome) in Swedish hatcheries, where reproduction is based on wild broodstock, with the exception of the years 1980–1984, when no or very low mortality was reported. Around 90% of the Baltic salmon stock is reared in hatcheries to compensate for the damming of rivers for hydroelectric power stations. However, larvae from wild spawning salmon have also been found to be affected in Sweden as well as in Finland (Soivio 1994; Karlström 1995). During the years 1992–1995, 57–87% of the female spawners at some Swedish hatcheries produced offspring with very high larval mortality. Just before death, the larvae exhibit lack of coordination, irregular swimming patterns, lethargy, and darkening of the skin. These signs have been correlated to low concentrations of thiamine (vitamin B_1) in the salmon eggs and larvae (Amcoff et al. 1996; Koski et al. 1996).

In North America, the early mortality syndrome (EMS) in several salmonid species in some of the Great Lakes (Lakes Michigan, Ontario, and Erie) and the Cayuga syndrome in landlocked Atlantic salmon in the Finger Lakes of New York State demonstrate similarities with the M74 syndrome in the Baltic salmon. The syndromes show similar clinical signs in the period before death. In Canada, in 1991, Fitzsimons conducted experiments during which he discovered that the mortality is related to low thiamine levels (Fitzsimons 1995). Affected larvae in these different locations have been treated successfully (as measured by lower mortality) with thiamine at the egg or larval stage (Bylund and Lerche 1995; Fitzsimons 1995; Åkerman et al. 1996b; Amcoff et al. 1996; Fisher et al. 1996; Koski et al. 1996). Thus, thiamine deficiency appears to be a common factor in these syndromes. The underlying reason for the low levels of thiamine is a crucial and important question that still needs to be answered.

In a previous report, comparisons were made of the reproductive success of cod from the Baltic Sea and the Barents Sea (Åkerman et al. 1996a). The results from that study indicate that the reproductive success of Baltic Sea cod was seriously impaired as a result of high mortality of the eggs and embryos. Elevated levels of DNA adducts were found in the cod offspring from the Baltic Sea before feeding, indicating a maternal transfer of xenobiotics (Ericson et al. 1996). In the present study, the results from a comparison of reproductive success are presented in more detail. Mortality rates of offspring from different females are presented, and frequencies of disorders in the larvae are illustrated. A comparison with mortality and disorders early in development in salmon offspring from the River Dalälven in Sweden, where the salmon are affected by the M74 syndrome, is also presented. Salmon were also treated with thiamine, by bathing of larvae or by nanoinjection of the newly fertilized eggs.

Materials and Methods

Cod

During the 1994 spawning season, comparative studies of the reproductive outcome from North East Arctic cod and Baltic cod were performed. North East Arctic cod were caught in the

TABLE 1.—Weight, length, condition factors, percentage of fertilized eggs, and number of fertilized eggs studied in Atlantic salmon during the 1994–1995 season (females A–F) and the 1995–1996 season (females G–L).

Female/male	Female weight (kg)	Female length (cm)	Condition factor[a]	Percentage of fertilized eggs	Number of fertilized eggs studied
A/1	10.8	101	1.05	43	77
A/2				44	88
B/1	12.8	103	1.17	98	210
B/2				99	192
B/3				98	196
B/4				98	253
C/3	8.2	89	1.16	96	158
C/4				96	130
D/4	10.2	96	1.15	96	211
D/5				6	14
E/5	6.8	88	1.00	29	65
E/6				63	192
F/6	8.2	91	1.09	21	47
F/7				99	201
G/8	13.5	108	1.07	81	116
H/9	6.9	85	1.12	87	126
I/10	7.2	82	1.31	92	133
J/11	6.2	84	1.05	95	136
K/12	9.5	93	1.18	87	153
L/13	10.5	98	1.12	64	111

[a] (Total weight in grams) ÷ (Total length in cubic centimeters) × 100.

Lofoten area by trawling during the spawning period (23–24 March). Mature cod were stripped by a slight pressure to the abdomen, and the eggs were fertilized immediately on the boat. Six females and 3 males were used in 12 different female–male combinations. Each egg batch contained eggs from one female fertilized by one male only. Immediately after fertilization and water hardening, the eggs were transported to the laboratory, where they were held in 34‰ seawater prepared from synthetic sea salt (hw Marinemix, Wiegandt, Germany) and distilled water. The use of synthetic seawater decreased the risk of contamination by biotic factors. The salinity used is the well-known concentration in the spawning area in Lofoten; at this salinity, fertilized eggs float and unfertilized and dead eggs sink to the bottom. From the eggs that remained buoyant at the blastula stage, 300 eggs were used for analyses. The egg batches were kept in a volume of 1 L and at a temperature of 6.5°C. The water was changed daily.

Baltic cod were caught by trawling during two sampling sessions (14 June and 11 July) north of the island Bornholm in the Baltic Sea. Mature cod were stripped and the eggs were fertilized immedi-

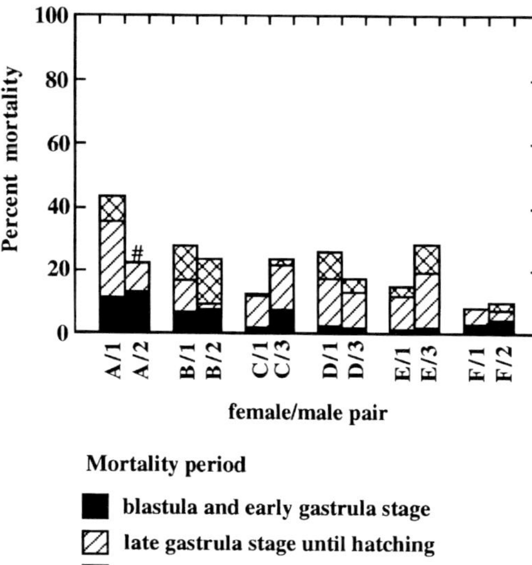

FIGURE 1.—Mortality at different periods in the offspring of six cod females (A–F) and three males (1–3) originating from Lofoten, Norway. The bars represent cumulative percentages of mortality at the different periods, calculated from the number of dead animals recorded during each period as a percentage of the number of fertilized eggs at the start (day 1).

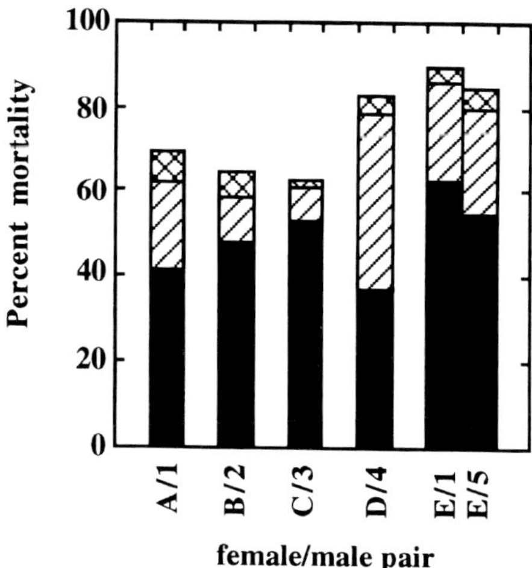

FIGURE 2.—Mortality at different periods in the offspring of five cod females (A–E) and five males (1–5) originating from our first sampling in the Baltic Sea. The percentages are calculated as described for Figure 1.

ately on the boat in the manner described above. The eggs were fertilized and held in 17‰ synthetic seawater prepared as described above. This salinity is optimal for Baltic cod egg development (Nissling and Westin 1991; Westin and Nissling 1991). From the first sampling session, 5 females and 5 males were investigated in 6 different batches; from the second sampling session, 11 females and 7 males were investigated in 11 different batches. Each egg batch contained eggs from one female fertilized by one male only. The number of eggs used in the investigation and the handling of eggs during development were the same as in the Lofoten investigation; the temperatures were 5.8 and 7.0–8.4°C, respectively, for the two sampling sessions.

Dead eggs, embryos, and larvae were removed daily and counted. When hatching was completed, the larvae were examined under a stereomicroscope (Wild M8, Heerbrugg, Switzerland; 6–50× magnification) and frequencies of disorders were recorded. Baltic cod larvae from the second sampling session were examined 2 d after hatching was completed, at 122 degree-days. Variables analyzed were severe disorders (larvae arrested in development combined with vertebrae and eye deformity), vertebrae deformity, disrupted yolk sac or edema in yolk sac, precipitate in yolk, and deformed or opalescent muscle. In total, 8,472 fertilized eggs were investigated; the survivors (3,542 individuals) were examined at 122 degree-days (newly hatched), and 205 were examined at 137 degree-days after fertilization.

Salmon

Studies of salmon reproductive outcome were performed during two seasons, 1994–1995 and 1995–1996. The eggs and sperm were obtained by stripping salmon from the River Dalälven, Sweden (Älvkarleby Fisheries Research Station). During these two reproductive seasons, 47 and 52%, respectively, of the mature female fish showed signs of the M74 syndrome. Hybrid fish (salmon and trout) were detected by starch gel electrophoresis of diagnostic enzymes (glucose-6-phosphate isomerase and phosphoglycometase) and were omitted from the experiments.

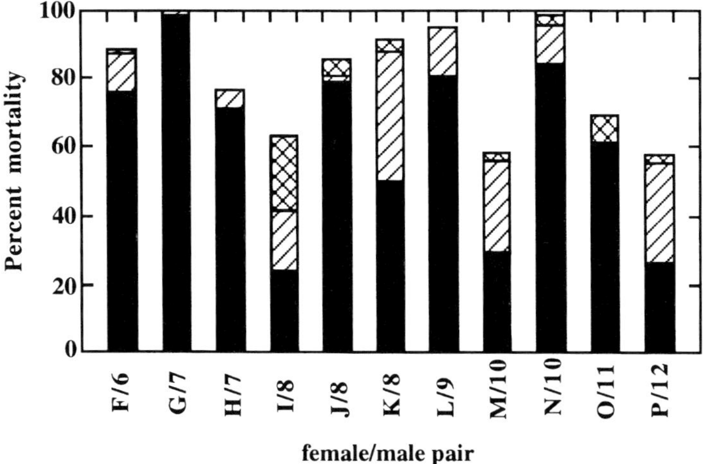

FIGURE 3.—Mortality at different periods in the offspring of 11 cod females (F–P) and 7 males (6–12) originating from our second sampling in the Baltic Sea. The percentages are calculated as described for Figure 1.

During the season 1994–1995, the offspring of six females and seven males were studied. The egg batch from each female was divided into two aliquots and fertilized with milt from two different males, one in each aliquot, except for one female whose egg batch was divided into four aliquots and fertilized with milt from four different males. After fertilization, the 14 egg batches, each containing around 200 eggs, were kept in separate aquariums supplied with running charcoal-filtered tap water from a nearby freshwater lake at an ambient temperature of 4.5–8.5°C until the 6 last weeks, when the temperature was increased to 9–13°C. Each aquarium held 2 L of water and had a water flow of 17 mL/min; thus, the turnover rate was 2 h. Mortality was recorded every second day during egg, larval, and juvenile development until 1,720 degree-days. During week 19 after fertilization, feeding with commercial food was started (Ewos EST 90, Sodertalje, Sweden).

Four weeks after hatching (100 degree-days), aliquots of larvae (30–40 larvae in each) from four family groups were treated by bathing once in thiamine hydrochloride (Sigma T-4625, Sigma Chemical Co., St. Louis, Missouri) at 400 mg/L for 1 h. Another four aliquots from the same family groups were treated for 2 h every third day for 3 weeks in thiamine hydrochloride at 200 mg/L. The pH change during these treatments was less than 0.1.

During the season 1995–1996, the offspring of six females and six males were studied. The entire egg batch from each female was fertilized by one male. After fertilization and water hardening, an aliquot of eggs from each female was placed in a 1% agarose gel in Petri dishes before they were put in separate aquariums as described above, now at an ambient temperature of 4.0–7.5°C. Four square Petri dishes, each holding 36 eggs, were used for each family pair. This method of placing the newly fertilized eggs in holes made in an agarose gel facilitates injections with fine glass capillaries into the eggs early in development and is known as the nanoinjection method (Åkerman and Balk 1995). Equally important, this method facilitates observation of embryonic development until hatching without disturbing the developmental process. The eggs in one Petri dish from each female were injected with 24–31 nL (0.02% of egg volume) of thiamine chloride solution (0.3 mol/L, pH adjusted to 6.4), and the eggs in one Petri dish from three of the females were

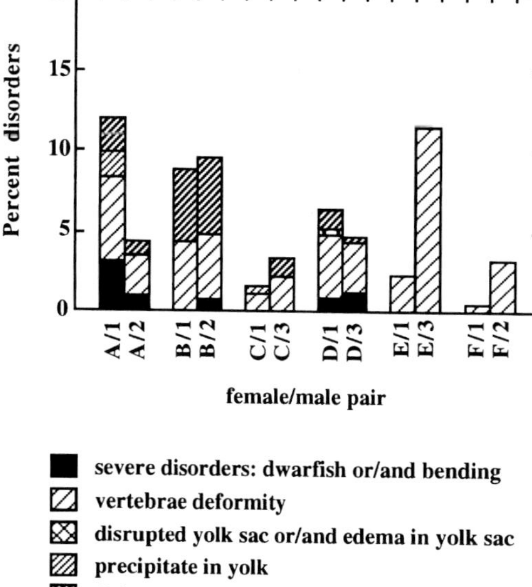

FIGURE 4.—Disorders recorded in newly hatched cod larvae from six females (A–F) and three males (1–3) originating from Lofoten, Norway. Females A–F and males 1–3 denote the corresponding female–male pairs as in Figure 1. The bars represent percentages of hatched larvae with various disorders. Larvae with more than one disorder are presented once, in the first group from below.

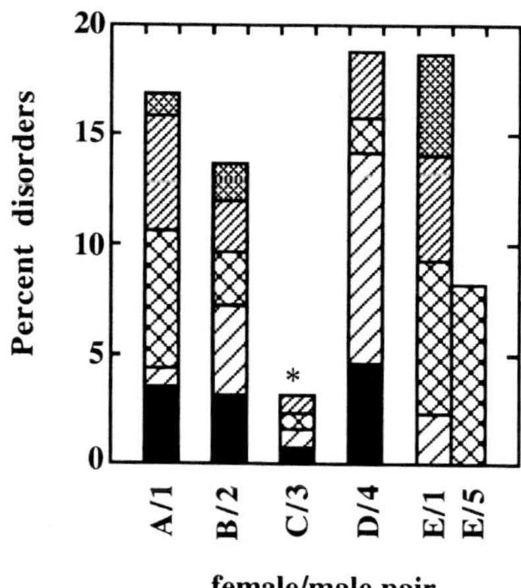

FIGURE 5.—Disorders recorded in newly hatched cod larvae from five females (A–E) and five males (1–5) originating from our first sampling in the Baltic Sea. Females A–E and males 1–5 denote the corresponding female–male pairs as in Figure 2. The percentages are calculated as described for Figure 4.

injected with 61–78 nL (0.05% of egg volume) of the same solution. After injection, the concentrations of thiamine in the eggs were increased by 52 and 130 nmol/g, respectively. Mortality was recorded every second day during egg, larval, and juvenile development until 940 degree-days. In all other respects, the eggs and larvae were handled and observed as described in the preceding season.

Immediately after hatching, the larvae were examined under a stereomicroscope (Wild M8; 6–50× magnification) and frequencies of disorders were recorded. Variables analyzed were vertebrae deformities, precipitate in the yolk, hemorrhages, and subcutaneous edema. All calculations of frequencies were made after disposal of unfertilized eggs.

The basic data for the salmon females used in these studies are shown in Table 1. For each female, the percentage of fertilized eggs with each male and the number of investigated eggs or embryos are also shown. The condition factor was calculated according to the formula [(total weight in grams) ÷ (total length in cubic centimeters) × 100]. In total, 3,878 salmon eggs were investigated for mortality during early development (until 940 or 1,720 degree-days). In addition, the survivors at hatch (2,432 individuals) were examined for disorders at the newly hatched stage.

Results

Cod

Mortality until hatching in the offspring of females and males caught in Lofoten ranged from 7 to 22%, except for one female–male combination whose offspring experienced 36% mortality (Figure 1). Mortality during the larval period ranged from 0.3 to 14%. The majority of deaths occurred during embryonic development. Mortality during the blastula and early gastrula stages was correlated to a greater extent to the female than to the male.

Mortality until hatching in the offspring of females and males caught in the first sampling session in the Baltic Sea ranged from 58 to 86%. Mortality was most

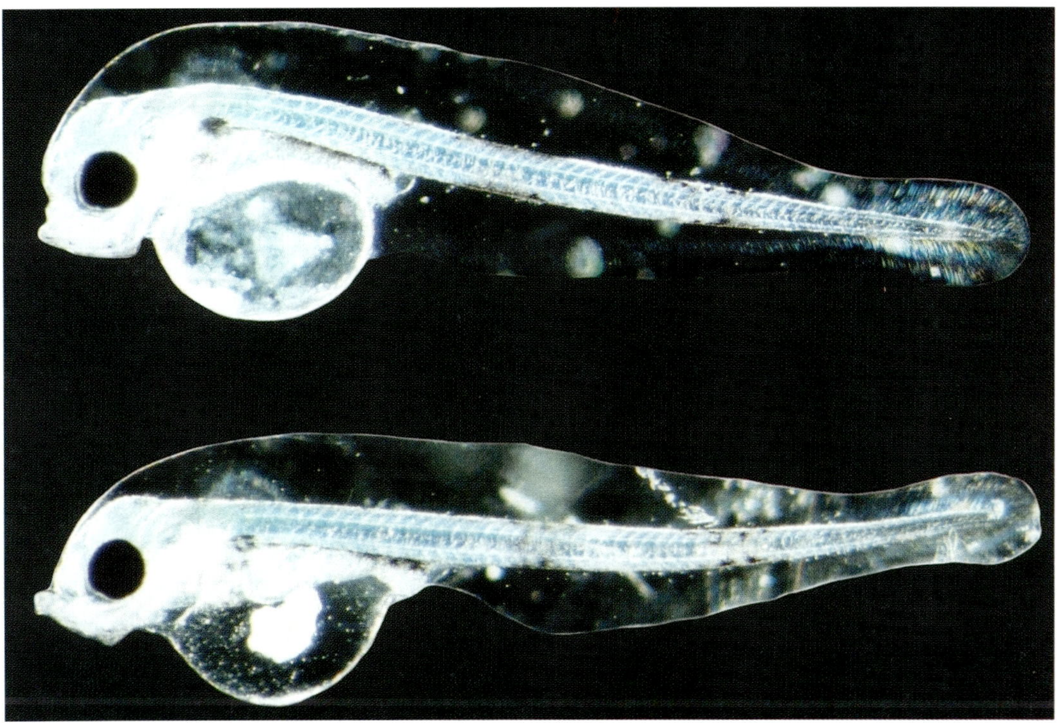

FIGURE 6.—Larvae from cod originating from the Baltic Sea. The upper larva has a precipitate in the yolk and the lower larva has a disrupted yolk sac. These kinds of disorders occur frequently in newly hatched cod larvae from the Baltic Sea (see Figures 5 and 8).

pronounced during the blastula and early gastrula stages (Figure 2). During the embryonic period (late gastrula until hatch), a relatively large difference in mortality was observed between females. The larval mortality was not greater than 7%. Only minor differences in mortality were observed between the egg batches from female E fertilized by male 1 or male 5.

The offspring of the females investigated from the second sampling session in the Baltic Sea showed a mortality range before hatching of 42–100% (Figure 3). As in the first sampling, the highest frequency of mortality occurred during early development, except in the egg batches from three females, I, M, and P, in which the frequencies were less than 30%. At the end of yolk sac consumption, however, the mortality reached almost 60% in these batches.

The major disorders in newly hatched larvae originating from Lofoten were vertebrae deformity and weak tail curvature (Figure 4). Vertebrae deformity was mostly expressed as curvature of the tail that affected swimming behavior. The larvae in the group with weak tail curvature showed normal swimming behavior. The frequencies of these two disorders differed depending on the male used, although egg batches from different females had the strongest influence.

The major disorders in newly hatched larvae originating from the Baltic Sea were vertebrae deformity and different kinds of abnormalities in the yolk sac, such as disrupted yolk sac, edema in the yolk sac, and precipitate in the yolk. Deformed or opalescent muscle was also frequently observed (Figure 5). Examples of abnormalities in the yolk sac are shown in Figures 6 and 7.

The larvae from the second sampling session in the Baltic Sea were investigated at a later stage of development, when only a minor part of the yolk remained. Vertebrae deformity together with disrupted yolk sac or edema were the main disorders (Figure 8).

Only small differences were found in the disorders seen in the fish from the first and second sampling sessions in the Baltic Sea. Offspring of cod originating from Lofoten showed no disrupted yolk sacs or edema and very rare occurrence of precipitate in the yolk, which were observed frequently in the offspring of cod originating from the Baltic Sea.

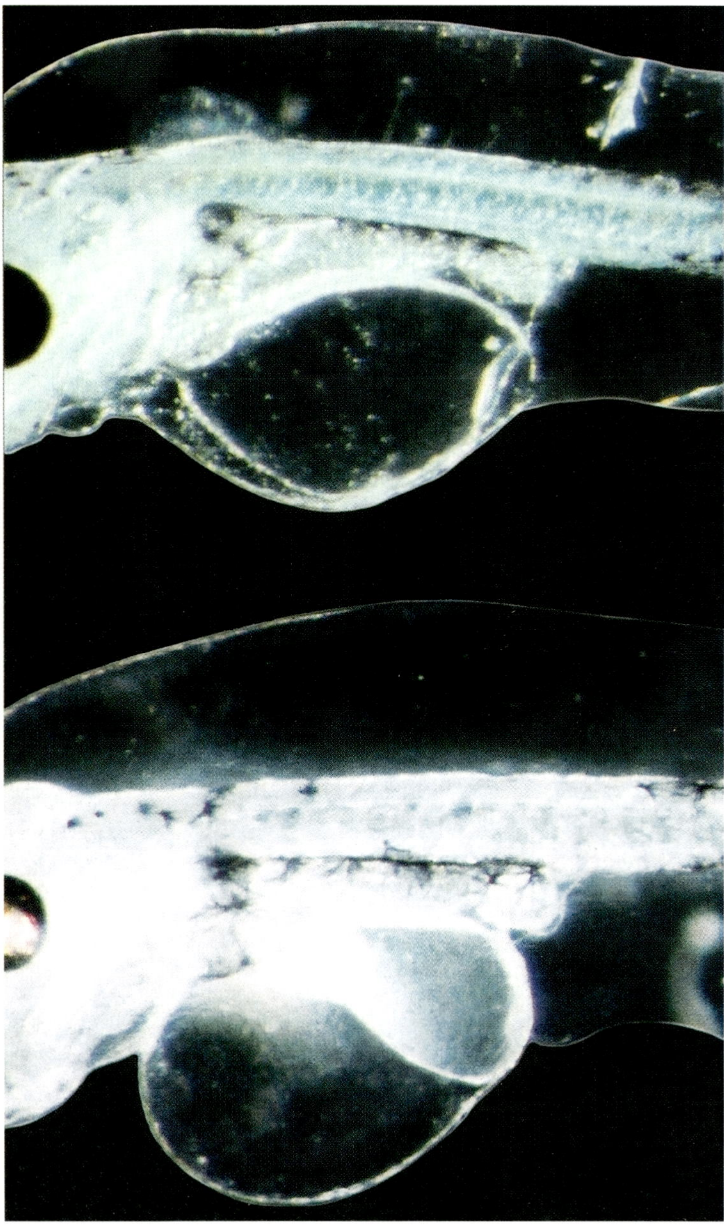

FIGURE 7.—Detail of yolk sacs in cod larvae originating from the Baltic Sea. The upper larva shows a normal yolk sac and the lower larva shows a large edema in the yolk sac. Edema in the yolk sac occurs frequently in newly hatched cod larvae from the Baltic Sea (see Figures 5 and 8).

Salmon

Mortality during different periods in the offspring of six females fertilized by seven males during the season 1994–1995 is shown in Figure 9. Early mortality was seen in the offspring of two females. Approximately 50% of the eggs or embryos from female A died before hatching, that is, about 20% during the first 4 weeks after fertilization and about 30% during embryonic development (weeks 5–12). High early mortality was also seen in the offspring of female E fertilized by male 6. In many embryos that died before hatching, the blastopore was not closed, and the embryos were very small, with severe vertebrae deformities (Figure 10). For two of the females, D and C, the larvae died during the later part of yolk sac absorption after showing signs such as lethargy and abnormal swimming. The larvae from female D experienced almost total mortality just before swim-up, and the larvae from female C experienced almost

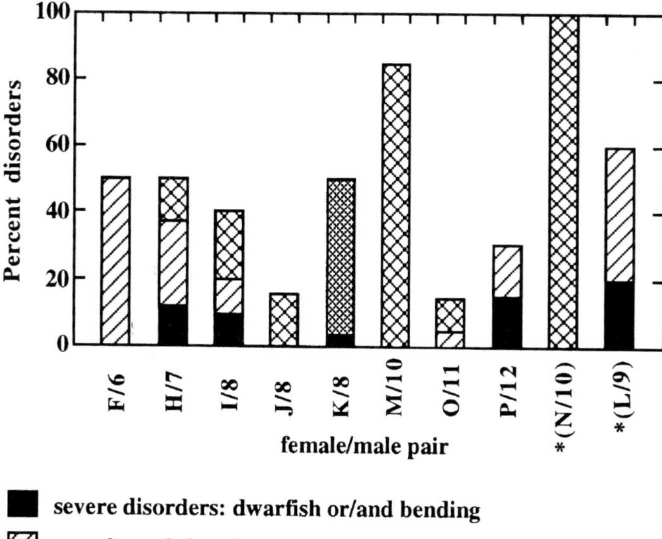

FIGURE 8.—Disorders recorded in cod larvae at 122 degree-days from 10 females (F and H–P) and 7 males (6–12) originating from our second sampling in the Baltic Sea. Females F and H–P and males 6–12 denote the corresponding female–male pairs as in Figure 3. The percentages are calculated as described for Figure 4.

total mortality just after swim-up. In the larval groups from females B and F, mortality started late, at weeks 24–28, which was several weeks after the start of feeding (week 19). Mortality of the remaining offspring of female A and the offspring of female F and male 7 started even later, during weeks 29–33. Before they died, they showed the same signs of lethargy and abnormal swimming that were seen in the larvae of females D and C.

Figure 9 also shows the influence of the different males used. In most cases, the mortality time curve obtained was correlated to the specific female with no or little influence from the male. However, for some family pairings, the male definitely influenced the mortality over time. For instance, for the eggs from female E, male 6 produced drastically earlier mortality compared with male 5. Also, for the eggs from female F, male 6 produced earlier mortality, in this case compared with male 7.

Thiamine treatment by bathing aliquots of larvae from four family pairs during weeks 16–18 delayed the onset of mortality in a dose-dependent manner (Figure 11). Untreated larvae from female D and male 4 experienced their major mortality during weeks 16–18. One treatment (400 mg/L for 1 h) during week 16 shifted the mortality to occur mainly during weeks 19–23. Repeated treatments (200 mg/L for 2 h) during weeks 16–18 shifted the mortality period even further, to weeks 29–33. Larvae from female F and male 7 experienced comparatively late mortality when left untreated, most occurring during weeks 24–28. One treatment shifted the major mortality to the last period studied, weeks 29–33, whereas repeated treatments protected the larvae during this period. The larvae from untreated females B and C experienced mortality at an intermediate period compared with the larvae from females D and F. For larvae from females B and C, only repeated treatments shifted the mortality to a later period, weeks 29–33. This was especially pronounced for larvae from female B.

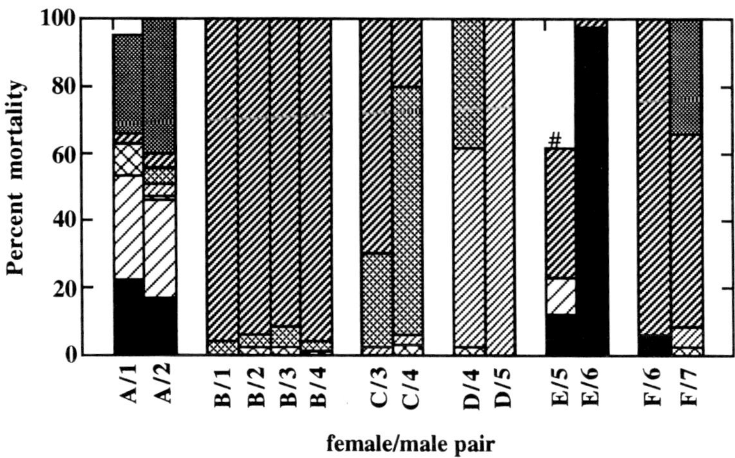

FIGURE 9.—Mortality at different periods in the offspring of six salmon females (A–F) and seven males (1–7) during the 1994–1995 season. The first period starts at fertilization (week 0) and the last period ends after 34 weeks or 1,720 degree-days. The percentages are calculated as described for Figure 1.

During the season 1995–1996, six different family pairs were investigated. In general, the mortality occurred comparatively earlier during development than in the season 1994–1995. The offspring of one female, L, experienced early mortality: 30% during the first weeks after fertilization (weeks 0–5) and another 30% during the embryonic period (weeks 6–16; Figure 12). The larval mortality for females H, I, J, and K occurred after the appearance of signs such as lethargy and abnormal swimming. The offspring of three of these females, H, I, and J, developed the signs when approximately only one-third to one-half of the yolk sac was consumed. For female L, the larval mortality during weeks 19–24 was not preceded by signs of lethargy. These larvae suffered from severe vertebrae deformity (see below). The offspring of female G showed very low overall mortality for the whole study period of 24 weeks. At 24 weeks, almost all of the oil in the yolk had been consumed.

In addition to the mortality in the untreated groups, Figure 12 also shows the results from the thiamine injections into the eggs immediately after fertilization by the nanoinjection method. Two dosages were investigated, 52 and 130 nmol/g. Both concentrations prevented larval mortality until the end (almost all oil consumed) of the experiment for the offspring of females H, I, J, and K. In some of the egg batches, however, thiamine caused a tendency toward increased early mortality. This was especially true for eggs from the relatively unaffected (low mortality) female G at the 130 nmol/g dose of thiamine.

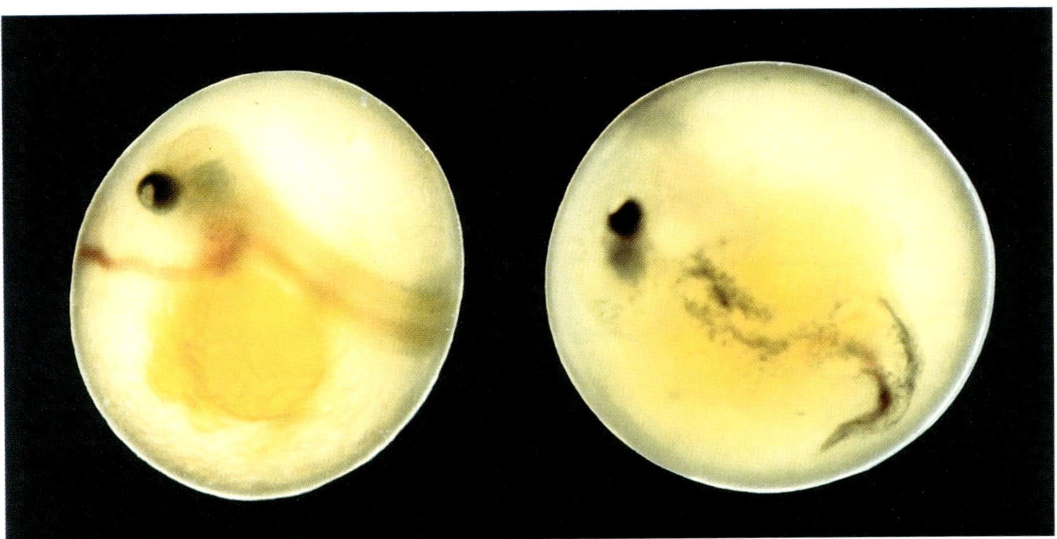

FIGURE 10.—Eggs from Atlantic salmon originating from the Baltic Sea. In the egg at left, the embryo has developed normally. In the egg at right, the embryo has developed severe disorders and will die before hatching. This kind of embryo was seen in the offspring of females A, F, and L (see Figures 9 and 12).

Blood disorders (Figure 13), such as hemorrhage in the head and areas of arrested blood cell circulation in the head or yolk sac vascular system, and precipitate in the yolk sac (Figure 14) were the major disorders in the newly hatched 1995 larvae. For blood disorders, a frequency of around 15–25% seems to be common. Examples of the most frequently seen type of hemorrhage, which occurs in the head, are shown in Figure 15. The larvae from female A showed the highest percentage of blood disorders, affecting 30–50% of the larvae. This was correlated to increased mortality before hatch (see above). The males that were used to fertilize the eggs may influence the frequency of disorders to some extent. Male 3 increased the frequency of blood disorders in larvae from female C and the frequency of edema in larvae from female B compared with male 4. An example of edema in the yolk sac is shown in Figure 16. Male 7 increased the frequency of blood disorders in larvae from female F compared with male 6. Larvae with high frequencies of blood disorders also seem to have high frequencies of precipitate in the yolk. The different males affected the frequency of precipitate by around 20% in the offspring of four females (Figure 14). The precipitate observed immediately after hatching was situated along the blood vessels; later in development, but before larval mortality, the precipitate was observed around the oil droplets situated near the yolk sac membrane (Figure 17).

Blood disorders and precipitate in the yolk were also the major disorders in the newly hatched 1996 larvae. For blood disorders, a frequency of 15–30% was seen in most of the larval groups (Figure 18). The frequency of precipitate was highest in larvae from females G and L (not shown). One group of larvae experienced a high degree (80%) of severe vertebrae deformities. This was correlated to a high level of early mortality (see above).

Injection of thiamine into the eggs at the newly fertilized stage had little influence on total disorder frequencies. A slight but consistent decrease in disorders was observed in larvae injected with thiamine at 52 nmol/g compared with control larvae (except those from female L).

Untreated larvae investigated at 21–24 weeks during the season 1995–1996 that showed signs of lethargy and abnormal swimming before death also exhibited dark pigmentation. Other disorders occurred sporadically within family groups. The most frequent disorder was precipitate in the yolk, but the amount differed between individual larvae in the same family group. Precipitate in the yolk is sometimes described as white precipitate or opalescent yolk. The appearance is different depending on the direction of light (from above or below) during observation or photography (see Figure 19). Exophthalmia was also frequent in all larvae groups

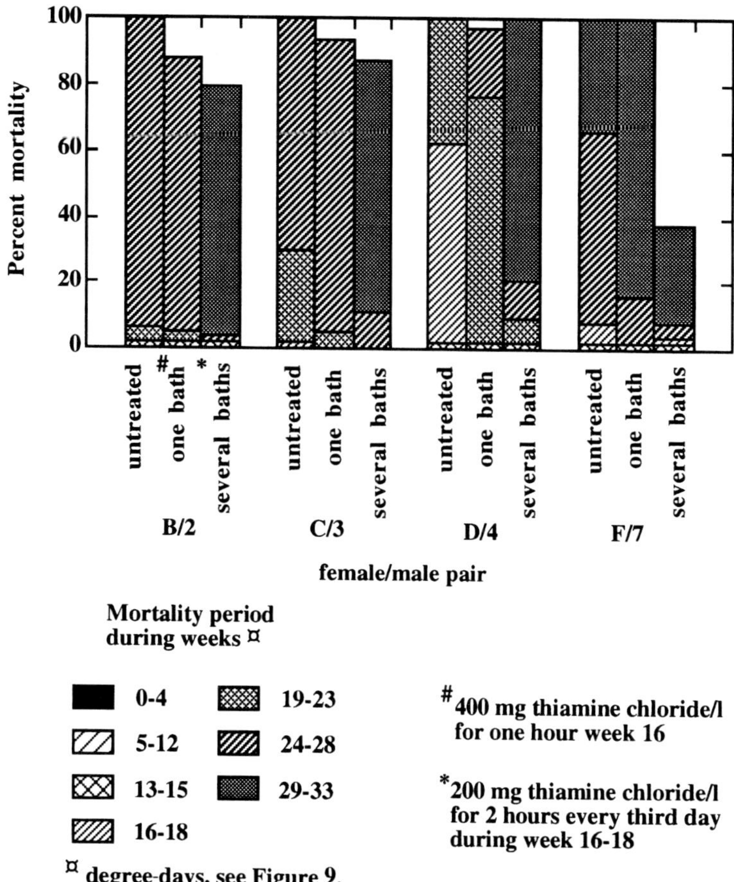

FIGURE 11.—Mortality at different periods after thiamine treatment in the larvae from four female–male pairs during the 1994–1995 season. Treatment consisted of bathing aliquots in thiamine hydrochloride. Females B–D and F and males 2–4 and 7 denote the corresponding female–male pairs as in Figure 9. The percentages are calculated as described for Figure 1.

but to a different extent in different groups. In every family group, some larvae had disorders such as hemorrhages in the head, cessation of blood flow in different tissues, and subcutaneous edema in the yolk sac. Some larvae had pale livers and some had pale yolk oil.

Discussion

The purpose of this investigation was to compare and carefully analyze mortality over time and mortality frequency together with the frequency of various kinds of disorders in both salmon and cod. Disorders were studied with the aim of obtaining data on variables that might be specific for the later development of yolk sac mortality and that might provide clues to the underlying reasons for impairment among offspring. It was decided to investigate the occurrence of disorders just after hatch. This period was selected to avoid disorders that occur near the previously described time of larval death (Bengsston et al. 1994), which could diminish the value of information concerning a cause and effect relationship in larval mortality.

Mortality among yolk sac larvae of salmon in a number of different rivers draining into the Baltic Sea has been described in previous studies (Bengtsson et al. 1994; Norrgren et al. 1994). The high mortality occurs at a specific time, that is, at a developmental stage when about two-thirds of the yolk sac is consumed (Norrgren et al. 1994; Bylund and Lerche 1995). In contrast to the disorders that occur near the time of high larval mortality, it has been argued that disorders that occur during the earlier stages of development generally are limited or absent. However, lower levels of the carotenoids, es-

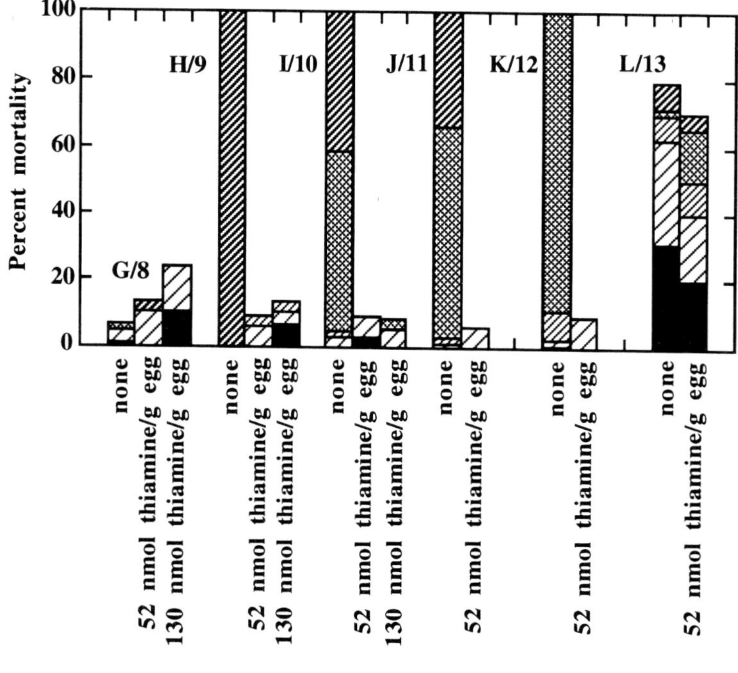

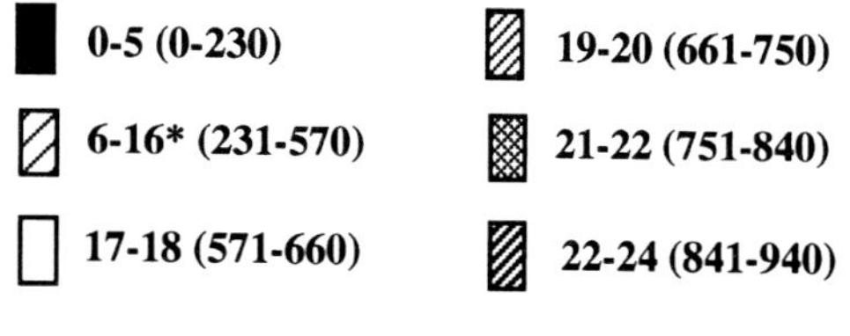

FIGURE 12.—Mortality at different periods in the offspring of six salmon females (G–L) and six males (8–13) during the 1995–1996 season. The second and third bars in each group show mortality in eggs and larvae that were nanoinjected with thiamine (52 or 130 nmol/g) in the yolk immediately after fertilization; the first bar in each group shows mortality in the noninjected control group (none). The first period starts at fertilization (week 0) and the last period ends after 25 weeks or 940 degree-days. The percentages are calculated as in Figure 1.

pecially astaxanthin, have been described in batches of eggs that subsequently develop high larval mortality (Lignell 1994; Pettersson and Lignell 1996).

The reproductive success of the Baltic cod was investigated in parallel with that of cod from the Lofoten area. The reason for this is that we are uncertain if there are healthy cod still to be found in the Baltic Sea. Lofoten is located in the northern part of Norway near the spawning grounds of the North East Arctic cod, which have their feeding areas in the relatively unpolluted Barents Sea. This cod stock is exposed to significantly lower concentrations of anthropogenic substances than the cod living in the Baltic Sea (Jensen et al. 1972; Koistinen 1990; Falandysz 1994; Falandysz et al. 1994). Obviously mature cod were caught in the field during their optimal spawning periods for the two areas (Lofoten and the Baltic Sea). Stripping (with a slight pressure) and fertilization were performed immediately on the boat. This might be a special advantage of this study compared with previous studies, because no selection of parent animals occurred as a result of mortality. Cod caught by trawling exhibit high mortality levels in several handling situations, such as during ship transport to the harbor, during land transport to

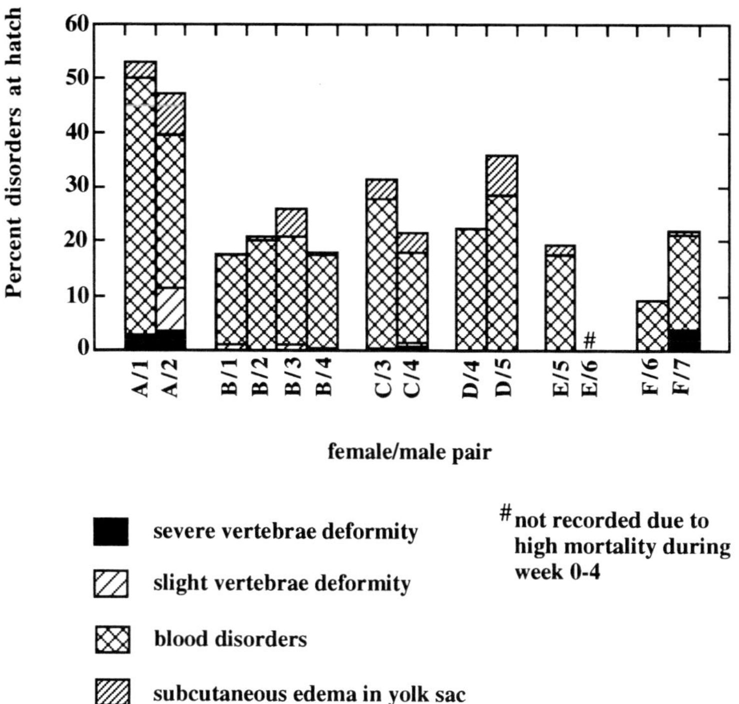

FIGURE 13.—Disorders recorded at hatch in salmon larvae from six females (A–F) and seven males (1–7) during the 1994–1995 season. Females A–F and males 1–7 denote the corresponding female–male pairs as in Figure 9. The percentages are calculated as in Figure 4.

the laboratory, and while staying in basins at the laboratory before producing gametes. This mortality might seriously influence the quality of the offspring produced when the cod are subsequently stripped for mature gametes and artificial fertilization or when they are allowed to spawn freely in the basins. The quality of the offspring in such experiments might be unnaturally high compared with that in the field, because there is a risk that some of the inferior animals will be eliminated as a result of mortality. For instance, fish with low thiamine contents have been reported to show increased sensitivity to handling (Boonyaratpalin and Wanakowat 1993). There is also a possibility that individuals in poor health do not develop mature gonads in the laboratory situation, which would further decrease the influence of affected fish. Together or in isolation, these factors could affect any analysis of the difference in offspring quality when cod originating from different areas are compared.

Cod and salmon are two teleost species very different in several respects, such as reproduction, behavior, and phylogenic origin. It has been hypothesized that substances of anthropogenic origin might be, at least in part, responsible for the observed reproductive impairment in these species. Therefore, it is highly relevant that they both feed, to a large degree, on the same prey in the Baltic Sea (Uzars 1994; Ikonen 1996). Consequently, we looked for possible similarities and dissimilarities between the two species.

The offspring of 3 or 4 of the 12 investigated salmon females experienced mortality during the period previously described as typical for the M74 syndrome (i.e., when around two-thirds of the yolk sac has been consumed) (Bengtsson et al. 1994; Norrgren et al. 1994). The larvae from 3 females experienced mortality when only one-third to one-half of the yolk was consumed, and the larvae from 3 or 4 females experienced mortality rather late in development. Remarkably, the offspring of 3 of the

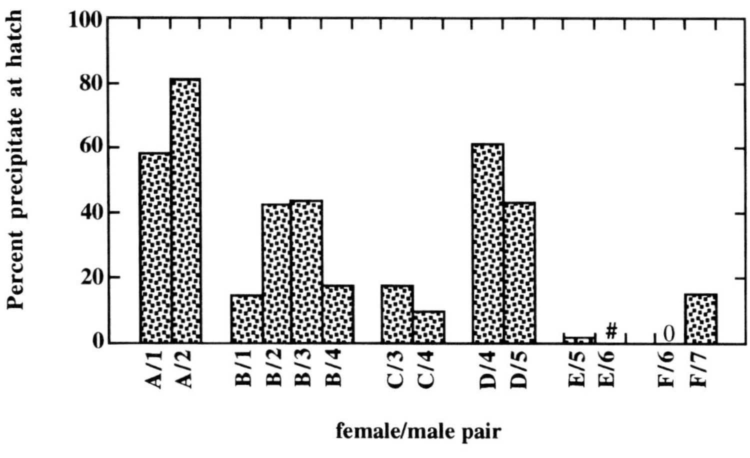

FIGURE 14.—Precipitate in the yolk seen at hatch in salmon larvae from six females (A–F) and seven males (1–7) during the 1994–1995 season. The larvae may also have other kinds of disorders, which are presented in Figure 13. Females A–F and males 1–7 denote the corresponding female–male pairs as in Figure 9.

12 females experienced a high level of mortality very early in development, before hatch. In summary, among the investigated females, mortality was found to occur from the first period (0–250 degree-days) to a period of more than 1,720 degree-days, which was several weeks after the start of feeding. These results are not in agreement with those of previous reports (Börjeson et al. 1994) on the occurrence of mortality in offspring of salmon originating from the Baltic Sea. However, they are in agreement with a recent presentation (Lundström et al. 1996), in which parts of these results were also presented in preliminary form (Åkerman et al. 1996b). Early mortality is not reported from Swedish hatcheries but is reported in connection with EMS in coho salmon *Oncorhynchus kisutch* from Lake Michigan (Marcquenski 1996).

No correlation of mortality to female size ($r = -0.61$) or condition factor ($r = 0.21$) could be seen among the 12 investigated salmon females. The sample size, however, might be too small to observe such a correlation. Karlsson et al. (1996) observed no differences in mortality among females of different ages during the 1994–1995 season. For female cod, no correlation between mortality and size or condition factor was observed, as previously presented (Åkerman et al. 1996a).

The larval mortality associated with the M74 syndrome is considered to be female dependent. The results from the season 1994–1995, when each female was fertilized by two or four different males, indicate some influence from the male with regard to both time when mortality occurred and the number and degree of disorders. The male might influence the expression of enzyme levels for metabolism of anthropogenic substances as well as exert other genetic influences.

The total frequency of disorders in salmon offspring at hatch was not correlated to mortality during the different periods. However, a high percentage of disorders, more than 40%, was correlated to a high mortality before hatch.

Injection of thiamine at 52 or 130 nmol/g had a very pronounced effect in newly fertilized eggs that otherwise showed 100% mortality during the larval period. A concentration of 52 nmol/g was found to be enough to prevent mortality almost completely. This rather high concentration corresponds to a level reported to occur in coho salmon eggs (65.8 nmol/g) from Lake Superior that do not develop EMS (Marcquenski 1996). However, for the egg batch from female L, which showed high mortality during the embryonic stage, the effect of 52 nmol/g was minor. The egg batches from females G, H, I, J, and K showed a decrease in disorders at hatch of only

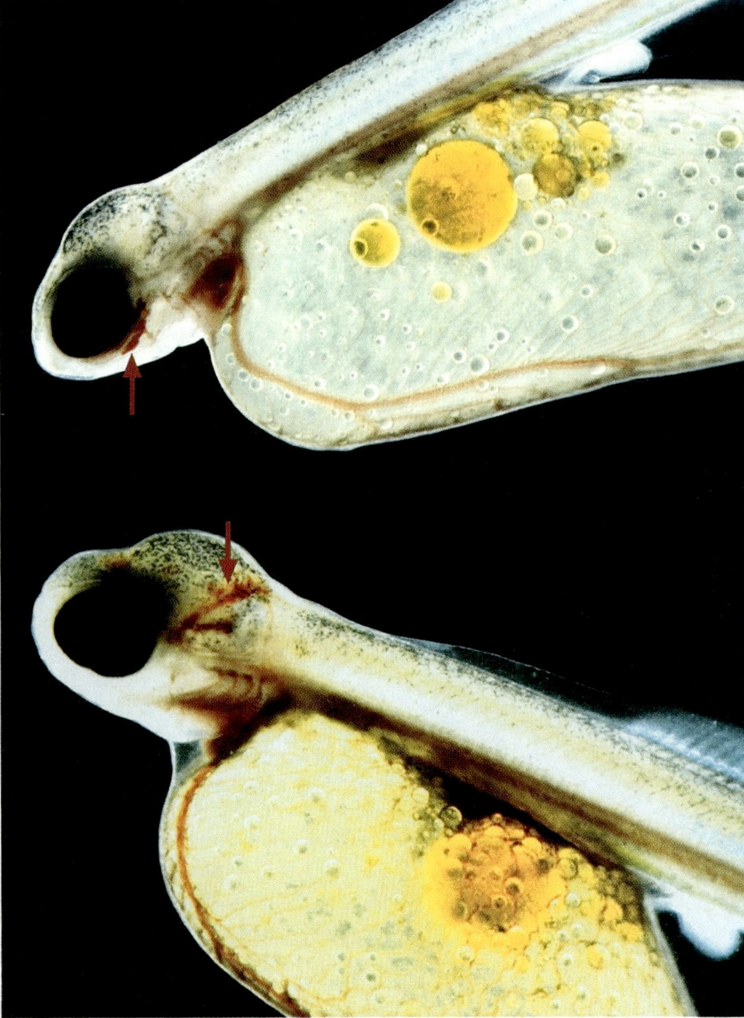

FIGURE 15.—Larvae from Atlantic salmon originating from The Baltic Sea. The arrows show hemorrhages in the head. This type of blood disorder occurs frequently in newly hatched salmon larvae (see Figures 13 and 18).

15–50% compared with noninjected eggs. The higher dose, 130 nmol/g, which was used in only a few egg batches, did not result in a decreased incidence of disorders at hatch.

The 12 cod family pairs from the Lofoten area showed a mortality of around 20%. Such low mortality was not found in any of the investigated family pairs from the Baltic Sea, where the mortality in most cases was around 80%. The high mortality recorded in the Baltic cod eggs agrees with results reported by Wieland et al. (1994), Pickova et al. (1996), and Mellergaard (1996). Wieland et al. reported that the average survival until hatching was around 30%. The spawning cod in that investigation were caught in the Bornholm basin, and incubation of the eggs started immediately on the boat, as in the present investigation. High rates of malformed embryos have been recorded in pelagic fish eggs (cod, plaice *Pleuronectes platessa*, flounder *Platichthys flesus*) sampled by plankton net in different areas of the Baltic Sea (Grauman 1986; Westernhagen et al. 1988). Some of the malformations reported in these investigations, such as a variety of vertebrae curvatures and irregular cell cleavages, resemble those seen in our Baltic cod egg batches before death.

In cod offspring from Lofoten, the total frequency of disorders at hatch was around or, in most cases, less than 10%. In the offspring from the Baltic Sea analyzed at hatch, the corresponding frequency was higher (Student's t-test, $P < 0.05$), around 15%, except for one group that showed a frequency of less than 5% (female C and male 3). However, when all of the larval groups were examined

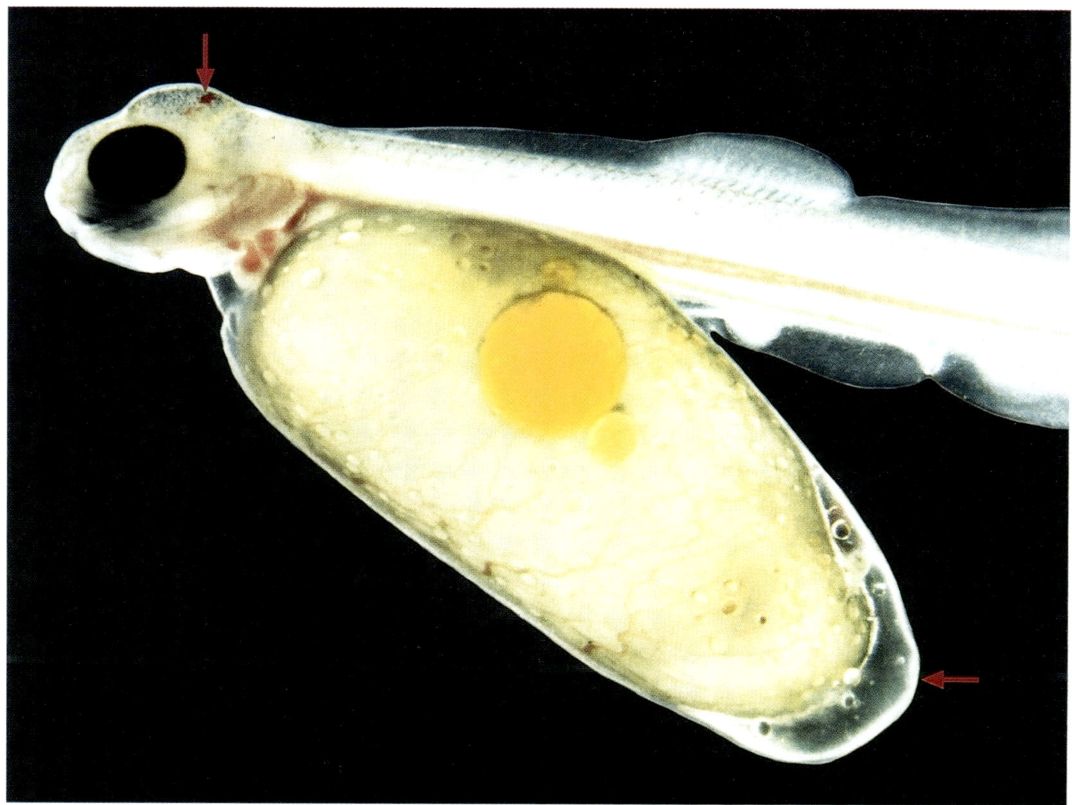

FIGURE 16.—A larva from Atlantic salmon originating from the Baltic Sea. The arrows show a small hemorrhage in the head and a subcutaneous edema in the yolk sac. This kind of disorder occurs frequently in newly hatched salmon larvae (see Figures 13 and 18).

after consumption of the yolk (results not presented), this low-frequency group was arrested in development and had consumed only a minor part of the yolk.

The frequencies of mortality during different periods and the kinds of disorders found in salmon and cod in this study differ in many respects. However, there are also some striking similarities, despite the large "biological" difference between these two species. For instance, larvae from the salmon females A and L experienced mortality during developmental stages similar to larvae from the cod females I, M, and P. In salmon, the results strongly indicate that there might be more than one kind of reproductive disorder. One is connected to thiamine deficiency and occurs at various stages of yolk sac consumption. The other is not directly connected to a thiamine deficiency and occurs mainly at earlier stages of development. This type shows similarities with reproductive disorders occurring in cod in the Baltic Sea. The prevailing hypothesis is that anthropogenic substances could be the underlying cause of the reproductive disorders in both of these species. It is tempting to speculate that what we are observing might be different responses on the dose axis among salmon females and that cod in general are in the more exposed or more sensitive response "area" relative to salmon.

The conclusions of the present study are summarized below.

1. Both salmon and cod from the Baltic Sea are affected by mainly female-associated mortality and disorders among their offspring.
2. Females of both salmon and cod from the Baltic Sea produce offspring that experience early mortality.

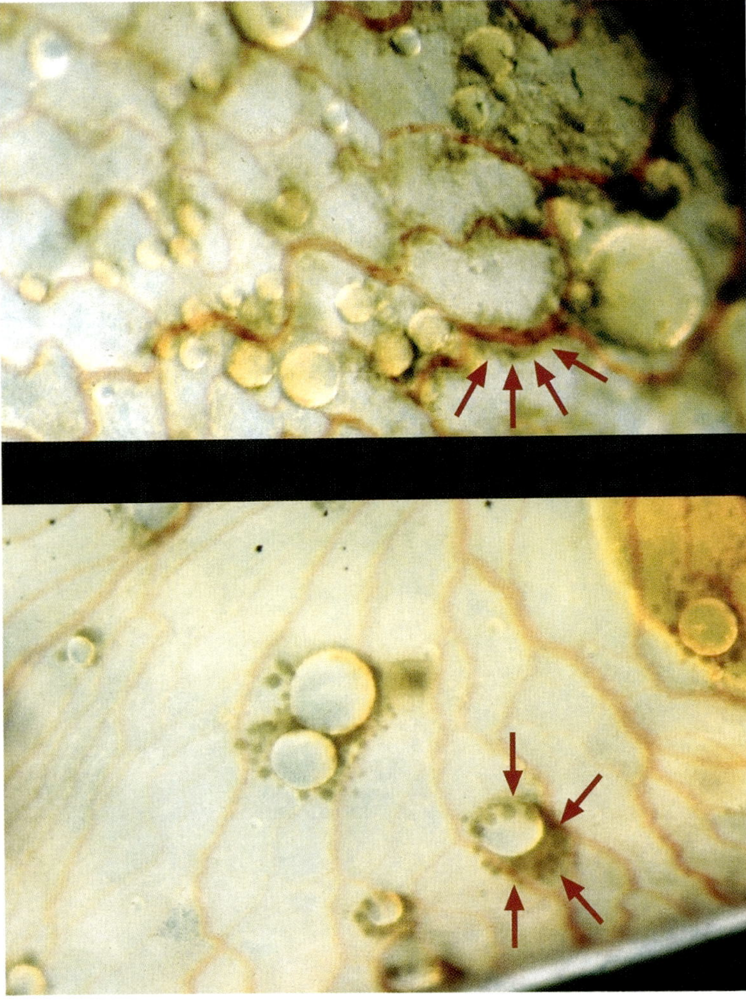

FIGURE 17.—Detail of yolk sacs in larvae from Atlantic salmon originating from the Baltic Sea. The upper larva has precipitate situated along the blood vessels (arrows). This kind of precipitate occurs frequently in newly hatched larvae (see Figure 14). The lower larva was photographed later in development but before larval mortality. At this stage, the precipitate (not recorded in these studies) can be observed around the oil droplets situated near the yolk sac membrane (arrows).

3. A major proportion of the salmon experience thiamine deficiency-dependent mortality. However, this mortality is not correlated to a specific stage of yolk sac consumption.

4. Cod exhibit a number of disorders at hatch, such as vertebrae deformity, disrupted yolk sac or subcutaneous edema in the yolk sac, and precipitate in the yolk.

5. Salmon exhibit a number of disorders at hatch, such as vertebrae deformity, blood disorders, subcutaneous edema in the yolk sac, and precipitate in the yolk.

6. Disorders at hatch in salmon offspring are not correlated to later thiamine deficiency-dependent mortality. Treatment of newly fertilized eggs by thiamine injection had only a minor influence on the frequency of disorders at hatch, whereas the treatment completely protected the larvae from later thiamine deficiency-dependent mortality. This indicates that other factors, in addition to thiamine deficiency, are involved in the disorders during development.

7. Both salmon and cod from the Baltic Sea exhibit disorders that might have similar biochemical mechanisms, because the formation of precipitates and edema in the yolk sac occurs in both species.

Acknowledgments

This study was partly supported by a grant from the World Wide Fund for Nature. We thank Torstein Pedersen (Norwegian College of Fishery Science, University of Tromsø, Norway) and

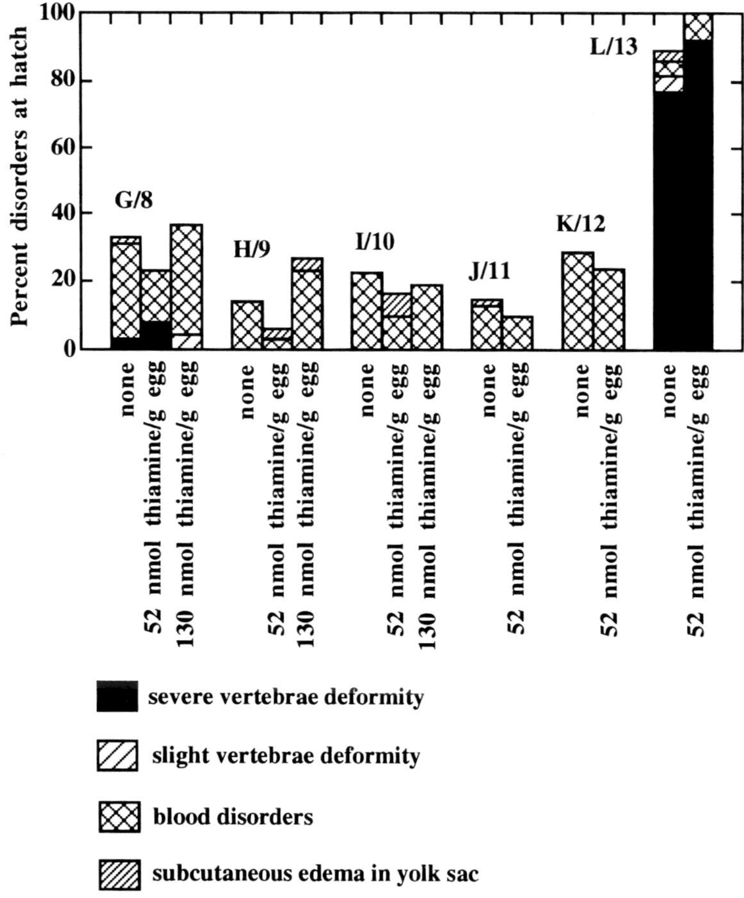

FIGURE 18.—Disorders recorded at hatch in salmon larvae from six females (G–L) and six males (8–13) during the 1995–1996 season. The second and the third bars in each group show disorders in larvae that were nanoinjected with thiamine (52 or 130 nmol/g) in the yolk immediately after fertilization; the first bar in each group shows disorders in the noninjected control group (none). Females G–L and males 8–13 denote the corresponding female–male pairs as in Figure 12. The percentages are calculated as in Figure 4.

Ronnie Nilsson (National Board of Fisheries, Baltic Sea Research Station, Karlskrona, Sweden) for allowing us to participate in their cod surveys. We also thank Bjarne Ragnarsson (National Board of Fisheries, Fisheries Research Station, Älvkarleby, Sweden) for supplying salmon eggs. Hans Börjeson (Swedish Salmon Research Institute, Älvkarleby, Sweden) is acknowledged for valuable help during this study.

References

Åkerman, G., and L. Balk. 1995. A reliable and improved methodology to expose fish in the early embryonic stage. Marine Environmental Research 39(1–4):155–158.

Åkerman, G., and five coauthors. 1996a. Comparison of reproductive success of cod, *Gadus morhua*, from the Barents Sea and Baltic Sea. Marine Environmental Research 42(1–4):139–144.

Åkerman, G., and six coauthors. 1996b. Studies of reproductive disorders in cod (*Gadus morhua*) and salmon (*Salmo salar*), using biomarkers, indicative environmental pollution as the common cause. Pages 63–64 *in* Bengtsson et al. (1996).

Amcoff, P., L. Norrgren, H. Börjeson, and J. Lindeberg. 1996. Lowered concentration of thiamine (vitamin B1) in M74-affected feral Baltic salmon (*Salmo salar*). Pages 38–39 *in* Bengtsson et al. (1996).

Bengtsson, B.-E., C. Hill, and S. Nellbring, editors. 1996. Report from the second workshop on reproduction disturbances in fish. Swedish Environmental Protection Agency Report 4534, Stockholm.

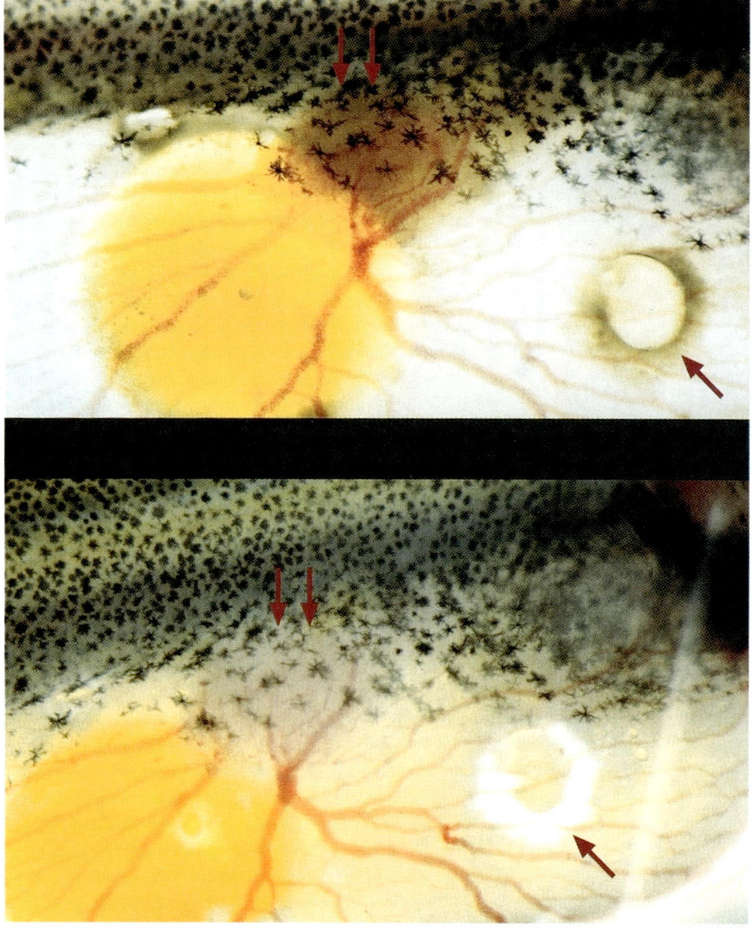

FIGURE 19.—The same salmon yolk sac photographed with light from two different directions (from above and below). The liver (arrows) has quite a different appearance, and different interpretations might occur. Precipitates in the yolk (arrow) are sometimes described as white precipitates, opalescent yolk, or opalescences in the yolk. It is obvious that identical disorders can be described and interpreted differently.

Bengtsson, B.-E., and six coauthors. 1994. Reproductive disturbances in Baltic fish. Swedish Environmental Protection Agency Report 4319, Stockholm.

Bignert, A., and six coauthors. 1993. The need for adequate biological sampling in ecotoxicological investigations: a retrospective study of twenty years pollution monitoring. Science of the Total Environment 128:121–139.

Boonyaratpalin, M., and J. Wanakowat, editors. 1993. Effect of thiamine, riboflavin, pantothenic acid and inositol on growth, feed efficiency and mortality of juvenile seabass. Volume 61. Fish nutrition in practice. Paris-France Institut National de la Recherche Agronomique, Paris.

Bylund, G., and O. Lerche. 1995. Thiamine therapy of M 74 affected fry of Atlantic salmon *Salmo salar*. Bulletin of the European Association of Fish Pathologists 15(3):93–97.

Börjeson, H., L. Norrgren, T. Andersson, and P-A. Bergqvist. 1994. The Baltic salmon—situation in the past and today. Pages 14–25 *in* Norrgren (1994).

Ericson, G., G. Åkerman, B. Liewenborg, and L. Balk. 1996. Comparison of DNA damage in the early life stages of cod, (*Gadus morhua*), originating from the Barents Sea and the Baltic Sea. Marine Environmental Research 42(1–4):119–123.

Falandysz, J. 1994. Polychlorinated biphenyl concentrations in cod-liver oil: evidence of a steady-state condition of these compounds in the Baltic area oils and levels noted in Atlantic oils. Archives of Environmental Contamination and Toxicology 27:266–271.

Falandysz, J., K. Kannan, S. Tanabe, and R. Tatsukawa. 1994. Organochlorine pesticides and polychlorinated biphenyls in cod-liver oils: North Atlantic, Norwegian Sea, North Sea and Baltic Sea. Ambio 23(4–5):288–293.

Fisher, J. P., J. D. Fitzsimons, G. F. Combs, Jr., and J. M. Spitsbergen. 1996. Naturally occurring thiamine deficiency causing reproductive failure in Finger Lakes Atlantic salmon and Great Lakes lake trout. Transactions of the American Fisheries Society 125:167–178.

Fitzsimons, J. 1995. The effect of B-vitamins on a swim-up syndrome in Lake Ontario lake trout. Journal of Great Lakes Research 21(Supplement 1):286–289.

Grauman, G. B. 1986. Morphological anomalies in the Baltic sea fishes at early stages of ontogenesis. Pages 282–291 *in* Symposium on ecological investigations of the Baltic Sea environment. Ekologija Baltijskogo morja, Gidrometoizdat, Leningrad.

Ikonen, E. 1996. Feeding of salmon during the spawning run, preliminary information. Pages 47–48 *in* Bengtsson et al. (1996).

Jensen, S., A. G. Johnels, M. Olsson, and G. Otterlind. 1972. DDT and PCB in herring and cod from the Baltic, the Kattegat and the Skagerrak. Ambio Special Report 1:36–38.

Karlsson, L., E. Pettersson, M. Hedenskog, H. Börjeson, and R. Eriksson. 1996. Biological factors affecting the incidence of M74. Page 25 *in* Bengtsson et al. (1996).

Karlström, Ö. 1995. Salmon parr (*Salmo salar* L.) production and spawning stocks in Baltic salmon rivers in Northern Sweden 1976–94. ICES (International Council for the Exploration of the Sea) CM M:23.

Karås, P., E. Neuman, and O. Sandström. 1991. Effects of a pulp mill effluent on the population dynamics of perch, *Perca fluviatilis*. Canadian Journal of Fisheries and Aquatic Sciences 48:28–34.

Koistinen, J. 1990. Residues of planar polychloroaromatic compounds in Baltic fish and seal. Chemosphere 20:1043–1048.

Koski, P., M. Pakarinen, and A. Soivio. 1996. A dose-response study of thiamine hydrochloride bathing for the prevention of yolk-sac mortality in Baltic salmon fry (M74 syndrome). Page 46 *in* Bengtsson et al. (1996).

Larsson, P.-O. 1994. Recent development of the cod stocks around Sweden and possible reproduction disturbances. Pages 26–34 *in* Norrgren (1994).

Larsson, P., S. Hamrin, and L. Okla. 1991. Factors determining the uptake of persistent pollutants on an eel population (*Anguilla anguilla* L.). Environmental Pollution 69:39–50.

Lignell, Å. 1994. Astaxanthin in yolk sac fry from feral Baltic salmon. Pages 94–96 *in* Norrgren (1994).

Lundström, J., L. Norrgren, and H. Börjeson. 1996. Clinical and morphological studies of Baltic salmon yolk-sac fry suffering from the M 74 syndrome. Pages 26–27 *in* Bengtsson et al. (1996).

Marcquenski, S.V. 1996. Characterization of early mortality syndrome (EMS) in salmonids from the Great Lakes. Pages 73–75 *in* Bengtsson et al. (1996).

Mellergaard, S. 1996. Are M-74-like problems involved in recruitment failure in Baltic cod? Pages 61–62 *in* Bengtsson et al. (1996).

Moriarty, C. 1990. European catches of elver of 1928–1988. Internationale Revue gesamten Hydrobiologie 75:701–706.

Nissling, A. and L. Westin. 1991. Egg mortality and hatching rate of Baltic cod (*Gadus morhua*) in different salinities. Marine Biology 111:29–32.

Norrgren, L., editor. 1994. Reproduction disturbances in fish. Swedish Environmental Protection Agency Report 4346, Uppsala.

Norrgren, L., B.-E. Bengtsson, and H. Börjeson. 1994. Summary of the workshop "reproduction disturbances in fish." Pages 7–11 *in* Norrgren (1994).

Pettersson, A., and Å. Lignell. 1996. Decreased astaxanthin levels in the Baltic salmon and the M74 syndrome. Pages 28–29 *in* Bengtsson et al. (1996).

Pickova, J., P. Dutta, A. Kiessling, and P.-O. Larsson. 1996. Fatty acid composition in fertilized eggs of cod (*Gadus morhua*) originating from the Baltic Sea and the Skagerrak. Pages 71–72 *in* Bengtsson et al. (1996).

Pulliainen, E., K. Korhonen, K. Kankaanranta, and K. Mäki. 1992. Non-spawning burbot on the northern coast of the Bothnian bay. Ambio 21:170–175.

Soivio, A. 1994. Reproductive disturbances of wild broodfish in Finland. Pages 38–39 *in* Norrgren (1994).

Uzars, D. 1994. Feeding of cod (*Gadus morhua callarias* L.) in the central Baltic in relation to environmental changes. ICES Marine Science Symposium 198:612–623.

Westernhagen, H., V. Dethlefsen, P. Cameron, J. Berg, and G. Furstenberg. 1988. Developmental defects in pelagic fish embryos from the western Baltic. Helgoländer Meeresuntersuchungen 42:13–36.

Westin, L., and A. Nissling. 1991. Effects of salinity on spermatozoa motility, percentage of fertilized eggs and egg development of Baltic cod (*Gadus morhua*), and implications for cod stock fluctuations in the Baltic. Marine Biology 108:5–9.

Wieland, K., U. Waller, and D. Schnack. 1994. Development of Baltic cod eggs at different levels of temperature and oxygen content. Dana 10:163–177.

American Fisheries Society Symposium 21:62–72, 1998

Clinical and Pathological Studies of Baltic Salmon Suffering from Yolk Sac Fry Mortality

JENNY LUNDSTRÖM[1]
Department of Pathology, Faculty of Veterinary Medicine
Swedish University of Agricultural Sciences, Box 7028, S-750 07 Uppsala, Sweden

HANS BÖRJESON
Swedish Salmon Research Institute, Forskarstigen, S-814 94 Älvkarleby, Sweden

LEIF NORRGREN
Department of Pathology, Faculty of Veterinary Medicine
Swedish University of Agricultural Sciences

Abstract.—Feral stocks of Baltic salmon *Salmo salar* suffer from a yolk sac fry mortality syndrome designated M74. This study showed that M74 is family dependent, with a 100% mortality within affected family groups. Differences between family groups were noted with regard to the age when the disease was manifested, and accordingly, the groups were categorized into those with early, intermediate, or late development of disease. Family groups with early development of disease had a short survival time, and after 5–10 d the whole family group was dead. Family groups with late development of disease survived for a longer period. Three consecutive stages of M74, preclinical, clinical, and terminal, are described. No clinical symptoms of disease can be seen in the newly hatched fry. During development, the yolk sac fry progressively pass through the preclinical stage and enter the clinical stage, which is characterized by aggravating neurological symptoms. In the terminal stage, the majority of symptoms might be secondary to the low heart rate that develops during the disease. The gross pathological characteristics of M74 include a distended gallbladder, a pale spleen, and a yolk sac precipitate. Yolk sac fry with M74 also have diminished yolk absorption and faster consumption of the pigments in the yolk sac fat droplet. To further elucidate the pathogenesis of M74 and to determine the involvement of nutritional and toxicological factors, future work must include both histological and functional studies of tissues with regard to the symptoms and gross pathological characteristics of M74. However, because there is heterogenicity between family groups that develop M74, careful selection of experimental samples is necessary and should include categorization of each family group and definition of the stage of disease at sampling.

The Baltic Sea, one of the world's largest brackish-water seas, is inhabited by unique populations of anadromous Atlantic salmon *Salmo salar*, the Baltic salmon. They were physically separated from the Atlantic stocks after the last ice period, when the Baltic Sea, because of the elevation of the land, was temporarily separated from the Atlantic Ocean for about 2,000 years (Karlsson and Karlström 1994). During the 20th century, the Baltic salmon has faced increasing challenges to its survival. A majority of the spawning grounds have been destroyed as a result of extensive building of hydroelectric power plants. Today, only 20 rivers have natural spawning populations of the Baltic salmon, compared with about 60 at the beginning of this century (Ackefors et al. 1991). In Sweden, salmon compensatory hatcheries were established in all rivers with hydroelectric power stations during the 1950s. In these rivers, feral spawners returning from their feeding grounds in the Baltic Sea are caught and stripped and the roe is fertilized with milt from feral males.

In 1974, a specific form of yolk sac fry mortality was noted in the salmon hatchery of Bergeforsen on the River Indalsälven. Because roe from individual females was incubated separately, it was noted that the disease was family dependent, resulting in total mortality of the affected family groups. The disease was designated M74 because M stands for "Miljö" (the Swedish word for environment) and 74 stands for the year in which it was first observed (Anonymous 1994).

Since 1974, the disease has been identified, with fluctuating frequency, in all Swedish compensatory salmon hatcheries breeding salmon smolts from feral spawners (Börjeson and Norrgren 1997). There are strong indications that M74 also affects the natural spawning populations; electrofishing has shown a low abundance of parr in Swedish rivers after years with high frequencies of M74 (Karlsson and

[1]To whom correspondence should be addressed.

Karlström 1994). Therefore, the disease is a major threat to the natural spawning populations and, thus, to the biological diversity of the Baltic salmon.

Several attempts have been made to determine the cause of M74. The disease has been correlated to a pale color of the roe, which suggests low levels of carotenoids (Börjeson and Norrgren 1997). Furthermore, induction of the hepatic cytochrome P450 system has been shown in both females whose progeny are affected by M74 and in the yolk sac fry (Norrgren et al. 1993). Recently, Amcoff et al. (1998a, this volume) reported low concentrations of thiamine (vitamin B_1) in both roe and yolk sac fry that developed the disease. Treatment of roe and yolk sac fry with thiamine resulted in improved rates of survival (Amcoff et al. 1998b, this volume). Parasitological, bacteriological, and virological examinations of affected yolk sac fry and females producing affected fry in Finland and Sweden have revealed no causative agents (Anonymous 1994). Chemical analyses of metal concentrations in roe have shown no differences between viable family groups and family groups that develop M74 (Norrgren et al. 1993).

Early life stage mortality in progeny from feral broodstocks of coho salmon *Oncorhynchus kisutch* was first recorded in the Great Lakes of North America in 1968 (Johnson and Pecor 1969). Similar mortalities have also been seen in progeny from feral broodstocks of other salmonid species in the area: lake trout *Salvelinus namaycush* (Mac et al. 1985), chinook salmon *O. tshawytscha* (Giesy et al. 1986; Mac 1988), steelhead *O. mykiss* (Skea et al. 1985), and brown trout *Salmo trutta* (Marcquenski 1996). The mortality occurs at swim-up, when the food source changes from endogenous yolk stores to an exogenous diet. The clinical description is similar among different species, and includes loss of equilibrium, swimming in a spiral pattern, lethary, dark pigmentation, hyperexcitability, tetanus, hemorrhages, and hydrocephalus. Because mortality rates vary between different family groups, a female-dependent factor has been suggested in the etiology. Several possible agents, such as rearing techniques, genetic factors, and infections, have been excluded as the cause of the syndrome (Marcquenski 1996). There are indications that environmental contaminants could be involved, but there is no link to any specific known contaminant (Mac 1988). Ecological and nutritional factors have also been considered because of the changes in food webs that have occurred in the Great Lakes. One food item for the salmonids in the Great Lakes is the alewife *Alosa pseudoharengus*, an exotic species containing high levels of thiaminase (Gnaedinger 1964). Recent work shows the involvement of thiamine in early mortality syndrome (EMS); the thiamine content was lower in roe samples from lake trout females whose progeny developed swim-up syndrome mortality (Fisher et al. 1996). Thiamine treatment has also been shown to reduce the incidence of mortality in Lake Ontario lake trout suffering from swim-up mortality (Fitzsimons 1995).

Another disease similar to M74, the Cayuga syndrome, has recently been described in landlocked Atlantic salmon in the Finger Lakes of New York State. The disease, which is associated with the ova, appears 2–4 weeks before yolk absorption is completed and results in 98–100% mortality within affected family groups (Fisher et al. 1995a). Because afflicted yolk sac fry have reduced tissue concentrations of thiamine and show complete recovery after thiamine treatment, a thiamine deficiency attributable to extensive feeding on alewife has been proposed as the cause of the disease (Fisher et al. 1996).

The main objective of this study is to describe the clinical symptoms and gross pathological characteristics of M74. This will enable us to compare our findings with descriptions of early life stage mortality syndromes of salmonids in North America.

Methods

Source of Fish and Husbandry

This investigation is based mainly on yolk sac fry sampled during the spring of 1996. An additional study of yolk sac absorption was conducted on yolk sac fry sampled in 1995. Sexually maturing feral salmon were caught in a salmon trap during spawning migration in their native river (River Dalälven). During the captivity period, the fish were kept at the salmon rearing station in Älvkarleby in indoor pools continuously supplied with river water. In October and November, females were stripped and the roe from each female was fertilized with milt from one feral male. The roe from each female was incubated separately so that the development of each family group could be followed, and all samples were supplied with river water of ambient temperature. The mean temperatures during the months concerned were as follows: November, 1.2°C (SD, 1.8); December, 0.09°C (0.04); January, 0.10°C (0.02); February, 0.08°C (0.01); March, 0.15°C (0.04); and April, 1.2°C (1.0). At the eyed stage, subsamples (N = 200–250) of roe from 27 family groups were transferred to the Swedish University of Agricultural Sciences, Uppsala, where the roe was incubated in stainless steel mesh cages (14 × 10 × 6 cm) in a flow-through system supplied with aerated groundwater. The flow rate in the incubation tank was 2.5 L/min, giving a turnover time of approximately 20 min. The water temperature was 10 ± 1°C, and oxygen saturation was 70–80% throughout the study period.

Clinical Symptoms and Gross Pathological Findings

All family groups were visually inspected daily in the cages from hatching, approximately 170 centigrade degree-days (d.d.) after fertilization, to 750–800 d.d. Variables studied included swimming behavior, skin pigmentation, hemorrhages, ascites, yolk sac precipitates, and gill color. In addition, more extensive studies were made on subsamples from each family group at different stages of development. On each occasion, 5–10 fry from each family group were anesthetized in a buffered solution of MS-222 (100 mg/L) for 60 s. However, fry in a terminal, lethargic stage of disease were not anesthetized before observation because of their poor condition. The observations were made under a Wild Photomacroskop M400 (Leica, Heerbrugg, Switzerland) at 63× magnification. Variables studied included heart rate, blood filling of the yolk sac vein, retrograde blood flow in the yolk sac vein, gill color, skin pigmentation, gasping, hemorrhages (intracranial, skin, yolk sac, retrobulbar), ascites, yolk sac precipitates, exophthalmos, volume of bile, blood filling of the spleen, blood congestion in the trunk muscles, and malformations (curvature of the notochord). The findings were graded in half steps from 0 to 3, where 0 indicated no change or occurrence and 3 indicated considerable change or occurrence. Family groups in the same stage of the disease and of approximately the same age were grouped together, and means and standard deviations were calculated for each studied variable. The heart rates of viable yolk sac fry and yolk sac fry that developed M74 from the same age group were compared using the Mann–Whitney *U*-test.

Pigmentation of the Yolk Sac Fat Droplet

Yolk sac fry afflicted with M74 (*N* = 41, from 13 family groups) and viable yolk sac fry (*N* = 19, from 6 family groups) were studied and photographed under a Wild Photomacroskop M400 (Kodachrome 64 ASA) at 63× magnification at two different ages. The evaluations were made blindly using the photographs and without knowledge of the clinical status of the fry. The pigmentation of the fat droplet was graded in half steps from 0 to 3, where 0 indicated a very pale, translucent pigmentation and 3 indicated a strong orange pigmentation. Means and standard deviations were determined for the different groups (viable 250 d.d., viable 350 d.d., M74 250 d.d., and M74 350 d.d.).

Yolk Sac Absorption

Yolk sac fry with M74 (*N* = 81, from 5 family groups) and viable yolk sac fry (*N* = 39, from 3 family groups) were studied from hatching until swim-up. Sampling was performed at different stages of development, and the yolk sac fry were anesthetized and fixed in neutral buffered formalin. The yolk sac was removed from the body and dried separately for 24 h at 60°C and then for 3 h at 100°C. The dry weight was determined, and a yolk sac index (YSI) was calculated for each yolk sac fry [yolk sac dry weight ÷ (fry body dry weight + yolk sac dry weight)]. Mean YSI values and standard deviations were determined for yolk sac fry representing two age groups, at hatching and 250–300 d.d. posthatch, and viable fry and yolk sac fry with M74 from the same age group were compared using the Mann–Whitney *U*-test.

Results

Incidence of the Disease

In the samples studied, 18 of 27 family groups developed M74, for an incidence of approximately 67%. In the family groups that developed M74, 100% mortality among the yolk sac fry was recorded.

Clinical Symptoms and Gross Pathological Findings

Propagation of the disease.—The clinical propagation of M74 can be described as follows. In the preclinical stage of the disease, increased motor activity is observed together with an impaired sense of locality, manifested by a diminished inclination among the yolk sac fry to orient themselves toward the corners of the cages (Figure 1). Later, in family groups with early or intermediate development of the disease (see below), a characteristic swimming behavior is noted, with sudden swimming toward the water surface, during which the fry turns itself around

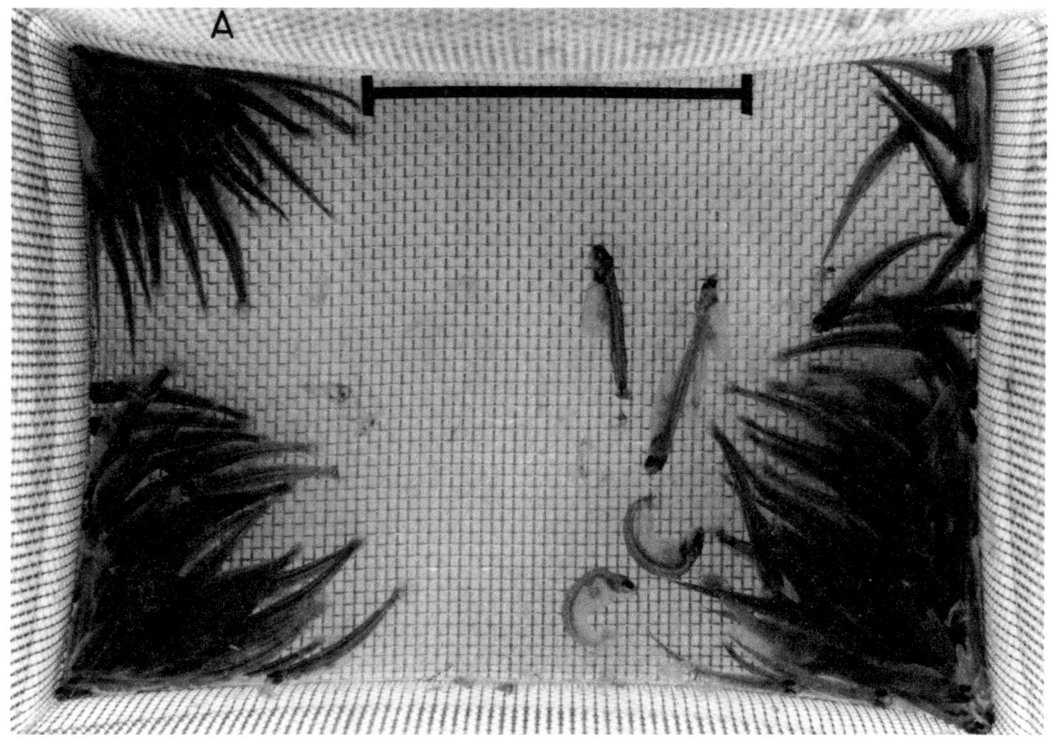

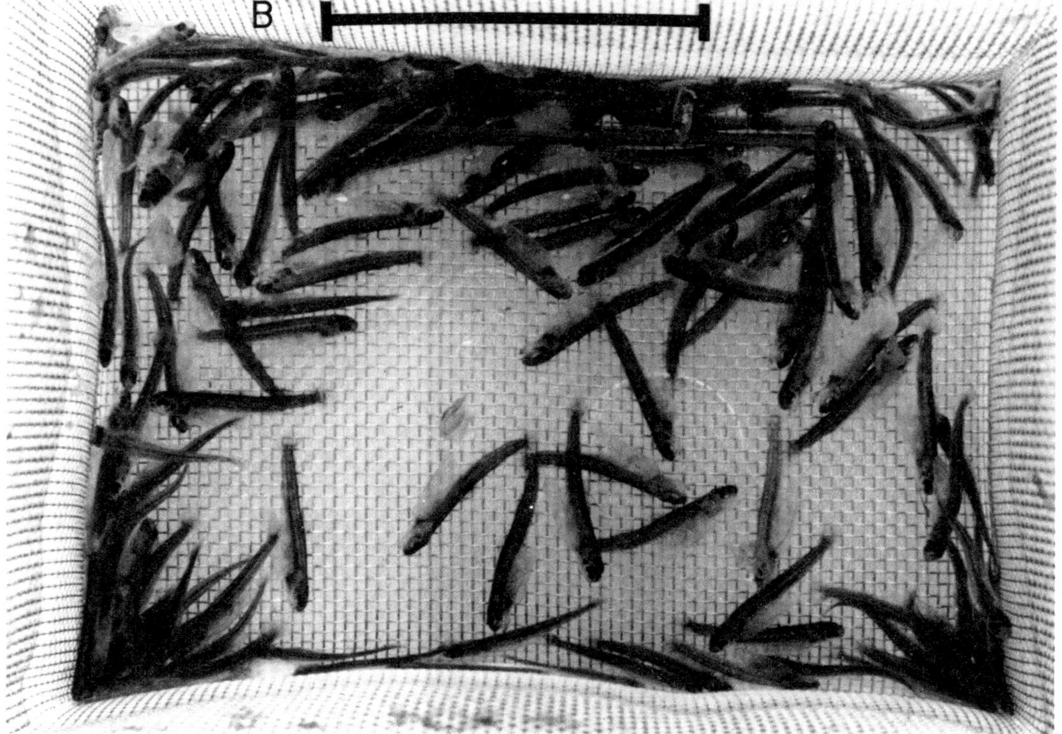

FIGURE 1.—(**A**) Family group developing normally. (**B**) Family group developing M74. Bar equals 5 cm.

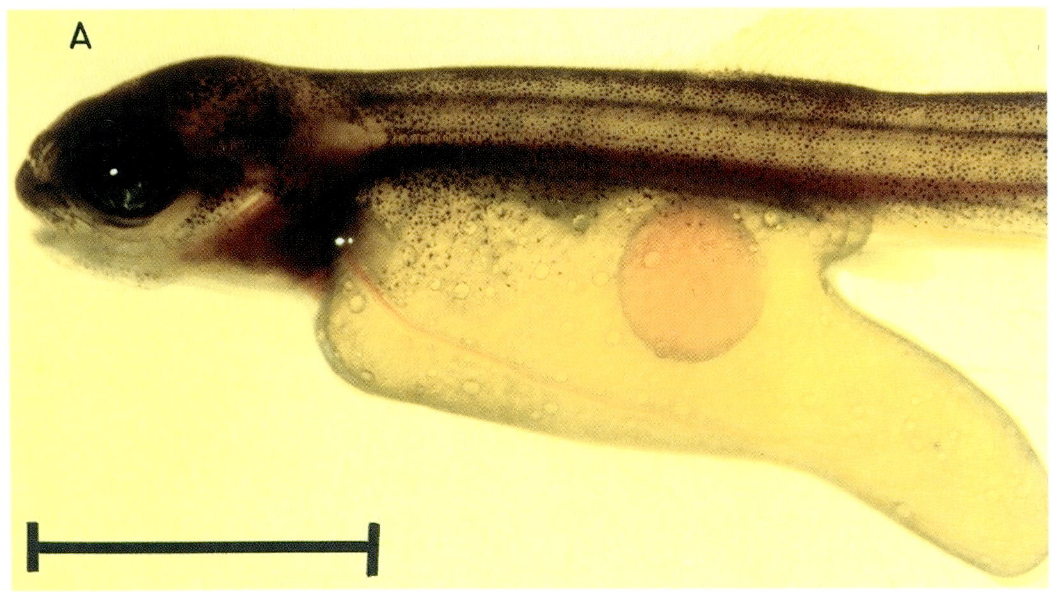

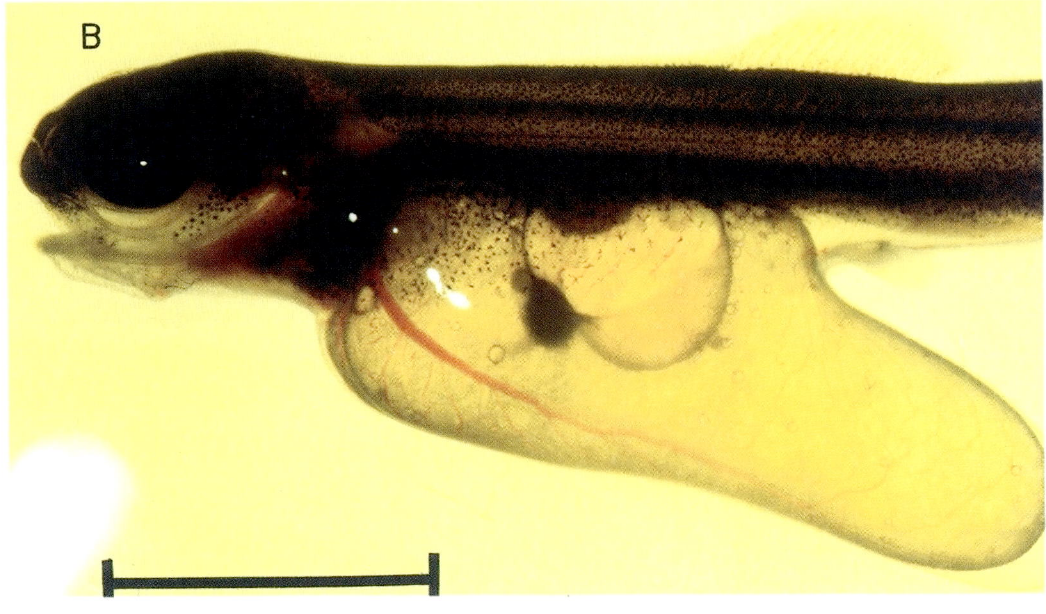

FIGURE 2.—(**A**) Normal yolk sac fry. (**B**) Yolk sac fry with M74. Note the pale pigmentation of the yolk sac fat droplet and the precipitate in the yolk sac. Bar equals 0.5 cm.

on its longitudinal axis and then slowly sinks to the bottom. At this stage, the family group is considered to be in the clinical stage of the disease. Other symptoms seen are dark pigmentation of the skin, flared operculae, and in many of the fry in the family group a white precipitate in the yolk sac, located adjacent to the fat droplet, is noted (Figure 2). The yolk sac fry also exhibit signs of increasing lack of coordination. The terminal stage of the disease is characterized by lethargy alternating with sudden outbreaks of swimming and seizures. In family groups that developed the disease at a very young age, a sudden whitening of the liver was noted a few days before death.

According to the patterns of the propagation of M74, family groups were categorized into those with early, intermediate, or late development of the disease (Table 1). Onset of disease was defined as the age when the family group entered the clinical stage of the disease. Family groups with early development had a short survival time, and the yolk sac fry died at a relatively young age. Family groups with late development of the disease survived for a longer period, with the last deaths recorded during the late yolk sac period.

Heart rate.—No differences in heart rate were recorded between viable yolk sac fry and yolk sac fry in the preclinical stage of M74. However, during the propagation of the disease, the heart rate decreased, and in yolk sac fry in the terminal stage of the disease, the heart rate was about one-third of the heart rate in the viable fry (Table 2).

Gross pathological findings.—Data on the gross pathological findings are shown in Tables 3–5. The main findings during the clinical stage of the disease were a white precipitate in the yolk sac located adjacent to the fat droplet, a small and pale spleen, and a distended gallbladder. A distended gallbladder was also seen in viable fry at

TABLE 1.—Categorization of the family groups that developed M74. Ages are expressed as degree-days after fertilization.

Variable	Category		
	Early	Intermediate	Late
Number of family groups	4	9	5
Age at onset	326–359	349–492	447–631
Age at last deaths	391–447	472–585	606–797
Duration of disease (d.d.)	47–96	108–181	136–231

TABLE 2.—Heart rate at different stages of the disease. Disease stages of yolk sac fry are M74 pc, preclinical stage; M74c, clinical stage; and M74t, terminal stage. Ages are expressed as degree-days after fertilization. Values are shown as means ± SD.

Status	Age	Number of family groups	Number of fry	Heart rate (beats per minute)
Viable	345–354	6	19	115 ± 19
M74pc	345–354	7	21	121 ± 18
M74c	393–454	6	31	72 ± 22[a]
M74t	353–416	5	31	40 ± 20[a]

[a] $P < 0.001$ compared with viable fry.

the swim-up stage. The terminal stage of the disease was additionally characterized by blood congestion and exophthalmos.

Pigmentation of the Yolk Sac Fat Droplet

At age 250 d.d., the pigmentation of the yolk sac fat droplet was similar in both viable and M74-affected family groups. However, at age 350 d.d., decreased pigmentation was noted in family groups that developed M74 (Figure 3).

Yolk Sac Absorption

During development, a progressive decrease in the YSI was recorded in both viable and M74-affected yolk sac fry (Figure 4). At hatching, viable yolk sac fry showed a slightly higher YSI compared with fry that developed M74. At age 250–300 d.d. after hatching, viable yolk sac fry had a lower YSI, showing better absorption of the yolk than yolk sac fry with M74 (Figure 4).

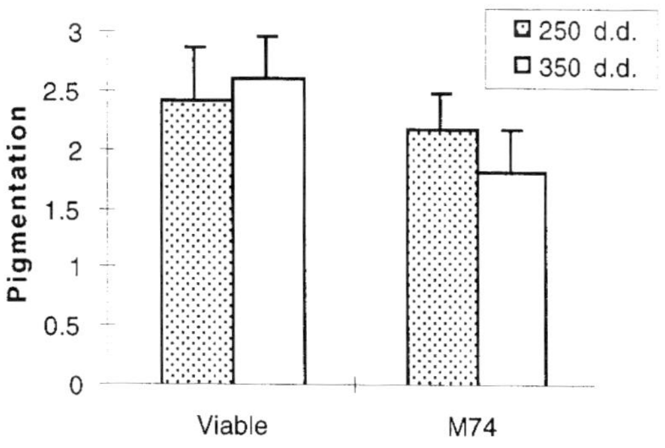

FIGURE 3.—Pigmentation of the yolk sac fat droplet. Values are shown as means + SD. Pigmentation ranges from pale, translucent (0) to strong, orange (3). Ages are expressed as degree-days (d.d.) after fertilization.

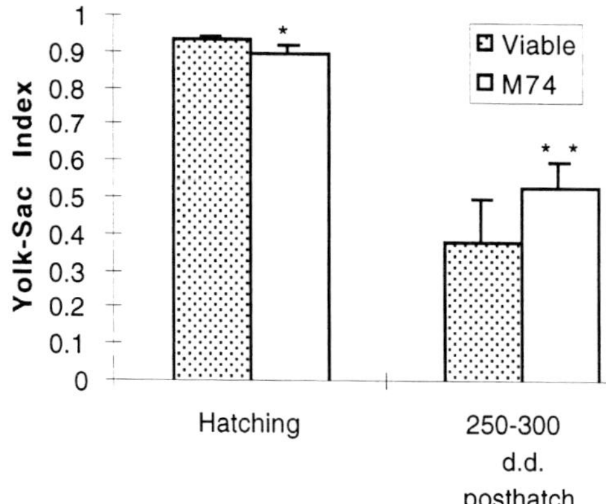

FIGURE 4.—Yolk sac index in viable fry and fry that developed M74. Values are shown as means + SD. Asterisks indicate $P < 0.05$ (*) and $P < 0.01$ (**) compared with the viable fry of the same age class. Ages are expressed as degree-days (d.d.) after hatching.

Discussion

This study confirms earlier results showing that M74 is a disease linked to certain family groups (Börjeson and Norrgren 1997). We have defined three different stages of M74: preclinical, clinical, and terminal. No clinical symptoms of disease can be seen in the newly hatched fry. During the posthatch period, the yolk sac fry progressively pass through the preclinical stage and enter the clinical stage. During this period, the neurological symptoms become aggravated and other symptoms, such as dark pigmentation of the skin and the presence of yolk sac precipitates, are seen. In the terminal stage, the majority of additional symptoms might be secondary to circulatory disturbances attributable to the low heart rate that develops during the disease.

Because the disease is manifested at different ages in different family groups, the groups were categorized as those with early, intermediate, or late development of the disease. Family groups with early development of the disease exhibit a short clinical stage, and after 5–10 d the whole family group is dead. This is in contrast to the longer survival time (2–3 weeks) seen in yolk sac fry with late development of the disease. Yolk sac fry with M74 showed decreased yolk absorption compared with viable yolk sac fry. This has also been noted in yolk sac fry with the Cayuga syndrome (Fisher et al. 1995b). Poor absorption of yolk has been reported in a variety of conditions. Several abiotic factors, such as temperature, oxygen tension, ammonia concentration, and suboptimal or supraoptimal salinity, influence the

TABLE 3.—Gross pathological findings in yolk sac fry aged 345–454 degree-days after fertilization. The results are shown as means ± SD (only variables with differences found are shown). The findings are graded in half steps, where 0 indicates no change or occurrence and 3 indicates considerable change or occurrence. Viable, fry from family groups that did not develop M74; M74pc, individuals in the preclinical stage of M74; M74c, individuals in the clinical stage of M74; M74t, individuals in the terminal stage of M74. Ages are expressed as degree-days after fertilization.

Variable	Status			
	Viable	M74pc	M74c	M74t
Age	345–354	345–354	393–454	353–416
Family groups (*N*)	6	7	6	5
Individuals (*N*)	30	35	57	51
Skin pigment	1.9 ± 0.5	2.5 ± 0.4	2.7 ± 0.3	2.4 ± 0.6
Ascites	0.12 ± 0.2	0.21 ± 0.3	0.34 ± 0.5	0.32 ± 0.4
Yolk sac precipitate	0.02 ± 0.1	0.07 ± 0.2	1.1 ± 0.8	0.85 ± 0.8
Exophthalmos	0.02 ± 0.1	0	1.5 ± 0.7	1.5 ± 1.2
Bile (volume)	0.02 ± 0.1	0.44 ± 0.6	2.2 ± 0.8	2.3 ± 0.8
Blood filling				
Yolk sac vein	1.4 ± 0.8	1.7 ± 0.6	1.8 ± 0.4	2.0 ± 0.6
Gills	1.6 ± 0.6	2.0 ± 0.4	2.0 ± 0.4	1.4 ± 0.8
Pale spleen	0.59 ± 0.7	1.0 ± 0.9	2.9 ± 0.2	2.6 ± 0.6
Blood congestion				
Muscle	0	0	0	0.6 ± 0.8
Retrobulbar	0.07 ± 0.4	0	0.02 ± 0.1	0.3 ± 0.6
Gasping	0.15 ± 0.3	0.13 ± 0.3	1.6 ± 0.8	2.1 ± 1.0

TABLE 4.—Gross pathological findings in yolk sac fry aged 452–584 degree-days after fertilization. The results are shown as means ± SD (only variables with differences found are shown). The findings are graded in half steps, where 0 indicates no change or occurrence and 3 indicates considerable change or occurrence. Viable, fry from family groups that did not develop M74; M74c, individuals in the clinical stage of M74; M74t, individuals in the terminal stage of M74. Ages are expressed as degree-days after fertilization.

Variable	Status				
	Viable	M74c	M74c	M74t	M74t
Age	461–501	461–494	501–584	452–454	501–506
Family groups (N)	6	6	9	2	3
Individuals (N)	55	53	69	17	7
Skin pigment	1.8 ± 0.6	2.7 ± 0.4	2.8 ± 0.3	2.7 ± 0.3	2.8 ± 0.4
Ascites	0.02 ± 0.1	0	0.04 ± 0.4	0	0
Yolk sac precipitate	0.04 ± 0.2	0.61 ± 0.6	1.2 ± 0.7	1.2 ± 0.8	1.6 ± 0.5
Exophthalmos	0.02 ± 0.1	1.3 ± 0.6	1.6 ± 0.8	2.5 ± 0.5	2.4 ± 0.5
Bile (volume)	0.87 ± 0.6	2.3 ± 0.7	2.2 ± 0.8	2.8 ± 0.3	2.8 ± 0.4
Blood filling					
Yolk sac vein	0.85 ± 0.9	1.3 ± 0.5	1.5 ± 0.7	1.5 ± 0.4	1.2 ± 0.6
Gills	1.5 ± 0.0	2.0 ± 0.3	1.9 ± 0.5	0.91 ± 0.3	0.64 ± 0.2
Pale spleen	0.04 ± 0.2	2.7 ± 0.8	2.3 ± 1.0	3.0 ± 0	3.0 ± 0
Blood congestion					
Muscle	0	0	0.1 ± 0.2	1.0 ± 0.7	0.14 ± 0.4
Retrobulbar	0	0.03 ± 0.2	0	0.59 ± 0.8	0.21 ± 0.6
Gasping	0.41 ± 0.5	1.5 ± 0.7	1.1 ± 0.8	1.9 ± 0.7	2.1 ± 0.7

rate of absorption (Heming and Buddington 1988). However, these factors can be disregarded in this study because all family groups were kept under the same rearing conditions. Sublethal concentrations of toxic xenobiotics reduce the absorption of yolk (Crawford and Guarino 1985). Among the endogenous substances that influence yolk absorption, thyroid hormones have an enhancing effect (Tagawa and Hirano 1987). At the yolk sac stage, most thyroid hormone is present in the yolk in the form of thyroxine and is suggested to be a result of maternal transfer (Brown et al. 1987).

The most obvious gross pathological signs seen in connection with M74 are a distended gallbladder, a pale spleen, and a yolk sac precipitate. A distended gallbladder could be the result of high production of bile, inadequate reabsorption of water and electrolytes, or depressed emptying mechanisms. Factors that control the production and secretion of bile in fish are not well understood (Sargent et al. 1989). Many fish species have been reported to excrete certain xenobiotics through the bile (Guarino 1991). However, because distended gallbladders were also seen in viable fry at the late yolk sac stage, it might indicate nutritional stress caused by diminished absorption of yolk.

The fish spleen has been proposed to have an important function as a blood-storing organ, and release of erythrocytes from in vitro perfused cod *Gadus morhua* spleen after stimulation with noradrenaline and acetylcholine has been reported (Fänge and Nilsson 1985). The pale spleens seen in individuals with M74 might thus indicate a release of erythrocytes.

A precipitate in the yolk sac has been reported in Atlantic salmon yolk sac fry afflicted with the Cayuga syndrome (Fisher et al. 1995b). The suggested cause of this is acidosis resulting from the increased pyruvate and lactate levels seen in connection with thiamine deficiency (Fisher et al. 1995b).

At a young age (250 d.d.), only a slight difference was seen in the pigmentation of the yolk sac fat drop between viable yolk sac fry and yolk sac fry in the preclinical stage of M74. During development, faster consumption of the pigments was recorded in fry afflicted with M74, indicating that a mechanism involving consumption of carotenoids is involved in the pathogenesis of the disease.

The clinical course of M74 shows many similarities with that of EMS and the Cayuga syndrome. However, there are major differences in the ages at

TABLE 5.—Gross pathological findings in yolk sac fry aged 745–785 degree-days. The results are shown as means ± SD (only variables with differences found are shown). The findings are graded in half steps, where 0 indicates no change or occurrence and 3 indicates considerable change or occurrence. Viable, fry from family groups that did not develop M74; M74c, individuals in the clinical stage of M74; ND, not detectable because of the pigmentation of the skin overlying the yolk sac. Ages are expressed as degree-days after fertilization.

Variable	Status	
	Viable	M74c
Age	745–785	770–774
Family groups (*N*)	4	2
Individuals (*N*)	40	14
Skin pigment	1.2 ± 0.4	2.6 ± 0.6
Ascites	0	0
Yolk sac precipitate	0.10 ± 0.3	1.1 ± 0.9
Exophthalmos	0	2.2 ± 1
Bile (volume)	2.3 ± 0.7	2.6 ± 0.5
Blood filling		
Yolk sac vein	ND	ND
Gills	1.5 ± 0.4	1.8 ± 0.4
Pale spleen	0	0.77 ± 1.0
Blood congestion		
Muscle	0	0
Retrobulbar	0	0
Gasping	0.19 ± 0.5	0.46 ± 0.8

which the diseases become apparent. Early mortality syndrome is usually manifested around swim-up, although a shift toward earlier life stages has been noted. In the Cayuga syndrome, symptoms appear at 540–730 d.d. (Fisher et al. 1995b), compared with 330–630 d.d. in M74. This difference might be partly attributable to the low temperature regimen used during rearing of the roe from Baltic salmon.

The neurological symptoms of M74 described in the present study are similar to the symptoms of EMS (Marcquenski 1996) and the Cayuga syndrome (Fisher et al. 1995b). The proposed cause of these syndromes is thiamine deficiency. In experimental studies on rainbow trout (*Oncorhynchus mykiss*) with thiamine-depleted food, similar neurological disturbances have been induced (Morito et al. 1986). In both EMS and the Cayuga syndrome, feeding on alewife has been proposed as an important factor in the development of disease. This exotic species colonized the Great Lakes at the end of the 19th century and thereby changed the salmonid food webs. In the Baltic Sea, no colonization by a foreign forage species for the salmon has occurred. However, in recent decades, an increase in Baltic sprat *Sprattus sprattus* and herring *Clupea harengus* has been recorded, probably as a result of the decreasing stocks of the most important top predator in the Baltic, the Baltic cod *Gadus morhua* (Rudstam et al. 1994). Both sprat and herring contain thiaminase (Deutsch and Hasler 1943; Angelsea and Jackson 1985), and reduced competition between cod and salmon might have changed the feeding habits of the Baltic salmon.

A correlation between pale roe and the development of M74 was observed as early as 1976. This has been confirmed by biochemical analyses showing low concentrations of carotenoids in pale roe (Börjeson and Norrgren 1997) and a higher incidence of M74 in roe with low levels of astaxanthin (Pettersson and Lignell 1998, this volume). Because carotenoids are important components of the salmon's defense system, diminished levels might lead to an increased susceptibility to anthropogenic substances (Pettersson and Lignell 1998). Consequently, even though there is at present a trend with decreasing levels of known organic pollutants in Baltic Sea biota, that is, herring (Olsson and Reutergårdh 1986) and guillemot *Uria aalge* (Bignert et al. 1995), the possible involvement of a toxicological component in the etiology of M74 should not be ignored. Recently, a strong connection was shown between M74 and the concentrations of the most frequently detected polychlorinated dibenzofurans and coplanar PCBs in muscle tissue of the female fish (Vuorinen et al. 1997).

To further elucidate the pathogenesis of M74 and to determine the involvement of both nutritional and toxicological factors, future work must include both histological and functional studies of tissues with regard to the symptoms and gross pathological findings characteristic of M74. However, because of the heterogeneity between family groups that develop M74 described in the present paper, careful selection of the experimental samples is necessary and should include categorization of each family group and definition of the stage of disease at sampling.

Acknowledgments

This study was supported by the Swedish Council for Forestry and Agricultural Research and the Swedish Environmental Protection Agency. We also acknowledge the National Board of Fisheries in Älvkarleby for supplying the roe.

References

Ackefors, H., N. Johansson, and B. Wahlberg. 1991. The Swedish compensatory programme for salmon in the Baltic: an action plan with biological and economical implications. ICES (International Council for the Exploration of the Sea) Marine Science Symposia 192:109–119.

Amcoff, P., H. Börjeson, R. Eriksson, and L. Norrgren. 1998b. Effects of thiamine treatments on survival of M74-affected feral Baltic salmon. Pages 31–40 *in* G. McDonald, J. D. Fitzsimons, and D. C. Honeyfield, editors. Early life stage mortality syndrome in fishes of the Great Lakes and Baltic Sea. American Fisheries Society, Symposium 21, Bethesda, Maryland.

Amcoff, P., H. Börjeson, J. Lindeberg, and L. Norrgren. 1998a. Thiamine concentrations in feral Baltic salmon exhibiting the M74 syndrome. Pages 82–89 *in* G. McDonald, J. D. Fitzsimons, and D. C. Honeyfield, editors. Early life stage mortality syndrome in fishes of the Great Lakes and Baltic Sea. American Fisheries Society, Symposium 21, Bethesda, Maryland.

Anglesea, J. D., and A. J. Jackson. 1985. Thiaminase activity in fish silage and moist fish feed. Animal Feed Science and Technology 13:39–46.

Anonymous. 1994. Report of the study group on occurrence of M-74 in fish stocks. ICES (International Council for the Exploration of the Sea) Council Meeting 1994/Environment:9.

Bignert, A., and five coauthors. 1995. Time-related factors influence the concentrations of sDDT, PCBs and shell parameters in eggs of Baltic guillemot (*Uria aalge*), 1861–1989. Environmental Pollution 89:27–36.

Brown, C. L., C. V. Sullivan, H. A. Bern, and W. W. Dickhoff. 1987. Occurrence of thyroid hormones in early developmental stages of teleost fish. Pages 332–345 *in* M. J. Dadswell and five coeditors. Common strategies of anadromous and catadromous fishes. American Fisheries Society, Symposium 1, Bethesda, Maryland.

Börjeson, H., and L. Norrgren. 1997. M74 syndrome: a review of potential etiological factors. Pages 153–166 *in* R. M. Rolland, M. Gilbertson, and R. E. Peterson, editors. Chemically induced alterations in functional development and reproduction of fishes. SETAC (Society for Environmental Toxicology and Chemistry), Pensacola, Florida.

Crawford, R. B., and A. M. Guarino. 1985. Effects of environmental toxicants on development of a teleost embryo. Journal of Environmental Pathology and Toxicology 6:185–194.

Deutsch, H. F., and A. D. Hasler. 1943. Distribution of a vitamin B_1 destructive enzyme in fish. Proceedings of the Society for Experimental Biology and Medicine 53:63–65.

Fänge, R., and S. Nilsson. 1985. The fish spleen: structure and function. Experientia 41:152–158.

Fisher, J. P., J. D. Fitzsimons, G. F. Combs, Jr., and J. M. Spitsbergen. 1996. Naturally occurring thiamine deficiency causing reproductive failure in Finger Lakes Atlantic salmon and Great Lakes trout. Transactions of the American Fisheries Society 125:167–178.

Fisher, J. P., and six coauthors. 1995a. Reproductive failure of landlocked Atlantic salmon from New York's Finger Lakes: investigations into the etiology and epidemiology of the "Cayuga syndrome." Journal of Aquatic Animal Health 7:81–94.

Fisher, J. P., J. M. Spitsbergen, and T. Iamonte. 1995b. Pathological and behavioral manifestations of the "Cayuga syndrome," a thiamine deficiency in larval landlocked Atlantic salmon. Journal of Aquatic Animal Health 7:269–283.

Fitzsimons, J. D. 1995. The effect of B-vitamins on a swim-up syndrome in Lake Ontario lake trout. Journal of Great Lakes Research 21(Supplement 1):286–289.

Giesy, J. P., J. Newsted, and D. L. Garling. 1986. Relationships between chlorinated hydrocarbon concentrations and rearing mortality of chinook salmon (*Oncorhynchus tshawytscha*) eggs from Lake Michigan. Journal of Great Lakes Research 12:83–98.

Gnaedinger, R. H. 1964. Thiaminase activity in fish: an improved assay method. Fishery Industrial Research 2:55–59.

Guarino, A. M. 1991. Regulatory and scientific roles for biodistribution studies in aquatic species. Veterinary and Human Toxicology 33(Supplement 1):54–59.

Heming, T. A., and R. K. Buddington. 1988. Yolk absorption in embryonic and larval fishes. Pages 408–446 *in* W. S. Hoar and D. J. Randall, editors. Fish physiology, volume XI. Academic Press, New York.

Johnson, H. E., and C. Pecor. 1969. Coho salmon mortality and D.D.T in Lake Michigan. Transactions of the North American Wildlife and Natural Resources Conference 34:159–166.

Karlsson, L., and Ö. Karlström. 1994. The Baltic salmon (*Salmo salar* L.): its history, present situation and future. Dana 10:61–85.

Mac, J. M. 1988. Toxic substances and survival of lake Michigan salmonids: field and laboratory approaches. Pages 390–401 *in* M. S. Evans, editor. Toxic contaminants and ecosystem health: a Great Lakes focus. Wiley, New York.

Mac, J. M., C. C. Edsall, and J. G. Seelye. 1985. Survival of lake trout eggs and fry reared in water from the upper Great Lakes. Journal of Great Lakes Research 11:520–529.

Marcquenski, S. V. 1996. Characterization of early mortality syndrome (EMS) in salmonids from the Great Lakes. Pages 73–75 *in* B.-E. Bengtsson, C. Hill, and S. Nellbring, editors. Report from the second workshop on reproduction disturbances in fish. Swedish Environmental Protection Agency Report 4534, Stockholm.

Morito, C. L. H., D. H. Conrad, and J. W. Hilton. 1986. The thiamine deficiency signs and requirement of rainbow trout (*Salmo gairdneri*, Richardson). Fish Physiology and Biochemistry 1:93–104.

Norrgren, L., T. Andersson, P.-A. Bergquist, and I. Björklund. 1993. Chemical, physiological and morphological studies of feral Baltic salmon (*Salmo salar*) suffering from abnormal fry mortality. Environmental Toxicology and Chemistry 12:2065–2075.

Olsson, M., and L. Reutergårdh. 1986. DDT and PCB pollution trends in the Swedish aquatic environment. Ambio 15:103–109.

Pettersson, A., and Å Lignell. 1998. Low astaxanthin levels in Baltic salmon exhibiting the M74 syndrome. Pages 26–30 *in* G. McDonald, J. D. Fitzsimons, and D. C. Honeyfield, editors. Early life stage mortality syndrome in fishes of the Great Lakes and Baltic Sea. American Fisheries Society, Symposium 21, Bethesda, Maryland.

Rudstam, L. G., G. Aneer, and M. Hildén. 1994. Top-down control in the pelagic Baltic ecosystem. Dana 10:105–129.

Sargent, J., R. J. Henderson, and D. R. Tocher. 1989.The lipids. Pages 153–218 *in* J. E. Halver, editor. Fish nutrition. Academic Press, New York.

Skea, J. C., J. Symula, and J. Miccoli. 1985. Separating starvation losses from other early feeding fry mortality in steelhead trout *Salmo gairdneri*, chinook salmon *Oncorhynchus tshawytscha*, and lake trout *Salvelinus namaycush*. Bulletin of Environmental Contamination and Toxicology 35:82–91.

Tagawa, M., and T. Hirano. 1987. Presence of thyroxine in eggs and changes in its content during early development of chum salmon, *Oncorhynchus keta*. General and Comparative Endocrinology 68:129–135.

Vuorinen P. J., and six coauthors. 1997. The M74 syndrome of Baltic salmon (*Salmo salar*) and organochlorine concentrations in the muscle of female salmon. Chemosphere 34:1151–1166.

American Fisheries Society Symposium 21:73–81, 1998

Thiamine Analysis in Fish Tissues[1]

SCOTT B. BROWN[2]
Department of Fisheries and Oceans, Winnipeg, Manitoba R3T 2N6, Canada

DALE C. HONEYFIELD
Biological Resources Division, U.S. Geological Survey
Research and Development Laboratory, Wellsboro, Pennsylvania 16901, USA

LENORE VANDENBYLLAARDT
Nore-Tech Laboratory Services, Anola, Manitoba R0E 0A0, Canada

Abstract.—Thiamine pyrophosphate, thiamine monophosphate, and thiamine were measured by reversed phase high-performance liquid chromatography in tissues of lake trout *Salvelinus namaycush* and alewife *Alosa pseudoharengus*. Mean assay sensitivity for thiamine and its phosphates was 0.012 pmol. Average recoveries of low and high doses of thiamine compounds added to tissue samples ranged from 91.4 to 104.5%. Average coefficients of variation for between assay reproducibility ranged from 4.8 to 12.8%. The predominant form of vitamin B_1 was unesterified thiamine in eggs and plasma of lake trout. Thiamine pyrophosphate was the predominant form in red blood cells, liver, muscle, and kidney. The stability of thiamine forms in fish tissues was temperature and species dependent. Thiamine levels were markedly depressed in lake trout collected from Lake Ontario relative to levels in fish captured from Lake 468 at the Experimental Lakes Area in northwestern Ontario.

Many physiological processes depend on adequate levels of vitamin B_1 (thiamine and its phosphorylated forms). Thiamine is a cofactor for several important enzymatic pathways in carbohydrate and amino acid metabolism, and it is vital for nerve function (Combs 1992). Thiamine deficiency in fish is characterized by poor appetite, muscle atrophy, convulsions, loss of equilibrium, edema, poor growth, and increased sensitivity to physical disturbance or light (Halver 1972; Morito et al. 1986). Low levels of egg thiamine are linked with the occurrence of a maternally related yolk sac and swim-up stage mortality in salmonids from the Finger Lakes (Fisher et al. 1996) and in the Laurentian Great Lakes (Fitzsimons 1995; Fitzsimons and Brown 1996). This type of mortality is widespread, affecting Atlantic salmon *Salmo salar*, lake trout *Salvelinus namaycush*, brown trout *Salmo trutta*, rainbow trout *Oncorhynchus mykiss*, coho salmon *O. kisutch*, and chinook salmon *O. tshawytscha* from various regions in the Great Lakes basin (Marcquenski 1996). The ailment has been referred to as Cayuga syndrome in the Atlantic salmon from the Finger Lakes region (Fisher et al. 1995) and early mortality syndrome (EMS) in the salmonids from the lower Great Lakes (Marcquenski 1996). Moreover, a similar thiamine-related embryonic mortality called M74 affects feral Atlantic salmon stocks in the Baltic Sea (Bylund and Lerche 1995; Johansson et al. 1995; Amcoff et al. 1996). To enhance the current understanding of these thiamine-related embryonic syndromes, it is essential to determine the cause(s) of the low levels of thiamine. An analytical method to measure quantities of thiamine and its active forms in various fish tissues and other biota is an important prerequisite to a quantitative description of thiamine dynamics in these syndromes.

In animal tissues, thiamine is found principally in its phosphorylated forms (Combs 1992), with the coenzyme, thiamine diphosphate, representing the predominant form (about 80%). In contrast, the major form of thiamine found in lake trout eggs from certain locations was free thiamine (this study). To detect and quantify thiamine and its different phosphorylated forms, these compounds were first extracted in trichloroacetic acid, converted to their respective thiochromes, and then assayed by reversed phase high-performance liquid chromatography (HPLC). The tissue extraction and assay procedures were modified from those described by Warnock (1982), Sanemori et al. (1980), and Kawasaki and Sanemori (1985). We used this protocol to assess the levels of thiamine in tissues of feral collections of lake trout from Lake Ontario, where EMS is known

[1] Portions of this publication were presented at the Second Workshop on Reproductive Disturbances in Fish, Stockholm, Sweden (1995).

[2] Present address: Environment Canada, Canada Centre for Inland Waters, 867 Lakeshore Road, Box 5050, Burlington, Ontario L7R 4A6, Canada.

to occur (Fitzsimons 1995), and at the Experimental Lakes Area in northwestern Ontario, where embryonic survival is high (Delorme 1995).

Methods

Fish Sampling and Sample Storage

Near spawning broodstock lake trout (weight, 850–3,320 g; length, 41–65 cm) were collected in September and October from Lake Ontario at Port Weller (near St. Catharines) and from Lake 468 at the Experimental Lakes Area, near Kenora in northwestern Ontario (Cleugh and Hauser 1971). Lake trout were captured either by gill nets examined for fish at 30-min intervals or by overnight trap net. Alewife *Alosa pseudoharengus* (weight, 14.2–33.2 g; length, 9.5–14.5 cm) were captured by trawl in the western basin of Lake Ontario. Only freshly caught live individuals were used for analysis. Before sampling, lake trout were anesthetized in water containing tricaine methanesulfonate (0.76 mmol/L) solution neutralized to ambient pH with ammonium hydroxide and NaCl (150 mmol/L) approximately isoosmotic with fish plasma. Immobilization was complete within 1–2 min. Blood was then removed from the caudal vessels using preheparinized 3- to 5-mL syringes with 18-gauge needles. Plasma and red blood cells were separated by centrifugation, placed into polyethylene vials, and immediately frozen on dry ice. Tissues were quickly dissected, weighed, packaged in Whirl-Pac® bags, and frozen between slabs of dry ice. Whole alewife specimens were quickly frozen. Samples were then transported to the laboratory on dry ice and stored at temperatures of less than −90°C. Samples were analyzed within 3 months of collection.

Reagents

Thiamine HCl (TH), thiamine pyrophosphate chloride (TPP), and thiamine monophosphate chloride (TMP) were obtained from ICN Biomedicals (Montreal, Quebec, Canada). American Chemical Society-grade sodium hydroxide, potassium ferricyanide, and trichloroacetic acid were purchased from Sigma Chemical Co. (Mississauga, Ontario, Canada). Potassium phosphate (HPLC-grade) was obtained from Fisher Scientific (Edmonton, Alberta, Canada). The distilled in glass *N,N*-Dimethylformamide (DMF) was obtained from Caledon (Edmonton, Alberta, Canada). We used distilled deionized water (DDW, MilliQ®, Millipore, Bedford, Massachusetts) to prepare stock solutions and buffers.

Apparatus

Gradient reversed phase chromatography was performed using a Hamilton PRP-1 column (150 × 4.1 mm; 5 mm mesh size; Alltech, Deerfield, Illinois) with attached guard column (25 × 2.3 mm; 12- to 20-mm mesh size) as stationary phase. The HPLC system consisted of two model 302 solvent pumps, a model 231 automatic sample injector, a model 704 system controller, and a four-channel model 620 data module (Gilson Medical Electronics, Middleton, Wisconsin). A Shimadzu (Columbia, Maryland) model RF-535 fluorometric detector was set at 375-nm excitation wavelength and 433-nm emission wavelength for thiochrome detection. The column thermostat was set at 30°C. The mobile phase consisted of 25 mM potassium phosphate (pH 8.4) and was applied for the first 4 min after sample injection. From 4 to 4.1 min, the mobile phase was changed to 3% DMF, 25 mM potassium phosphate (pH 8.4), and this was run until 8 min to elute thiamine pyrophosphate and thiamine monophosphate. Then between 8 and 8.1 min, the mobile phase was changed to 20% DMF, 25 mM potassium phosphate (pH 8.4) to elute thiamine. After 13.0 min, the mobile phase was returned to the initial conditions to equilibrate the column for the next sample. The flow rate was 1.0 mL/min and the total run time was 20 min.

Statistics

Significant differences between groups were determined by *t*-tests for independent samples or paired *t*-test for dependent samples using the Systat statistical package (Wilkinson et al. 1992).

Assay Procedure

The tissue extraction and assay procedures were modified from those described by Warnock (1982) and Kawasaki and Sanemori (1985). All thiamine standards were freshly prepared in DDW and used immediately. Aliquots of standards were subjected to the same extraction and washing procedures as the tissue samples.

Tissue Extraction

1. While tissue is frozen, finely chop approximately 500 mg and place it into a chilled, preweighed centrifuge tube. Reweigh the tube to obtain exact tissue weight.

2. Add 1.5 mL of ice-cold 2% trichloroacetic acid (TCA) and homogenize for 1–2 min either by hand or with a low-speed tissue grinder. Tis-

sue homogenization must be thorough and carefully conducted. Variable results will be obtained unless the close fitting homogenizer (0.02 cm difference between the diameter of pestle and the inside diameter of the tube) is used. If recovery of thiamine is low or variable, grind twice, once when tissue is placed in TCA and a second time after the boiling step. High-speed and ultrasonic homogenization caused losses and changes in the proportions of different thiamine compounds (Figure 1) and is not recommended.

3. Place tubes in a boiling water bath for 10 min, then remove tubes and briefly spin the mixture. Cool tubes for 10 min on ice. Preliminary experiments indicated an optimal heating time of between 5 and 10 min (Figure 2).

4. Add 1.5 mL of ice-cold 10% TCA. Homogenize sample briefly to mix.

5. Centrifuge the tubes at approximately 14,000 g for 15 min and transfer the supernatant to a clean container. The thiamine compounds in the sample supernatant are now stable for at least 72 h when stored at 4°C (Figure 3).

6. Wash the supernatant four times with an equal volume of ethyl acetate:hexane (3:2, volume per volume). This step removes most TCA and raises the pH of the supernatant to approximately 5.

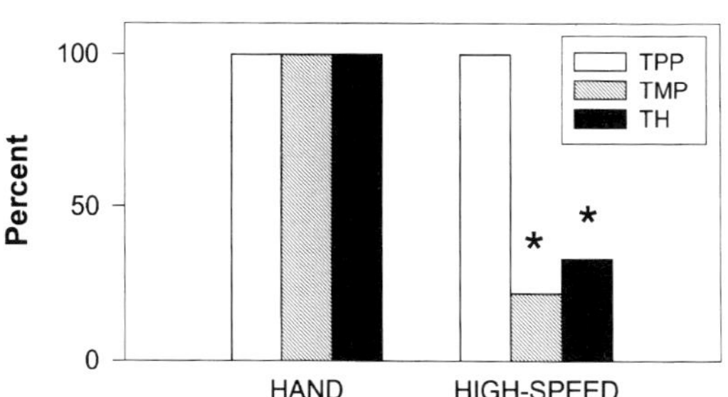

FIGURE 1.—The percentage recovery of thiamine pyrophosphate (TPP), thiamine monophosphate (TMP), and thiamine (TH) in red blood cells after hand or high-speed homogenization. Values are the mean of duplicate determinations from each of two samples. Asterisks indicate significant differences from hand homogenization.

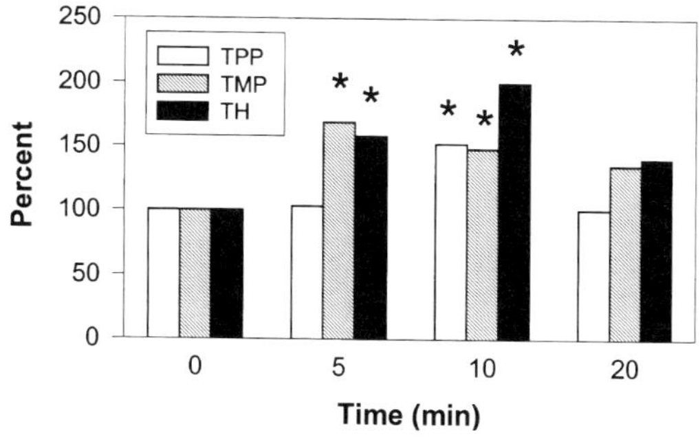

FIGURE 2.—The percentage recovery of thiamine pyrophosphate (TPP), thiamine monophosphate (TMP), and thiamine (TH) in eggs after heating at 100°C for up to 20 min. Values are the mean of duplicate determinations from each of two samples. Asterisks indicate differences from time 0.

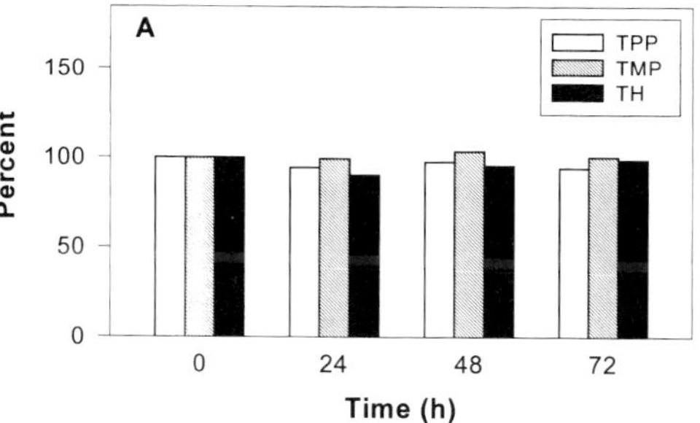

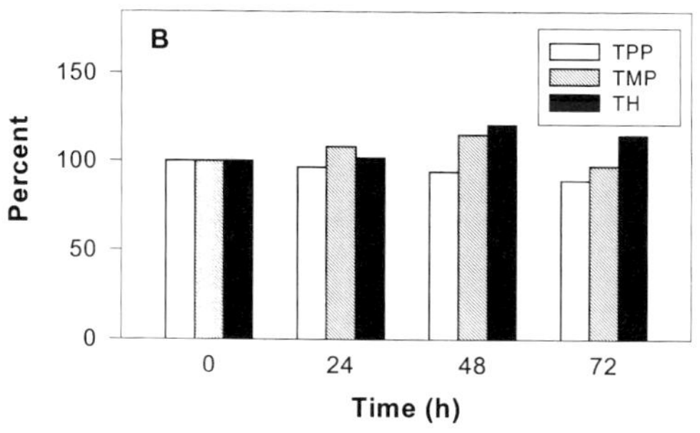

FIGURE 3.—The percentage recovery of thiamine pyrophosphate (TPP), thiamine monophosphate (TMP), and thiamine (TH) from extracted standards (**A**) and extracts of egg tissue (**B**) after storage of supernatants from the 10% TCA precipitation step at 4°C for up to 72 h. Values are the mean of duplicate determinations from each of two samples.

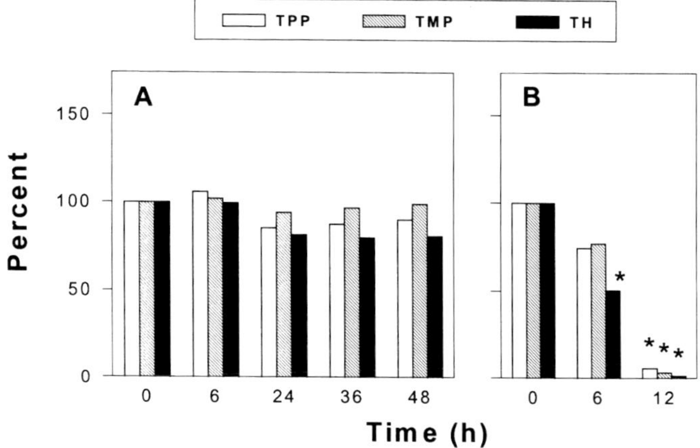

FIGURE 4.—The percentage recovery of thiamine pyrophosphate (TPP), thiamine monophosphate (TMP), and thiamine (TH) after room temperature storage of thiochrome solutions of samples in the dark (**A**) and in the light (**B**). Values are the mean of duplicate determinations from each of two samples. Asterisks indicate differences from time 0.

Thiochrome Preparation

1. Transfer 425 μL of the washed aqueous supernatant to a clean microcentrifuge tube and mix with 45 μL of 1.2 N NaOH and 30 μL of 0.1% potassium ferricyanide (prepared fresh daily). A final pH of greater than 8 is necessary for maximal fluorescence of thiochrome and its phosphates (Kawasaki and Sanemori 1985). When protected from light, alkaline solutions (approximately pH 9) of thiochrome were stable for 48 h (Figure 4).
2. Chromatograph the oxidized thiamine supernatant (20–100 μL) by reversed phase HPLC. Blanks are obtained by substituting distilled water for NaOH.

Results and Discussion

Assay Characteristics

Thiochrome fluorescence of extracted thiamine standards eluted with characteristic retention times that did not differ between preparations (Figure 5). Typical standard curves for phosphorylated thiamine

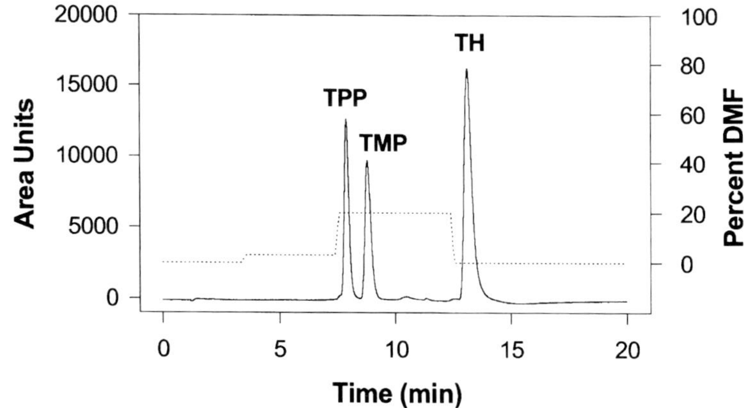

FIGURE 5.—The solid line indicates thiochrome fluorescence (375-nm excitation wavelength and 433-nm emission wavelength) after chromatography of a standard sample containing 8.4 pmol of thiamine pyrophosphate chloride (TPP), 10.3 pmol of thiamine monophosphate chloride (TMP), and 10.7 pmol of thiamine HCl (TH) on a Hamilton PRP-1 column (150 × 4.1 mm; 5-mm mesh size). The dotted line indicates the percentage of *N,N*-dimethylformamide (DMF) in the mobile phase (25 mM potassium phosphate, pH 8.4).

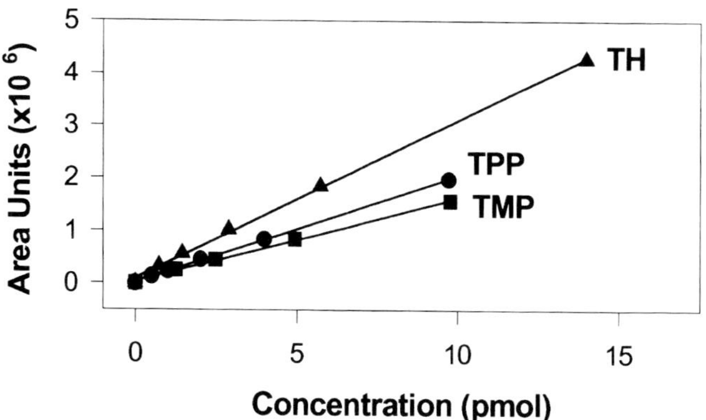

FIGURE 6.—Standard curves for thiamine pyrophosphate chloride (TPP), thiamine monophosphate chloride (TMP), and thiamine HCl (TH). Fluorescence detector response was linear ($r^2 = 0.99$ for TPP, TMP, and TH). Amounts injected ranged from 0.5 to 14.0 pmol. Values are the mean of triplicate determinations.

(TPP and TMP) and thiamine (TH) were linear ($r^2 \geq 0.99$; Figure 6). The detection limit for thiamine and its phosphates averaged 0.012 pmol per injection loop (20–100 μL). Dilutions of extracts of liver or egg tissue, ranging from 25 to 175 mg, gave parallel standard curves with $r^2 > 0.98$ for thiamine pyrophosphate, thiamine monophosphate, and thiamine in liver tissue and $r^2 > 0.96$ for thiamine pyrophosphate, thiamine monophosphate, and thiamine in eggs. Recovery of low (1 nmol/g) and high doses (50 nmol/g) of added thiamine compounds from 10 samples averaged 104.5 ± 2.8, 98.8 ± 1.9, and 91.4 ± 1.6% for thiamine pyrophosphate, thiamine monophosphate, and thiamine, respectively. Repeated measures (six repetitions) on extracts of the same egg homogenate or liver sample gave coefficients of variation of 8.1, 12.4, and 5.5% for thiamine pyrophosphate, thiamine monophosphate, and thiamine,

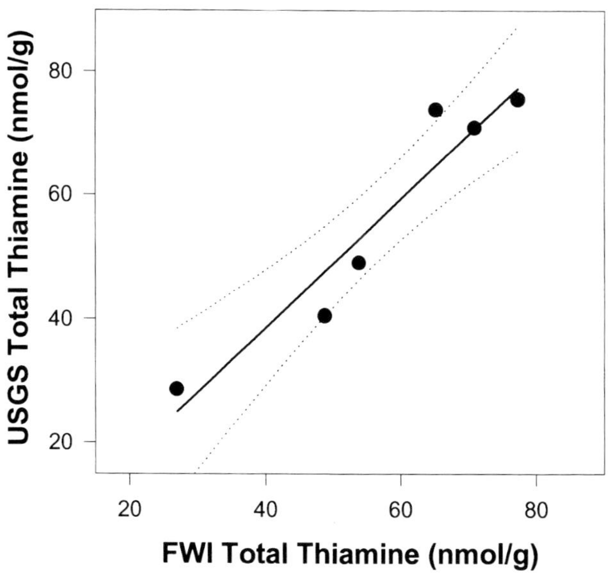

FIGURE 7.—The solid line shows the linear relationship ($r^2 = 0.916$, slope = 1.037) between total thiamine levels measured in six different lake trout egg samples at the U.S. Geological Survey Laboratory (USGS), Wellsboro, Pennsylvania, and at the Freshwater Institute Science Laboratory (FWI), Winnipeg, Manitoba. The dotted lines indicate the 95% confidence range.

respectively. Repeated measures (12 repetitions) on a tissue extract from a reference pool of lake trout eggs, analyzed on different days, gave coefficients of variation of 4.8, 7.8, and 12.8% for thiamine pyrophosphate, thiamine monophosphate, and thiamine, respectively. Using the protocol described above (see "Assay Procedure"), six different egg batches were measured at both the U.S. Geological Survey Research and Development Laboratory (Wellsboro, Pennsylvania) and the Freshwater Institute Science Laboratory (Winnipeg, Manitoba, Canada; Figure 7). The r^2-values for the correlation between laboratories were 0.928, 0.834, 0.924, and 0.916 for thiamine pyrophosphate, thiamine monophosphate, free thiamine, and total thiamine, respectively.

Stability of Thiamine in Fish Samples

The stability of thiamine forms in liver and muscle samples of trout and alewife were species and temperature dependent (Table 1). When liver tissue from lake trout was held at room temperature, the total thiamine levels were unchanged. Initially, thiamine pyrophosphate predominated; however, there was a gradual shift between the levels of thiamine pyrophosphate and free thiamine such that free thiamine was the predominant form after 24 h. When the tissues were maintained at 4°C, changes in the type of thiamine were not apparent in the first 4 h. After 24 h at 4°C, there was some evidence of conversion of thiamine monophosphate to free thiamine in trout liver. Maintaining muscle tissue from lake trout at room temperature resulted in lower thiamine pyrophosphate levels at 24 h. This decline was offset by a corresponding increase in the level of thiamine monophosphate. Samples of alewife muscle were unstable at room temperature, and the levels of all thiamine forms declined sharply after 1 h. Refrigeration at 4°C stabilized the total thiamine levels in alewife but did not prevent a shift from thiamine pyrophosphate to thiamine monophosphate after 4 h. Reanalysis of tissue samples stored at −90°C for 1 year gave results similar to those from fresh tissue. However, if the sample thaws and is refrozen, the analysis of extracts of the refrozen tissue will reflect losses and changes in the forms of thiamine present.

Although our information about thiamine stability was derived from laboratory experiments, the findings are relevant to thiamine measurements in fish collected in field surveys. Measurements in fish that were not freshly caught and sampled would lead to erroneous assessments of the proportions and quantities of the different thiamine forms. Species such as alewife and smelt that contain thiaminase activity (Gnaedinger 1964) seem particularly vulnerable. Furthermore, the degenerative changes occur at a faster rate when temperatures are higher. Appropriate protocols for collection and storage of the samples are critical. A procedure in which fresh samples from live specimens are quickly frozen is necessary to obtain an accurate representation of thiamine forms.

TABLE 1.—Percentage total thiamine compounds for thiamine pyrophosphate (TPP), thiamine monophosphate (TMP), and free thiamine (TH) and percentage recovery of total thiamine in liver or muscle samples held at 20 or 4°C for up to 24 h before analysis. Values represent the mean of duplicate measurements. Differences from 0 h are indicated by z.

Time	Percentage total thiamine			Percentage
	TPP	TMP	TH	recovery
	Lake trout liver (20°C)			
0 h	85.2	14.0	0.8	100.0
1 h	75.8	18.7	9.2	103.8
4 h	62.6z	12.4	24.2z	99.3
24 h	21.5z	7.1	83.9z	112.5
	Lake trout liver (4°C)			
0 h	81.9	17.0	1.1	100.0
1 h	88.3	20.1	2.7	111.1
4 h	85.7	21.6	5.4z	112.7
24 h	81.5	12.1	16.2z	109.9
	Lake trout muscle (20°C)			
0 h	86.6	12.6	0.9	100.0
1 h	81.1	9.6	0.5	91.2
4 h	92.0	15.6	1.2	108.8
24 h	23.2z	50.7z	6.5z	80.4z
	Alewife muscle (20°C)			
0 h	76.9	18.4	4.7	100.0
1 h	78.2	26.3	5.2	109.7
4 h	3.5z	7.8z	0.5z	11.8z
24 h	2.2z	0.0z	0.0z	2.2z
	Alewife muscle (4°C)			
0 h	71.2	24.3	4.5	100.0
1 h	70.2	35.6	2.6	108.5
4 h	53.7z	44.0z	3.1	100.8
24 h	23.4z	69.6z	6.7	99.6

Thiamine Levels in Lake Trout Tissues

Similar to sea urchin eggs (Shimada et al. 1993), in lake trout eggs the major form of thiamine was free thiamine (Figure 8A). Total thiamine levels in spawning female fish were lowest in plasma (Table 2). Although plasma levels of phosphorylated forms were detectable, free thiamine was the predominant form. Free thiamine may be able to cross cell membranes more readily than esterified forms (Combs 1992). Moreover, the possible presence of a female-specific vitamin transport protein for thiamine similar to that reported in birds and amphibians (Adiga and Murty 1983; White 1987) warrants investigation as a mechanism for the incorporation of the large amounts of free thiamine detected in oocytes. As is generally found in other animal species (Combs 1992), thiamine in red blood cells, liver, and kidney of lake trout was predominantly the metabolically functional enzyme cofactor (TPP; Figure 8B, Table 2). In female lake trout collected from Lake 468 at the Experimental Lakes Area, levels of total thiamine were comparable with levels reported in liver of feral bream *Abramis brama*, roach *Rutilis rutilus*, and pike *Esox lucius* (Malyarevskaya and Karasina 1992). Red blood cell and liver thiamine pyrophosphate levels of female lake trout from Lake 468 (Table 1) were also similar to concentrations reported for juvenile rainbow trout fed a commercial diet supplemented with thiamine (Masumoto et al. 1987). Depending on the tissue examined, total thiamine levels of lake trout collected from Lake Ontario were only 10–50% of concentrations found in fish from Lake 468 (Table 2). The low levels of thiamine found in red blood cells and liver from lake trout collected in Lake Ontario (Table 2) were comparable with those found in juvenile rainbow trout exhibiting overt signs of thiamine deficiency after consuming a thiamine-deficient diet (Masumoto et al. 1987). Levels of free thiamine in eggs showed the greatest difference between locations. The low thiamine levels found in salmonid eggs from areas in the Laurentian Great Lakes have been implicated as a possible cause of early mortality syndrome and recent reproductive failures (Fitzsimons 1995; Fisher et al. 1996; Marcquenski 1996).

Acknowledgments

This work was partially supported by the Fish Health Monitoring project in the Department of Fisheries and Oceans Toxic Chemicals Program. We thank John Fitzsimons for arranging the collection

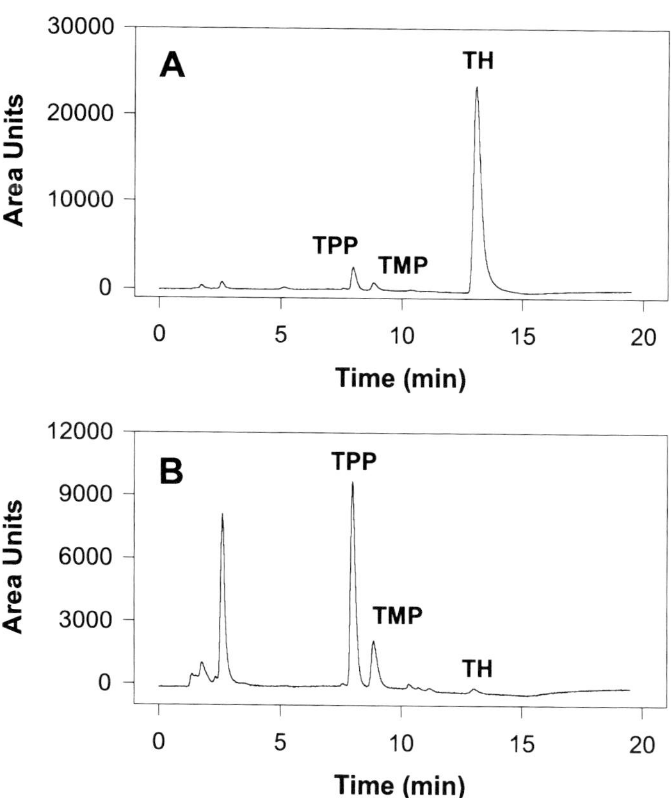

FIGURE 8.—Thiochrome fluorescence after chromatography of tissue extracts prepared from eggs (**A**) and liver (**B**) from a female lake trout captured in Lake 468 at the Experimental Lakes Area. Identified peaks co-elute with thiochromes of thiamine pyrophosphate chloride (TPP), thiamine monophosphate chloride (TMP), and thiamine HCl (TH).

TABLE 2.—Thiamine pyrophosphate (TPP), thiamine monophosphate (TMP), free thiamine (TH), and total thiamine (TTH) (nmol/g) in selected tissues of female lake trout collected from Lake 468 at the Experimental Lakes Area and from Lake Ontario near Port Weller. Values represent the mean (SE) of duplicate measurements from three or four fish.

	Lake 468				Lake Ontario			
Tissue	TPP	TMP	TH	TTH	TPP	TMP	TH	TTH
Eggs	1.843	0.840	16.954	19.637	0.723	0.353	0.951	2.027
	(0.068)	(0.013)	(0.197)	(0.278)	(0.076)	(0.090)	(0.544)	(0.706)
Plasma	0.036	0.039	0.072	0.148	0.013	0.024	0.036	0.073
	(0.010)	(0.018)	(0.013)	(0.035)	(0.004)	(0.005)	(0.003)	(0.009)
Red blood cells	1.170	0.168	0.038	1.376	0.213	0.104	0.080	0.398
	(0.184)	(0.046)	(0.004)	(0.217)	(0.036)	(0.041)	(0.010)	(0.078)
Liver	8.501	2.954	0.247	11.702	5.142	0.493	0.147	5.782
	(1.753)	(0.243)	(0.038)	(1.809)	(0.418)	(0.077)	(0.142)	(0.629)
Kidney	9.153	3.405	2.419	14.976	3.346	0.392	0.181	3.920
	(1.046)	(0.923)	(0.548)	(2.191)	(0.503)	(0.051)	(0.042)	(0.584)

of lake trout and alewife from Lake Ontario. We gratefully acknowledge the helpful criticisms of K. Mills, R. Hunt, and C. Haux on a previous version of the manuscript.

References

Adiga, P. R., and C. V. R. Murty. 1983. Vitamin carrier proteins during embryonic development in birds and mammals. Pages 111–136 *in* R. Porter and J. Whelan, editors. Molecular biology of egg maturation. Pitman Books, London.

Amcoff, P., L. Norrgren, H. Börjeson, and J. Lindeberg. 1996. Lowered concentrations of thiamine (vitamin B_1) in M74-affected feral Baltic salmon (*Salmo salar*). Pages 38–39 *in* B.-E. Bengtsson, C. Hill, and S. Nellbring, editors. Report from the second workshop on reproduction disturbances in fish. Swedish Environmental Protection Agency Report 4534, Stockholm.

Bylund, G., and O. Lerche. 1995. Thiamine therapy of M74 affected fry of Atlantic salmon, *Salmo salar*. Bulletin of the European Association of Fish Pathologists 15(3):93–97.

Cleugh, T. R., and B. W. Hauser. 1971. Results of an initial survey of the Experimental Lakes area, northwestern Ontario. Journal of the Fisheries Research Board of Canada 28:129–137.

Combs, G. F., Jr. 1992. The vitamins. Academic Press, San Diego, California.

Delorme, P. D. 1995. The effects of toxaphene, chlordane and 2,3,4,7,8-pentachlorodibenzofuran on lake trout and white sucker in an ecosystem experiment and the distribution and effects of 2,3,4,7,8-pentachlorodibenzofuran on white sucker and broodstock rainbow trout in laboratory experiments. Doctoral dissertation. University of Manitoba, Winnipeg.

Fisher, J. P., J. D. Fitzsimons, G. F. Combs, Jr., and J. M. Spitsbergen. 1996. Naturally occurring thiamine deficiency causing reproductive failure in Finger Lakes Atlantic salmon and Great Lakes lake trout. Transactions of the American Fisheries Society 125:167–178.

Fisher, J. P., and six coauthors. 1995. Reproductive failure of landlocked Atlantic salmon from New York's Finger Lakes: investigations into the etiology and epidemiology of the "Cayuga syndrome." Journal of Aquatic Animal Health 7:81–94.

Fitzsimons, J. D. 1995. The effect of B-vitamins on a swim-up syndrome in Lake Ontario lake trout. Journal of Great Lakes Research 21 (Supplement 1):286–289.

Fitzsimons, J. D., and S. B. Brown. 1996. Effect of diet on thiamine levels in Great Lakes lake trout and relationship with early mortality syndrome. Pages 76–78 *in* B.-E. Bengtsson, C. Hill, and S. Nellbring, editors. Report from the second workshop on reproduction disturbances in fish. Swedish Environmental Protection Agency Report 4534, Stockholm.

Gnaedinger, R. H. 1964. Thiaminase activity in fish: an improved assay method. Fishery Industrial Research 2:55–59.

Halver, J. E. 1972. The vitamins. Pages 29–103 *in* J. E. Halver, editor. Fish nutrition. Academic Press, New York.

Johansson, N., P. Jonsson, O. Svanberg, A. Södergren, and J. Thulin. 1995. Reproduction disorders in Baltic fish. Swedish Environmental Protection Agency Report 4347, Stockholm.

Kawasaki, T., and H. Sanemori. 1985. Vitamin B_1: thiamines. Modern Chromatographic Science Series 30:385–412.

Malyarevskaya, A. Y., and F. M. Karasina. 1992. Variations in levels of heavy metals and total thiamine in fishes. Hydrobiological Journal 28:17–24.

Marcquenski, S. V. 1996. Characterization of early mortality syndrome (EMS) in salmonids from the Great Lakes. Pages 73–75 *in* B.-E. Bengtsson, C. Hill, and S. Nellbring, editors. Report from the second workshop on reproduction disturbances in fish. Swedish Environmental Protection Agency Report 4534, Stockholm.

Masumoto, T., R. W. Hardy, and E. Casillas. 1987. Comparison of transketolase activity and thiamine pyrophosphate levels in erythrocytes and liver of rainbow trout (*Salmo gairdneri*) as indicators of thiamine status. Journal of Nutrition 117:1422–1426.

Morito, C. L. H., D. H. Conrad, and J. W. Hilton. 1986. The thiamine deficiency signs and requirement of rainbow trout (*Salmo gairdneri*, Richardson). Fish Physiology and Biochemistry 2:93–104.

Sanemori, H., H. Ueki, and T. Kawasaki. 1980. Reversed-phase high-performance liquid chromatographic analysis of thiamine phosphate esters at subpicomole levels. Analytical Biochemistry 107:451–455.

Shimada, K., S. Nakagawa, K. Hotta, T. Shibata, and T. Yagi. 1993. Effect of processing and storage on the fate of vitamins B_1, B_2 and B_6 and nicotinamide of sea urchin gonads. Journal of Agricultural and Food Chemistry 41:1021–1025.

Warnock, L. G. 1982. The measurement of erythrocyte thiamine pyrophosphate by high performance liquid chromatography. Analytical Biochemistry 126:394–397.

White, H. B., III. 1987. Vitamin-binding proteins in the nutrition of the avian embryo. Journal of Experimental Zoology (Supplement 1):53–63.

Wilkinson, L., M. Hill, J. P. Welna, and G. K. Birkenbeuel. 1992. Systat for Windows: statistics version 5. Systat Inc., Evanston, Illinois.

American Fisheries Society Symposium 21:82–89, 1998

Thiamine Concentrations in Feral Baltic Salmon Exhibiting the M74 Syndrome

PATRIC AMCOFF[1]
Department of Pathology, Faculty of Veterinary Medicine
Swedish University of Agricultural Sciences, Box 7028, S-750 07 Uppsala, Sweden

HANS BÖRJESON
Swedish Salmon Research Institute, S-814 94 Älvkarleby, Sweden

JOHAN LINDEBERG
National Food Administration, Box 622, S-751 26 Uppsala, Sweden

LEIF NORRGREN
Department of Pathology, Faculty of Veterinary Medicine
Swedish University of Agricultural Sciences

Abstract.—Since 1974, feral Baltic salmon *Salmo salar* populations have suffered from yolk sac fry mortality caused by the M74 syndrome. This syndrome affects yolk sac fry originating from specific females, and the mortality in affected family groups is usually 100%. Since 1990–1991, disturbances in the behavior of spawning migrating Baltic salmon have been observed. This study found a strong correlation between wiggling behavior in adult female Baltic salmon and the development of M74 in their offspring. Moreover, the ovarian thiamine concentrations in wiggling females were found to be significantly lower than those of females with normal behavior. In addition, eyed eggs and yolk sac fry that subsequently developed M74 contained only 13% (0.24 nmol/g) and 6% (0.11 nmol/g), respectively, of the thiamine concentrations detected in viable progeny sampled during the same periods. Eyed eggs with thiamine concentrations below a threshold limit interval of 0.36–0.77 nmol/g were found to have a high risk of developing M74 at the yolk sac fry stage.

Feral Baltic salmon *Salmo salar* are afflicted by abnormally high yolk sac fry mortality caused by a reproductive disorder known as the M74 syndrome. The syndrome was first observed in a Swedish compensatory rearing station along the Baltic coast in 1974. Occurrence of M74 mortality has fluctuated between rivers, and during the 1990s an increased mortality has been recorded (Börjeson and Norrgren 1997). The M74 syndrome is linked to the progeny of specific females, and mortality in affected family groups is usually 100%. Yolk sac fry that develop M74 are characterized by a wide variety of symptoms, including increased motor activity, abnormal swimming behavior with sudden movements toward the water surface, and, finally, lethargy and death. Hyperpigmentation of the skin, pale spleen, and white precipitates in the yolk sac are also common clinical signs. M74-related mortality is usually manifested during the middle and later parts of the yolk sac resorption process (Norrgren et al. 1993; Lundström et al. 1998, this volume), which spans a 4- to 6-week period depending on water temperature. Clinical signs and mortality rates associated with the M74 syndrome are similar to those observed in early mortality syndrome (EMS), which affects the progeny of several salmonid species in the Great Lakes basin of North America (Skea et al. 1985; Mac 1988; Fitzsimons et al. 1995). A similar reproductive disturbance affecting landlocked Atlantic salmon yolk sac fry in the Finger Lakes of New York State has been termed the Cayuga syndrome (CS; Fisher et al. 1995a, 1995b). Yolk sac fry with EMS and CS have reduced thiamine (vitamin B_1) concentrations (Fisher et al. 1995b; Brown et al. 1998, this volume).

Since 1990–1991, ascending spawning Baltic salmon of both sexes caught from June to September in Swedish rivers for compensatory rearing programs have displayed abnormal behavior such as wiggling, sideways swimming, and lack of coordination. The behavior often becomes more pronounced as spawning approaches in October and November, and in severe cases the fish die before stripping. This behavior resembles the neurological disturbances observed in thiamine-deficient farmed salmonids (Lehmitz and Spannhof 1977; Morito et al. 1986; Masumoto et al. 1987).

[1] To whom correspondence should be addressed.

The purpose of this investigation was to determine if the wiggling behavior in adult female Baltic salmon was associated with the development of M74 in their progeny and whether these females have lowered thiamine concentrations. Accordingly, hepatic and ovarian thiamine concentrations in wiggling and normally behaving females were measured, and their offspring were monitored for the development of M74. In addition, thiamine concentrations were analyzed in both eyed eggs and yolk sac fry that developed M74 and those that developed into normal progeny.

Methods

Fish Material

Relationship between the thiamine status of female Baltic salmon and their swimming behavior and occurrence of M74 in offspring of females displaying wiggling behavior.—In 1993, Baltic salmon from River Luleälven stock were caught in salmon traps during their spawning migration and transferred to indoor pools with flowing river water. In captivity (from July to November), some females showed abnormal swimming behavior that became accentuated as ovulation approached. The disturbance was characterized by wiggling, sideways swimming, a lack of coordination, and disturbances in swim bladder inflation that resulted in overinflation or underinflation and, in severe cases, death. Of 402 females, 103 manifested wiggling behavior during the captivity period, and of these wiggling individuals, 27 died before stripping was performed. Of the total number, 17 females (6 normal and 11 that displayed wiggling behavior) were randomly selected in early October, 2–4 weeks before ovulation, for studies of hepatic and ovarian thiamine concentrations. For each female, length and weight were measured. After anesthetization in MS-222® (Sandoz Ltd., Basel, Switzerland; 5 min in 140 mg/L) and decapitation, livers and ovaries were removed and weighed and then immediately frozen between slabs of dry ice and stored at −70°C in airtight plastic bags for a maximum of 2 months until thiamine analysis. The remaining 358 females were stripped in October and November. The egg batch from each female was fertilized with a mixture of milt from two males and incubated in separate hatching trays, where the progeny were monitored for development into normal or M74-affected yolk sac fry until swim-up. The temperature varied according to the natural fluctuation in the river, ranging from 0.1 to 12°C during the period from November to June. A condition factor (CF) was calculated [(body weight in grams ÷ length in cubic centimeters) × 100] for all sampled females. Also, liver (LSI) and gonadal (GSI) somatic indexes were calculated for the 17 females sampled [(weight of liver or ovaries in kilograms ÷ body weight in kilograms) × 100)].

Relationship between thiamine concentrations in Baltic salmon eyed eggs and yolk sac fry and occurrence of M74.—In 1994, as a follow-up to the study from 1993, feral spawning migrating female Baltic salmon (N = 45) of River Dalälven stock were caught (June–September) on their spawning run using salmon traps. Fish were kept in indoor pools with flowing river water until stripping, which was performed only on normally behaving females in November. The eggs of each female were fertilized with milt from two males and incubated in separate hatching trays, where the M74 mortality of each batch was monitored. The temperature from incubation to swim-up varied according to the natural fluctuation in the river, ranging from 0.1 to 15°C during the period from November to May. In March, eyed eggs from each family group were sampled for thiamine analysis. Prognostic hatching was performed by keeping 200 eggs from each family group in separate hatching trays at an elevated temperature (6.5°C) to advance the hatching date. This indicated that of the 45 groups of eggs, 31 developed M74 and 14 developed normally. Based on these results, eight normally developing groups and eight groups developing M74, all reared in river water at a lower temperature based on the fluctuation of the river, were sampled 1 week after hatching (60 posthatch centigrade degree-days) for thiamine analysis. In addition, offspring from farmed Baltic salmon (N = 3) sampled at the same times were analyzed. The eggs and yolk sac fry were frozen in liquid nitrogen and stored at −70°C in airtight plastic bags for a maximum of 2 months until thiamine analysis.

Thiamine Assay

Thiamine was extracted using acid and enzymatic hydrolysis based on the method of Roser et al. (1978). Each sample (3–15 g) was extracted using 0.1 M HCl at 121°C for 30 min. The extract was cooled to 23°C and the pH adjusted to 4.0 by adding 2.0 M sodium acetate buffer (pH 6.1). A suspension of taka-diastase in water was added to the extract at a concentration of 0.1 g/g of sample. After incubation at 45°C for 4 h, the extract was cooled to 23°C

TABLE 1.—Mean thiamine concentrations ± SD (nmol/g, wet weight) in livers and ovaries from wiggling (N = 11) and normally behaving (N = 6) feral female Baltic salmon. Significant differences between groups are indicated by different letters after the mean.

	Wiggling behavior	Normal behavior	Statistics
Body weight (kg)	8.6 ± 2.8	9.8 ± 4.1	NS
Length (cm)	91 ± 8.4	93 ± 11	NS
Condition factor[a]	1.1 ± 0.082	1.2 ± 0.18	NS
Hepatic thiamine (nmol/g)	4.8 ± 1.0	5.8 ± 1.1	NS
Liver somatic index[b]	1.3 ± 0.31	1.4 ± 0.20	NS
Ovarian thiamine (nmol/g)	0.27 ± 0.072 z	1.9 ± 2.5 y	$P \leq 0.001$
Gonadal somatic index[c]	19 ± 4.8	22 ± 1.5	NS

[a] (Body weight in grams) ÷ (Length in cubic centimeters) × 100.

[b] (Weight of liver in kilograms) ÷ (Body weight in kilograms) × 100.

[c] (Weight of ovaries in kilograms) ÷ (Body weight in kilograms) × 100.

and filtered through Munktell V120H folded paper (Munktell, Grycksbo, Sweden). The conversion efficiency of the taka-diastase preparation was checked by analysis of known amounts of thiamine and thiamine diphosphate added to different types of tissue samples (liver, egg, and yolk sac fry). The recovery of added thiamine and thiamine diphosphate was between 96 and 99%. The coefficient of variation (V = 0.012) of the method was determined by consecutive analysis of two different tissue samples. All samples were analyzed in duplicate and data are presented on a wet weight basis (ww). The thiamine in the extract was converted to the fluorescent thiochrome compound using an automated precolumn derivation technique. An ASPEC liquid-handling robot with a model 401 dilutor (Gilson, Villiers-le-Bel, France) was used to mix 2.0 mL of the sample extract with 1.1 mL of derivation reagent [3 mM $K_3Fe(CN)_6$ in 4 M NaOH]. A stream of air was used to ensure mixing, and the derived extract was subjected to high-performance liquid chromatography (HPLC) after 80 s. The HPLC system consisted of an LC-10AD pump, an RF-551 spectrofluorometric detector, a Chromatopac C-R5A integrator (all from Shimadzu, Tokyo, Japan), and a model 7010 injector (Rheodyne, Cotati, California) equipped with a 20-μL loop. The column (5 μm of packing material; 150 mm × 4.1 mm internal diameter) was a polymer-based PRP-1 (Hamilton Co., Reno, Nevada). The mobile phase was a 40% (volume per volume) mixture of methanol in water adjusted to pH 4.5 with acetic acid and degassed on an ultrasonic bath. The flow rate was 0.7 mL/min. All analytical work was performed in laboratories protected against ultraviolet radiation. Detection was performed at an excitation wavelength of 366 nm and an emission wavelength of 435 nm. Thiamine concentrations were calculated using external standards of thiamine that were subjected to the extraction and derivation steps described above. The thiamine standard was prepared daily in 0.01 M HCl and used immediately. Integrated peak areas were corrected for thiamine originating in the enzyme preparations by subtracting the peak areas of the blanks from the samples. Reference material was analyzed in parallel with the samples to ensure reliable results.

Chemicals

The thiamine HCl (96.6% dry weight) used in the thiamine analysis was supplied by Fluka (purum, no. 95160, lot 604066; Buchs, Switzerland). Taka-diastase was supplied by Pfaltz & Bauer (no. T00040, lot 045513; Chemicon, Stockholm, Sweden). All other chemicals were of analytical grade, and the water was of Milli-Q quality (Millipore).

Statistics

To test for differences in frequency of M74 between offspring of females with wiggling (N = 65) versus normal (N = 293) behavior, the χ^2 test was applied. To test for differences in weight and CF, the z-test for unpaired samples was used. To test for differences in thiamine concentrations, weight, length, CF, LSI, and GSI of the dissected females (N = 17) and when comparing thiamine concentrations between eggs and yolk sac fry developing into normal or M74-

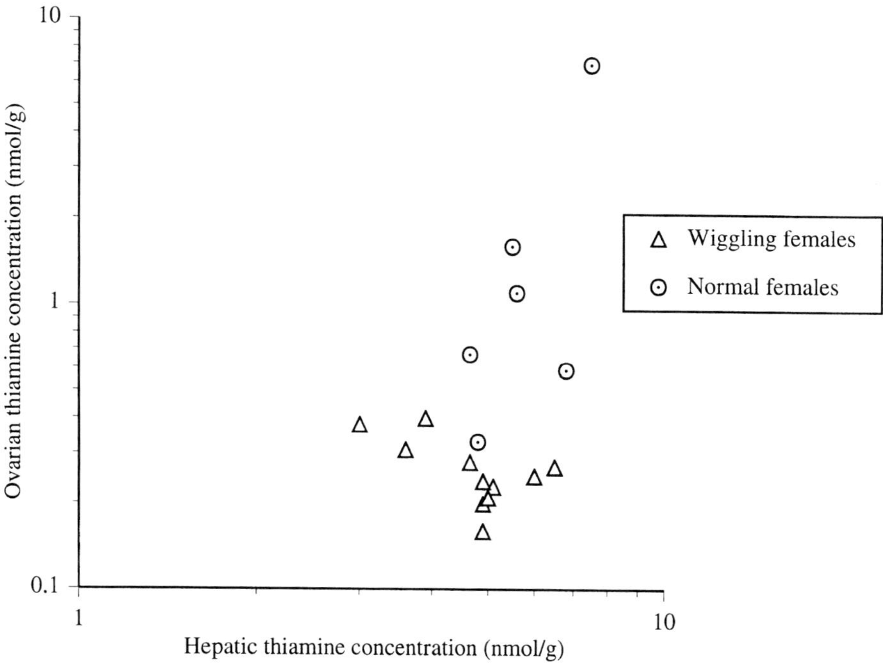

FIGURE 1.—Hepatic and ovarian thiamine concentrations (nmol/g, wet weight) in wiggling (N = 11) and normally behaving (N = 6) feral Baltic salmon females.

affected offspring, the two-tailed Mann–Whitney *U*-test was used. *P*-values as shown in Figure 2 are ≤0.05 (*) and ≤0.001 (***). In all testing, the work of Zar (1984) was consulted, and the statistics were analyzed in the StatView 4.5 data analysis system (Abacus Concepts, Inc., Berkeley, California).

Results

Relationship between the Thiamine Status of Female Baltic Salmon and Their Swimming Behavior and Occurrence of M74 in Offspring of Females Displaying Wiggling Behavior

In the study of M74 incidence in the offspring of a group of females (N = 358), the mean weights of wiggling (N = 65) and normal (N = 293) females were 11 ± 4.0 and 8.4 ± 3.4 kg, respectively (z = 4.31, $P \leq$ 0.001), whereas CF values were 1.22 ± 0.14 and 1.17 ± 0.13 (z = 2.88, $P \leq 0.01$). Of the females with wiggling or normal swimming behavior, 98% (N = 64) and 51% (N = 149; χ^2 = 46.1, $P \leq 0.001$) had progeny that developed M74. The total occurrence of M74 in the 358 females investigated was 60%, which was the highest M74 frequency ever observed in the River Luleälven salmon population.

In a subsample of wiggling (N = 11) and normal (N = 6) females, the weight, length, CF, LSI, and GSI were not significantly different between groups (Table 1). The mean hepatic thiamine concentrations of 4.8 and 5.8 nmol/g (ww), respectively, were not significantly different ($P > 0.05$). The mean thiamine concentration of 0.27 nmol/g (ww) in the ovaries of wiggling females was significantly less ($P \leq 0.001$) than the 1.9 nmol/g (ww) found in the ovaries of normal females (Figure 1).

Relationship between Thiamine Concentrations in Baltic Salmon Eyed Eggs and Yolk Sac Fry and Occurrence of M74

Eyed eggs from farmed Baltic salmon had a mean thiamine concentration (20 ± 10 nmol/g, ww) that was significantly greater than that of feral salmon whether or not they developed M74 ($P \leq 0.001$; Figure 2). The mean thiamine concentrations in eyed eggs from feral Baltic salmon developing into normal or M74-affected yolk sac fry (1.9 ± 2.1 and 0.24 ± 0.16 nmol/g, ww, respectively) were significantly different ($P \leq 0.001$). The lowest thiamine concentration detected among normal family groups (0.36 nmol/g, ww) was less than the highest thiamine content (0.77 nmol/g, ww) detected among family groups whose progeny developed

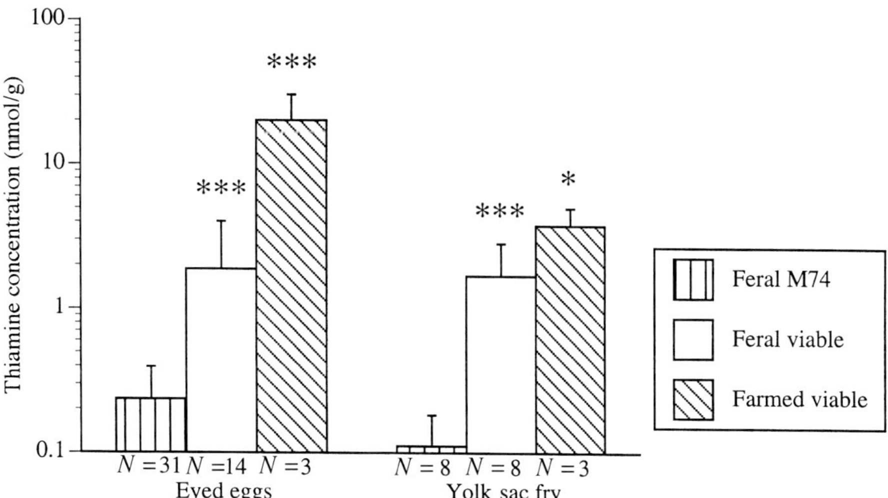

FIGURE 2.—Mean thiamine concentrations (± SD; nmol /g, wet weight) in eyed eggs and yolk sac fry from feral broodstock whose progeny developed M74 and from feral and farmed broodstock that had viable offspring. Significant differences between groups are indicated by the symbols * and *** representing $P \leq 0.05$ and $P \leq 0.001$, respectively.

M74. These results suggest a possible thiamine threshold limit interval in eggs for development of M74 of 0.36–0.77 nmol/g (ww).

All yolk sac fry in the M74-affected groups (N = 8) died, whereas those in the viable feral (N = 8) and farmed (N = 3) groups showed mean mortality from fertilization to swim-up of 7.6 and 5.3%, respectively (Figure 3). The mean thiamine concentration (3.7 ± 1.2 nmol/g, ww) found in farmed yolk sac fry was significantly higher than that of feral viable or M74 developing yolk sac fry ($P \leq 0.05$), whereas feral offspring that developed normally had a mean thiamine concentration of 1.7 ± 1.1 nmol/g (ww), which was significantly higher ($P \leq 0.001$) than the 0.12 ± 0.10 nmol/g (ww) found in yolk sac fry with M74. The lowest thiamine concentration in the viable feral group was 0.31 nmol/g (ww), and the highest thiamine content in M74-affected yolk sac fry was 0.34 nmol/g (ww). These findings suggest a thiamine threshold limit interval in yolk sac fry of 0.31–0.34 nmol/g (ww) for the development of M74.

Discussion

This study indicated a strong association between wiggling behavior in females and the occurrence of M74 in their offspring, although variability in the development of M74 in the progeny of females with normal behavior suggests that female behavior alone is not a good predictor of the potential of progeny to develop M74. We did find, however, that eyed egg thiamine concentrations from normally behaving females whose progeny developed M74 were significantly lower than eyed egg thiamine concentrations from normally behaving females whose progeny did not develop M74. Furthermore, the ovarian thiamine concentrations of wiggling females were significantly lower than those of females that behaved normally, suggesting that the wiggling behavior may be an indication of a hierarchical thiamine deficiency in which wiggling represents a severe thiamine deficit not only affecting the progeny but also the adult broodfish, which in severe cases die before stripping. The mean ovarian thiamine concentration (0.27 nmol/g), but not the mean hepatic thiamine concentration (4.8 nmol/g), was significantly lower in the wiggling females than in normal females. The large variation in ovarian thiamine concentration (1.9 ± 2.5 nmol/g) in the group of normally behaving females, which includes individuals with low ovarian thiamine content, may indicate the presence of females potentially producing M74-affected offspring. The normally behaving female with the lowest ovarian thiamine concentration (0.33 nmol/g) contained 4.8 nmol/g hepatic thiamine, whereas the highest ovarian thiamine concentrations detected in wiggling females (N = 2) were 0.38 and 0.40 nmol/g. The hepatic thiamine concentrations of these two wiggling females, however, were among the lowest found in all females (3.0 and 3.9 nmol/g). In a comparison of the ovarian thiamine contents in normally behaving females and the threshold limit interval of eyed eggs that later developed M74 (0.36–0.77 nmol/g) suggested in this study, three normally behaving females showed ovarian thiamine concentrations within or below (0.33–0.67 nmol/g) the

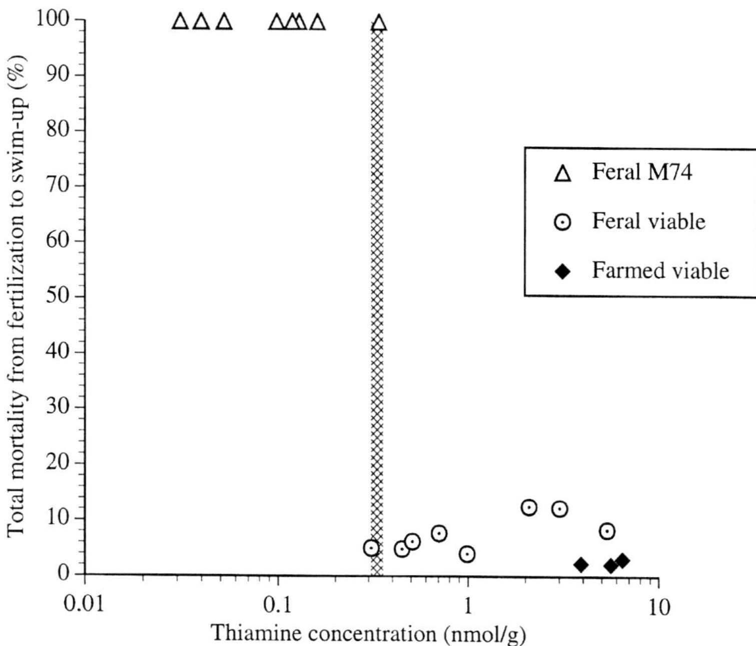

FIGURE 3.—Thiamine concentrations (nmol/g, wet weight) in yolk sac fry and mortality (%) from fertilization to swim-up in feral broodstock developing M74 (N = 8) and in feral (N = 8) and farmed viable (N = 3) broodstock. The shadowed area represents the suggested thiamine threshold limit interval of 0.31–0.34 nmol/g for development of M74 found in this study.

suggested threshold limit interval. Comparing thiamine concentrations of dissected ovaries with those of eyed eggs may be somewhat misleading because several factors may influence thiamine concentrations in ovaries and developing embryos, for example, the thiamine contents of ovarian follicle cells and connective tissues of the dissected ovaries may contribute to or reduce the ovarian thiamine concentration. In addition, during water hardening, as much as 25% (by weight) water may be incorporated into Baltic salmon eggs, subsequently causing a decline in thiamine concentration (Li et al. 1989). In rainbow trout *Oncorhynchus mykiss*, a natural reduction (<25%) of thiamine during development from fertilization to eyed egg has been shown (Sato et al. 1987), and in lake trout *Salvelinus namaycush*, a 50% reduction was observed between unfertilized eggs and swim-up fry (Brown et al. 1998). In view of these data, the probable outcome of the progeny of the three normally behaving females with the lowest ovarian thiamine concentrations (0.33–0.67 nmol/g) would be M74, because the loss of thiamine during embryo and yolk sac fry development may result in an acute thiamine deficiency.

If the etiology of M74, CS, and EMS is the same, a fair conformity in thiamine levels at comparable stages of development would be expected, especially for M74 and CS, because they affect the same species at the same developmental period, that is, during the yolk sac fry stage. In this study, a thiamine threshold limit interval of 0.36–0.77 nmol/g in eyed eggs of Baltic salmon was found. Fisher et al. (1996) showed that thiamine concentrations in unfertilized lake trout eggs of less than 0.77 nmol/g (<260 ng/g) were associated with increased mortality at swim-up, and Brown et al. (1998) found that unfertilized lake trout eggs with free thiamine concentrations of less than 0.8 nmol/g showed increased EMS mortality (67%). In Baltic salmon yolk sac fry developing M74, a thiamine threshold limit interval of 0.31–0.34 nmol/g was found in this study; Amcoff et al. (1998, this volume) suggested a threshold limit interval of 0.34–0.47 nmol/g in the same species. A slightly higher threshold limit interval of 0.37–0.69 nmol/g (124–234 ng/g) has been reported in Atlantic salmon yolk sac fry afflicted with CS (Fisher et al. 1996), and Brown et al. (1998) observed an increased EMS mortality (80%) in lake trout yolk sac fry containing thiamine diphosphate concentrations of less than 0.8 nmol/g (ww). The mean thiamine concentration in viable Baltic salmon yolk sac fry in this study was 1.7 nmol/g, which is very close to the mean thiamine concentration in viable Atlantic salmon yolk sac fry from Cayuga Lake (1.8 nmol/g [615 ng/g]; Fisher et al. 1996).

The relatively small variations in threshold limits between the different syndromes indicates similarities in susceptibility to low thiamine concentrations. Declines in thiamine content during the course of natural development have been recorded previously (Sato et al. 1987; Brown et al. 1998), suggesting that thiamine is required during embryo and yolk sac fry development in salmonids. In this study, a mean reduction in thiamine content (10–49%) between the eyed eggs and the yolk sac fry was observed in the feral family groups.

In EMS and CS, the associated low thiamine concentrations are hypothesized to be the result of extensive feeding on rainbow smelt *Osmerus mordax* or alewife *Alosa pseudoharengus* (Fisher et al. 1995a, 1995b, 1996; Fitzsimons 1995), both of which contain high concentrations of thiaminase, an enzyme that destroys thiamine and disrupts its coenzymatic activity (Gnaedinger 1964). Several of the salmonid species affected by EMS are, like their main prey, rainbow smelt and alewife, recent introductions to the Great Lakes area (Smith 1970; Leatherland 1993). However, the Baltic salmon and its most common prey, the clupeids Atlantic herring *Clupea harengus* and sprat *Sprattus sprattus*, are native Baltic species that have probably coexisted for several millennia. Sprat and herring also contain thiaminase (Suomalainen and Pihlgren 1955; Anglesea and Jackson 1985), but whether the thiaminase of these species has a negative effect on the thiamine status of the adult Baltic salmon is not yet known.

Another factor that might influence the thiamine status of the offspring is the female load of chloroorganics. Anthropogenic emissions of persistent organic compounds are widespread in the Baltic Sea (Bignert et al. 1995) as well as in several of the Great Lakes (Mac et al. 1993). In long-term feeding experiments with rats, DDT and PCBs gave rise to thiamine deficiency, implying a link between chloroorganic loading and metabolism of thiamine (Berdanier et al. 1975; Yagi et al. 1979). This thiamine deficiency may be a secondary effect of induced biotransformation systems such as the cytochrome P450 system (Pélissier et al. 1992). Elevated total hepatic cytochrome P450 levels have been observed in Baltic salmon females that produce M74-affected offspring compared with females that produce viable progeny (Norrgren et al. 1993). To clarify whether the cytochrome P450 system interacts with the thiamine in feral Baltic salmon, however, future investigations are necessary.

Despite the association we found between thiamine concentrations and M74, the cause of the M74 syndrome remains unknown. The finding that eggs with poor carotenoid pigmentation were associated with the development of M74 suggests an important role for the antioxidant astaxanthin during larval development (Börjeson and Norrgren 1997; Pettersson and Lignell 1998, this volume). Reduced concentrations of ubiquinone (vitamin Q) and α-tocopherol (vitamin E), also antioxidants, have been shown as well, further implicating a general oxidative stress situation in M74-affected individuals (Börjeson and Norrgren 1997).

The M74 syndrome may be the consequence of several deleterious factors in the Baltic salmon, such as loading of persistent organic compounds, free radical formation, induced biotransformation systems, and altered nutritional status. Nevertheless, the data presented here suggest that M74 may be a maternally transmitted thiamine deficiency. Additional studies of thiamine dynamics in different tissues of the adult fish and their progeny and of the interactions with contaminants are required to clarify the role and importance of thiamine in the development of M74.

Acknowledgments

This investigation was financed by grants from the FiRe group at the Swedish Environmental Protection Agency. The staff at the Heden and Västanå salmon hatcheries, Vattenfall AB, and at the rearing station of the National Board of Fisheries in Älvkarleby are acknowledged for providing data regarding wiggling broodfish and for assisting in the sampling of tissues for thiamine analysis.

References

Amcoff, P., H. Börjeson, R. Eriksson, and L. Norrgren. 1998. Effects of thiamine treatments on survival of M74-affected feral Baltic salmon. Pages 31–40 *in* McDonald et al. (1998).

Anglesea, J. D., and A. J. Jackson. 1985. Thiaminase activity in fish silage and moist fish feed. Animal Feed Science and Technology 13:39–46.

Berdanier, C. D., R. B. Tobin, R. C. Nielsen, M. A. Mehlman, and R. L. Veech. 1975. Effect of polychlorinated biphenyls and thiamine deficiency on liver metabolism in growing rats. Journal of Toxicology and Environmental Health 1:91–105.

Bignert, A., and five coauthors. 1995. Time-related factors influence the concentrations of sDDT, PCBs and shell parameters in eggs of Baltic guillemot, (*Uria aalge*) 1861–1989. Environmental Pollution 89:27–36.

Börjeson, H., and L. Norrgren. 1997. M74-syndrome: a review of potential etiological factors. Pages 153–166 *in* R. M. Rolland, M. Gilbertson, and R. E. Peterson, editors. Chemically induced alterations in functional development and reproduction in fishes. SETAC (Society of Environmental Toxicology and Chemistry), Pensacola, Florida.

Brown, S. B., J. D. Fitzsimons, V. P. Palace, and L. Vandenbyllaardt. 1998. Thiamine and early mortality syndrome in lake trout. Pages 18–25 *in* McDonald et al. (1998).

Fisher, J. P., J. D. Fitzsimons, G. F. Combs, Jr., and J. M. Spitsbergen. 1996. Naturally occurring thiamine deficiency causing reproductive failure in Finger Lakes Atlantic salmon and Great Lakes lake trout. Transactions of the American Fisheries Society 125:167–178.

Fisher, J. P., and six coauthors. 1995a. Reproductive failure of landlocked Atlantic salmon from New York's Finger Lakes: investigations into the etiology and epidemiology of the "Cayuga syndrome." Journal of Aquatic Animal Health 7:81–94.

Fisher, J. P., J. M. Spitsbergen, T. Iamonte, E. E. Little, and A. DeLonay. 1995b. Pathological and behavioral manifestations of the "Cayuga syndrome," a thiamine deficiency in larval landlocked Atlantic salmon. Journal of Aquatic Animal Health 7:269–283.

Fitzsimons, J. D. 1995. The effect of B-vitamins on a swim-up syndrome in Lake Ontario lake trout. Journal of Great Lakes Research 21(Supplement 1):286–289.

Fitzsimons, J. D., S. Huestis, and B. Williston. 1995. Occurrence of a swim-up syndrome in Lake Ontario lake trout in relation to contaminants and cultural practices. Journal of Great Lakes Research 21(Supplement 1):277–285.

Gnaedinger, R. H. 1964. Thiaminase activity in fish: an improved assay method. Fishery Industrial Research 2:55–59.

Leatherland, J. F. 1993. Field observations on reproductive and developmental dysfunction in introduced and native salmonids from the Great Lakes. Journal of Great Lakes Research 19:737–751.

Lehmitz, R., and L. Spannhof. 1977. Transketolase activity and thiamine deficiency in the kidney of rainbow trout (*Salmo gairdneri*) fed crude herring. Archiv fuer Tierernaehrung 27:287–295. (German; English summary.)

Li, X., E. Jenssen, and H. J. Fyhn. 1989. Effects of salinity on egg swelling in Atlantic salmon *Salmo salar*. Aquaculture 76:317–334.

Lundström, J., H. Börjeson, and L. Norrgren. 1998. Clinical and pathological studies of Baltic salmon suffering from yolk sac fry mortality. Pages 62–72 *in* McDonald et al. (1998).

Mac, M. J. 1988. Toxic substances and survival of Lake Michigan salmonids: field and laboratory approaches. Pages 389–401 *in* M. S. Evans, editor. Toxic contaminants and ecosystem health: a Great Lakes focus. Wiley, New York.

Mac, M. J., T. R. Schwartz, C. C. Edsall, and A. M. Frank. 1993. Polychlorinated biphenyls in Great Lakes lake trout and their eggs: relations to survival and congener composition 1979–1988. Journal of Great Lakes Research 19:752–765.

McDonald, G., J. D. Fitzsimons, and D. C. Honeyfield, editors. 1998. Early life stage mortality syndrome in fishes of the Great Lakes and Baltic Sea. American Fisheries Society, Symposium 21, Bethesda, Maryland.

Masumoto, T., R. W. Hardy, and E. Casillas. 1987. Comparison of transketolase activity and thiamine pyrophosphate levels in erythrocytes and liver of rainbow trout (*Salmo gairdneri*) as indicators of thiamine status. Journal of Nutrition 117:1422–1426.

Morito, C. L. H., D. H. Conrad, and J. W. Hilton. 1986. The thiamine deficiency signs and requirement of rainbow trout (*Salmo gairdneri*, Richardson). Fish Physiology and Biochemistry 1:93–104.

Norrgren, L., T. Andersson, P.-A. Bergqvist, and I. Björklund. 1993. Chemical, physiological and morphological studies of feral Baltic salmon (*Salmo salar*) suffering from abnormal fry mortality. Environmental Toxicology and Chemistry 12:2065–2075.

Pélissier, M.-A., and seven coauthors. 1992. Effect of prototypic polychlorinated biphenyls on hepatic and renal vitamin contents and on drug-metabolizing enzymes in rats fed diets containing low or high levels of retinyl palmitate. Food and Chemical Toxicology 30:723–729.

Pettersson, A., and Å. Lignell. 1998. Low astaxanthin levels in Baltic salmon exhibiting the M74 syndrome. Pages 26–30 *in* McDonald et al. (1998).

Roser, L., A. H. Andrist, W. H. Harrington, H. K. Naito, and D. Lonsdale. 1978. Determination of urinary thiamine by high-pressure liquid chromatography utilizing the thiochrome fluorescent method. Journal of Chromatography 146:43–53.

Sato, M., R. Yoshinaka, R. Kuroshima, H. Morimoto, and S. Ikeda. 1987. Changes in water soluble vitamin contents and transaminase activity of rainbow trout egg during development. Nippon Suisan Gakkaishi 53:795–799. (Japanese; English summary.)

Skea, J. C., J. Symula, and J. Miccoli. 1985. Separating starvation losses from other early feeding fry mortality in steelhead trout (*Salmo gairdneri*) chinook salmon (*Oncorhynchus tshawytscha*) and lake trout (*Salvelinus namaycush*). Bulletin of Environmental Contamination and Toxicology 35:82–91.

Smith, S. H. 1970. Species interactions of the alewife in the Great Lakes. Transactions of the American Fisheries Society 99:754–765.

Suomalainen, P., and A.-M. Pihlgren. 1955. On the thiaminase activity of fish and some other animals and on the preservation of thiaminase in silage made from fish. Acta Agralia Fennica 83:221–229.

Yagi, N., K. Kamohara, and Y. Itokawa. 1979. Thiamine deficiency induced by polychlorinated biphenyls (PCB) and dichlorodiphenyltrichloroethane (DDT) administration to rats. Journal of Environmental Pathology and Toxicology 2:1119–1125.

Zar, J. H., editor. 1984. Biostatistical analysis, second edition. Prentice-Hall, Inc., Englewood Cliffs, New Jersey.

American Fisheries Society Symposium 21:90–98, 1998

Thiamine Levels in Food Chains of the Great Lakes

JOHN D. FITZSIMONS
Department of Fisheries and Oceans, Bayfield Institute, 867 Lakeshore Road Burlington, Ontario L7R 4A6, Canada

SCOTT B. BROWN
Department of the Environment, 867 Lakeshore Road Burlington, Ontario L7R 4A6, Canada

LENORE VANDENBYLLAARDT
Department of Fisheries and Oceans, 501 University Crescent Winnipeg, Manitoba R3T 2N6, Canada

Abstract.—Thiamine concentrations in representative Great Lakes prey fish, including alewives *Alosa pseudoharengus*, rainbow smelt *Osmerus mordax*, slimy sculpin *Cottus cognatus*, bloater chub *Coregonus hoyi*, and lake herring *Coregonus artedi*, and their major dietary items, including mysids *Mysis relicta*, amphipods *Diporeia hoyi*, and net macroplankton, were measured to assess their potential involvement in depressed thiamine concentrations in lake trout *Salvelinus namaycush* of the Great Lakes. Mean thiamine concentrations in all biota were greater than the recommended dietary intake of 3.3 nmol/g for prevention of effects on growth, although the adequacy of these concentrations for reproduction is not known. Mean thiamine concentrations decreased in the order alewives > bloater chub, herring > smelt and differed from the order of associated egg thiamine concentrations published for lake trout feeding on these species (herring > alewives, smelt). As a result, these data strongly implicate the high thiaminase content, rather than the low thiamine content, of alewives and smelt as being responsible for the low egg thiamine concentrations of Great Lakes lake trout stocks that feed heavily on these species. Variations in thiamine content among prey species did not appear to be related to levels in their diet, because thiamine concentrations in *Mysis*, *Diporeia*, and macroplankton showed little consistency between group or between lake variation. There was no lake to lake variation in mean thiamine concentrations of prey species, but considerable within species variation occurred that was unrelated to size.

Recent studies have identified reduced thiamine concentrations in the eggs of some Great Lakes and inland lakes lake trout *Salvelinus namaycush* stocks that have been attributed to a possible thiaminase-rich diet (Fisher et al. 1996; Fitzsimons and Brown 1998, this volume). This thiaminase-rich diet consists of a high proportion of either alewives *Alosa pseudoharengus* or rainbow smelt *Osmerus mordax*, which contain high levels of thiaminase, in contrast to native species such as lake herring *Coregonus artedi* and slimy sculpin *Cottus cognatus*, which contain low levels of thiaminase (Deutsch and Hasler 1943; Nielands 1947; Gnaedinger 1964; Gnaedinger and Krzeczkowski 1966; Ji and Adelman 1998, this volume). Depressed egg thiamine concentrations in lake trout are of concern because concentrations below a threshold of 0.8 nmol/g (Brown et al. 1998a, this volume) are associated with a marked increase in a thiamine-responsive swim-up mortality called early mortality syndrome (EMS; Fitzsimons 1995; Fitzsimons et al. 1995; Fisher et al. 1996). The lower reproductive efficiency associated with EMS threatens lake trout restoration in the Great Lakes.

Reduced egg thiamine concentrations occur in lake trout from Lakes Ontario, Erie, Huron, and Michigan, where diets are composed almost entirely of either alewives or smelt (Madenjian et al. 1998; Rand and Stewart, in press; F. Cornelius, New York Department of Environmental Conservation [NYDEC], personal communication; J. Johnson, Michigan Department of Natural Resources, personal communication). In contrast, in Lake Superior, where the summer diet of nearshore lake trout is only 24% smelt and the remainder lake herring (58%) and other species (18%; M. Gallinat, Red Cliff Band of Lake Superior Chippewa Indians, personal communication), egg thiamine levels are 5 to 10 times higher and similar (Fitzsimons and Brown 1998) to those of offshore siscowet lake trout, whose diet is composed almost entirely of lake herring and no smelt (Fisher and Swanson 1996).

Several observations reveal that, despite the association between a thiaminase-rich diet and reduced thiamine concentrations in the eggs of lake trout and other salmonids (Marcquenski and Brown 1997; Hornung et al. 1998, this volume), other factors may

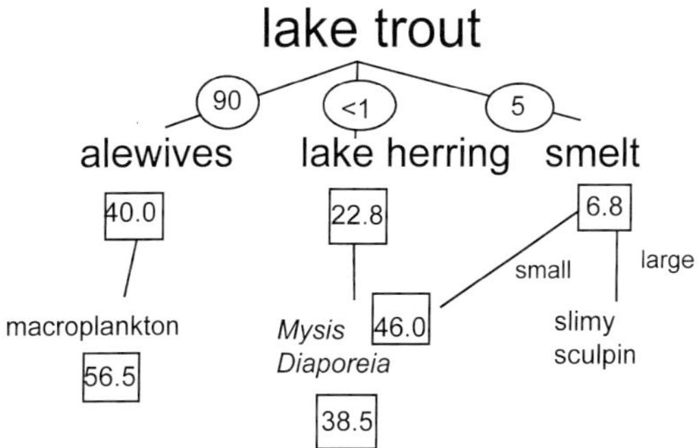

FIGURE 1.—Food web for Lake Ontario. Numbers in ovals indicate proportion of that prey item in the diet of lake trout. Numbers in squares indicate thiamine content on a dry weight basis.

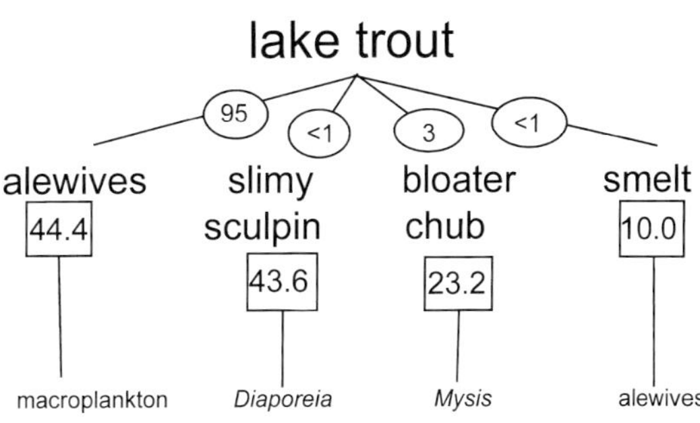

FIGURE 2.—Food web for Lake Michigan. Numbers in ovals indicate proportion of that prey item in the diet of lake trout. Numbers in squares indicate thiamine content on a dry weight basis.

also be involved. Acting alone or in concert with the thiaminase-rich diet, these other factors may reduce egg thiamine concentrations below a threshold level. For example, coho salmon *Oncorhynchus kisutch* have fed continuously and almost exclusively on alewives in Lake Michigan from 1960 to 1995 (Jude et al. 1987; M. Keniry, Wisconsin Department of Natural Resources, personal communication). Only in 1966 and 1989–1994, however, did epizootics of EMS occur in this species, the last of which was determined to be thiamine responsive based on the reversal of clinical signs with thiamine baths (Hornung et al. 1998). Lake Michigan lake trout experienced EMS in 1979–1981. Based on clinical signs (Fitzsimons et al. 1995; Fisher et al. 1996), this EMS was nearly identical to a thiamine-responsive early mortality syndrome described in lake trout from Lake Ontario (Mac and Edsall 1991; Fitzsimons 1995). In Lake Ontario, EMS occurred in 80% of females evaluated in 1990–1991, causing almost 50% mortality of swim-up fry, whereas in 1976–1981 only 5% mortality occurred (Symula et al. 1989; H. Simonin, NYDEC, personal communication). Wide fluctuations in the occurrence of thiamine-responsive EMS during times when the proportion of thiaminase-rich alewives in the diet remained constant, coupled with the relationship between egg thiamine concentration and EMS mortality, suggest a possible time-dependent change in the availability of thiamine to predators. Conceivably, dietary changes during periods of thiamine deposition to the egg, shifts in the thiamine or thiaminase content of individual prey (Ji and Adelman 1998), or changes in the amount of thiamine transferred up the food chain could explain these observations.

Thus, we provide documentation of thiamine concentrations at various trophic levels in Great Lakes food chains (see Figures 1 and 2) that lead to lake trout and Pacific salmon *Oncorhynchus* sp. and assess the adequacy of these species' thiamine levels in preventing thiamine deficiency. Moreover, we evaluate the relationship between lake to lake variation in lake trout egg thiamine concentrations and thiamine concentrations in their prey.

Methods

Collection Methods

Alewives, rainbow smelt, and lake herring were collected from offshore areas of eastern Lake Ontario, and alewives, bloater chub *Coregonus hoyi*, rainbow smelt, and slimy sculpin were collected from offshore areas of western Lake Michigan (Table 1, Figure 3). Within 30 min of capture, live individuals were frozen (−20°C) until the time of analysis. By quick freezing whole fish and sampling only the epaxial musculature, we assumed that the influence of the thiaminase in smelt and alewives on their thiamine content would be minimized (Brown et al. 1998b, this volume). Ji and Adelman (1998) reported that thiaminase activity in smelt and alewives was 6 to 10 times higher in the viscera than in the remaining carcass. Losses of thiamine from alewives, which we infer represent thiaminase activity, are also affected by temperature, because losses of thiamine declined to zero at subzero temperatures (Brown et al. 1998b).

Samples of *Mysis relicta*, *Diporeia hoyi*, and microcrustacean zooplankton were collected using the methods described by Kiriluk et al. (1995) from offshore zones of Lakes Superior, Huron, Erie, and

TABLE 1.—Summary of sample locations, dates, and collection methods for samples collected for thiamine analysis in the Great Lakes. See Figure 3 for precise geographic locations within specific lakes.

Lake	Sample	Location	Date	Collection method
Ontario	Alewife	Main Duck Island	8 August 1995	Trawl
	Lake herring	Main Duck Island	3 April 1995	Trawl
	Rainbow smelt	Main Duck Island	28 and 30 August 1995	Trawl
	Mysis	Cobourg	9 September 1994	Epibenthic sled
	Diporeia	Cobourg	9 September 1994	Epibenthic sled
	Macroplankton	Cobourg	9 September 1994	Plankton net
Erie	*Diporeia*	Port Dover	17 August 1992	Epibenthic sled
	Macroplankton	Pelee Island	21 June 1994	Plankton net
Huron	*Mysis*	Goderich	2 July 1992	Epibenthic sled
	Diporeia	Goderich	2 July 1992	Epibenthic sled
	Macroplankton	Goderich	2 July 1992	Plankton net
Michigan	Alewife	Waukegan	7 October 1995	Trawl
	Bloater chub	Waukegan	7 October 1995	Trawl
	Rainbow smelt	Waukegan	7 October 1995	Trawl
	Slimy sculpin	Waukegan	7 October 1995	Trawl
Superior	*Mysis*	Whitefish Bay	17 June 1992	Epibenthic sled
	Diporeia	Whitefish Bay	17 June 1992	Epibenthic sled
	Macroplankton	Whitefish Bay	17 June 1992	Plankton net

Ontario (Table 1, Figure 3). Briefly, samples of *Mysis* and *Diporeia* were collected with an epibenthic sled, separated immediately after sled retrieval, and stored in ointment tins on dry ice until transfer to a freezer and then stored at −80°C until analysis for thiamine. Zooplankton was collected with surface (approximately 1-m depth) hauls of plankton nets (153 μm), filtered with a weak vacuum to remove water, transferred to ointment tins, and stored at −80°C.

Thiamine Analysis

For fish, frozen subsamples were removed from the epaxial musculature posterior to the operculum just before analysis using the methods described by Brown et al. (1998b). All data were corrected for recoveries of each of the three forms: free thiamine, thiamine monophosphate, and thiamine pyrophosphate. Weights (to the nearest 0.1 g) and total lengths (to the nearest millimeter) were measured for all fish. Invertebrates were subsampled as whole organisms of approximately 0.5 g total weight while frozen and analyzed for thiamine as described above.

Statistics

Thiamine concentrations in fish were compared using either *t*-tests or analysis of variance with Student–Newman–Keuls' multiple-range test ($P <$ 0.05; Snedecor and Cochran 1967). To account for heteroscedasticity, data were logarithmically transformed before statistical analysis. The relationship between thiamine concentration and fish weight was estimated using linear regression ($\alpha < 0.05$).

Results

Fish

Total thiamine concentrations exhibited considerable between species variation but no significant within species or within subgenus variation (Table 2). The mean thiamine concentration in alewives from Lake Michigan (11.1 ± 1.3 nmol/g) did not differ ($t = -0.35$, $P = 0.73$) from that in alewives from Lake Ontario (10.0 ± 1.0 nmol/g), nor did mean concentration of thiamine in smelt from Lake Michigan (2.5 ± 0.4 nmol/g) differ ($t = 1.55$, $P = 0.14$) from that in smelt from Lake Ontario (1.7 ± 0.3 nmol/g). Similarly, the mean concentration of thiamine in bloater chub from Lake Michigan (5.8 ± 0.6 nmol/g) did not differ ($t = 0.11$, $P = 0.92$) from that in lake herring from Lake Ontario (5.7 ± 0.7 ng/g). Within Lake Michigan, mean thiamine concentrations in alewives and slimy sculpin (10.9 ± 1.0 ng/g), although not different ($t = 0.08$, $P = 0.91$) from each other, were higher ($F = 16.3$, $P < 0.0001$) than the mean concentration in bloater chub, which in turn was higher ($t = 4.47$, $P = 0.003$) than the mean

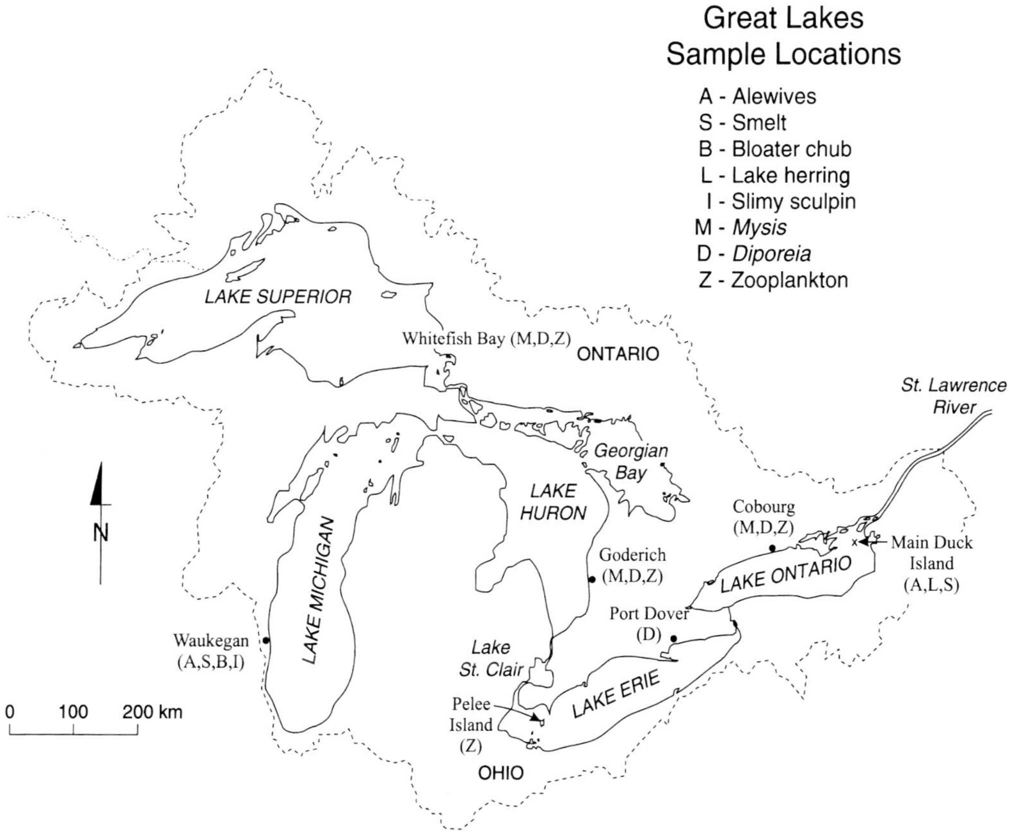

FIGURE 3.—Map of the Laurentian Great Lakes showing the locations of fish and invertebrate samples collected for thiamine analysis. The dotted line shows the limit of the Great Lakes drainage basin.

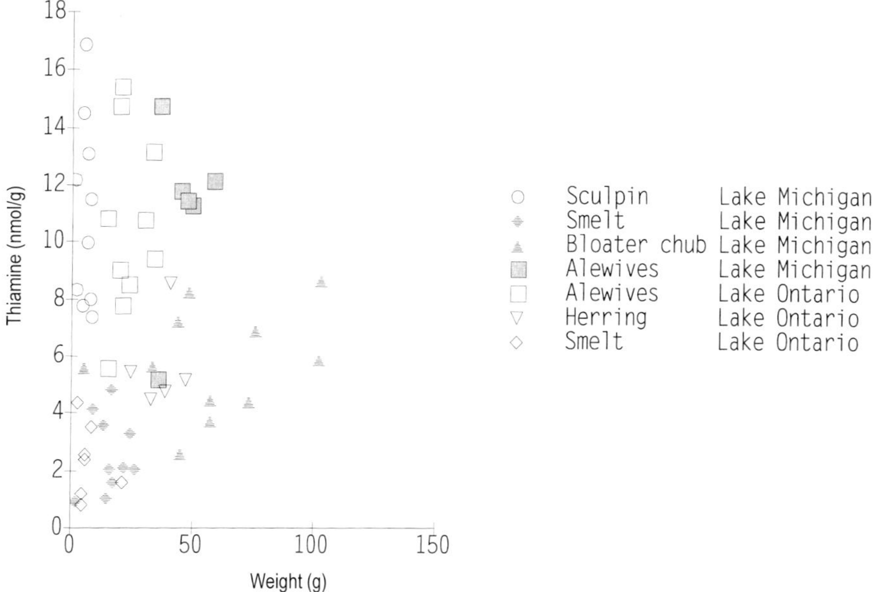

FIGURE 4.—Relationship between weight and thiamine concentration for prey fish from Lakes Ontario and Michigan. Open symbols are for Lake Ontario and closed symbols are for Lake Michigan.

TABLE 2.—Summary of lengths, weights, and concentrations of thiamine pyrophosphate (TPP), thiamine monophosphate (TMP), free thiamine (Free T), and total thiamine in prey fish from Lakes Ontario and Michigan. Values shown are means ± SE (*N*). Total thiamine concentrations are also provided on a dry weight basis using the dry to wet weight ratio of 0.25 to aid in comparison with the reported dietary requirement.

Lake	Species	Mean length (mm)	Mean wet weight (g)	TPP (nmol/g)	TMP (nmol/g)	Free T (nmol/g)	Total thiamine (nmol/g)	Total thiamine (dry weight)
Ontario	Alewife	15.2 ± 0.6 (6)	23.1 ± 2.0 (11)	7.0 ± 0.7 (11)	2.7 ± 0.4 (11)	0.2 ± 0.0 (11)	10.0 ± 1.0 (11)	40.0
	Rainbow smelt	16.3 ± 0.6 (5)	18.0 ± 4.2 (12)	1.3 ± 0.3 (13)	0.3 ± 0.0 (13)	0.1 ± 0.0 (13)	1.7 ± 0.3 (13)	6.8
	Lake herring	16.1 ± 0.6 (5)	36.6 ± 3.8 (5)	3.9 ± 0.4 (5)	1.6 ± 0.3 (5)	0.2 ± 0.1 (5)	5.7 ± 0.7 (5)	22.8
Michigan	Alewife	15.2 ± 0.6 (6)	44.8 ± 3.5 (6)	7.3 ± 1.0 (6)	3.4 ± 0.4 (6)	0.3 ± 0.0 (6)	11.1 ± 1.3 (6)	44.4
	Rainbow smelt	13.3 ± 0.5 (10)	16.2 ± 2.3 (10)	1.9 ± 0.3 (10)	0.5 ± 0.1 (10)	0.1 ± 0.0 (10)	2.5 ± 0.4 (10)	10.0
	Bloater chub		58.4 ± 8.7 (11)	2.9 ± 0.4 (11)	2.3 ± 0.2 (11)	0.6 ± 0.1 (11)	5.8 ± 0.6 (11)	23.2
	Slimy sculpin	6.1 ± 0.7 (5)	5.2 ± 0.8 (10)	5.7 ± 0.6 (10)	3.7 ± 0.3 (10)	1.5 ± 0.1 (10)	10.9 ± 0.1 (10)	43.6

concentration in smelt. In a similar manner, the mean concentration of thiamine in alewives from Lake Ontario was higher ($t = 3.19$, $P = 0.007$) than that in lake herring, which was in turn higher ($t = 5.83$, $P = 0.0001$) than the mean concentration in smelt from this lake. Although variations in the thiamine content of individual species within a location existed, none could be attributed to length or weight (Figure 4).

Invertebrates

Mean thiamine concentrations for *Mysis*, *Diporeia*, and zooplankton of 8.1 ± 0.6, 5.9 ± 0.7, and 6.1 ± 1.3 nmol/g (Tables 3 and 4) across all lakes sampled were similar to each other and were intermediate to those observed in fish. No obvious between lake or between group variation occurred in either total thiamine concentration or predominance of one of the three forms of thiamine. We were limited, however, by the preliminary nature of the analyses, which involved only a single sample per lake per group.

Discussion

Thiamine concentrations in all fish and invertebrates appear adequate to support the growth of trout based on nutritionally balanced test diets. Morito et al. (1986) reported a dietary requirement of 3.3 nmol/g dry weight for trout. Although this was only about one-tenth of the requirement (33–40 nmol/g) cited by Halver (1989), his recommendation was based on the work of Phillips et al. (1945), who used fluke-infested beef liver as the major component of the thiamine-deficient test diet. Using dry to wet

TABLE 3.—Summary of concentrations (nmol/g) of thiamine pyrophosphate (TPP), thiamine monophosphate (TMP), free thiamine (Free T), and total thiamine in *Mysis*, *Diporeia*, and macroplankton from the Great Lakes. Results represent a single sample. Total thiamine concentrations are also provided on a dry weight basis using the dry to wet weight ratios of 0.161, 0.143, and 0.138 for *Mysis* , *Diporeia*, and macroplankton to aid in comparison with the reported dietary requirement.

Lake	Sample	TPP	TMP	Free T	Total thiamine	Total thiamine (dry weight)
Ontario	*Mysis*	3.7	3.3	0.4	7.4	46.0
	Diporeia	3.5	1.5	0.5	5.5	38.5
	Macroplankton	2.4	2.5	2.9	7.8	56.5
Erie	*Diporeia*	5.6	1.9	0.4	7.9	5.2
	Macroplankton	1.5	1.7	3.1	6.3	45.7
Huron	*Mysis*	5.3	4.3	0.3	9.9	61.5
	Diporeia	3.4	1.5	0.5	5.3	37.1
	Macroplankton	2.9	4.4	0.7	8.0	58.0
Superior	*Mysis*	5.2	2.8	0.3	8.3	51.6
	Diporeia	3.3	0.6	0.7	4.6	32.2
	Macroplankton	0.4	1.4	0.4	2.3	16.7

TABLE 4.—Summary of mean concentrations (nmol/g) of thiamine pyrophosphate (TPP), thiamine monophosphate (TMP), free thiamine (Free T), and total thiamine in *Mysis*, *Diporeia*, and macroplankton in the Great Lakes based on Lakes Ontario, Erie, Huron, and Superior. Values shown are means ± SE (*N*). Total thiamine concentrations are also provided on a dry weight basis using the dry to wet weight ratios of 0.161, 0.143, and 0.138 for *Mysis*, *Diaporeia*, and macroplankton to aid in comparison with the reported dietary requirement.

Sample	TPP	TMP	Free T	Total thiamine	Total thiamine (dry weight)
Mysis	4.0 ± 0.8 (3)	3.4 ± 0.3 (3)	0.8 ± 0.4 (3)	8.1 ± 0.6 (3)	50.3
Diaporeia	4.0 ± 0.6 (4)	1.4 ± 0.3 (4)	0.5 ± 0.1 (4)	5.9 ± 0.7 (4)	41.3
Macroplankton	1.8 ± 0.5 (4)	2.5 ± 0.7 (4)	1.8 ± 0.7 (4)	6.1 ± 1.3 (4)	44.2

weight ratios of 0.25 for fish (Borgmann and Whittle 1983) and 0.161 for *Mysis*, 0.143 for *Diporeia*, and 0.138 for zooplankton (Borgmann and Whittle 1994), total thiamine levels on a dry weight basis observed in this study (see Tables 1–3) were all above the 3 nmol/g limit. Therefore, if growth requirements are an adequate predictor of thiamine needs, the reduced thiamine levels documented by Fitzsimons and Brown (1998) for Great Lakes lake trout cannot be attributed to an inadequate supply of thiamine in their diet.

We do not know, however, if the dietary requirement for thiamine is higher for reproduction than for growth. With ascorbic acid, also a water-soluble vitamin, Blom and Dabrowski (1995) reported that the National Research Council's recommended dietary level of 50 mg of ascorbic acid per kilogram of diet for rainbow trout *Oncorhynchus mykiss*, established on the basis of juvenile growth, was inadequate for broodstock fish. To optimize tissue ascorbic acid levels and achieve maximum reproductive success, values eight times this established norm were necessary (Blom and Dabrowski 1995). Thiamine deficiencies documented in eggs of lake trout from Lake Erie and Atlantic salmon *Salmo salar* from the Finger Lakes of New York State (Fisher et al. 1996) appear to occur without any pronounced effect on adult growth (Cornelius et al. 1995; J. Fisher, University of Connecticut, personal communication). This suggests that reproduction may require more thiamine than growth, although the extent of this difference is unknown. This requirement may increase during oogenesis, especially given that the turnover time in lake trout appears relatively short (estimated at 40 d; Ji et al. 1998, this volume).

Regardless of what the requirement for reproduction is, thiamine levels in alewives, on the basis of muscle levels, are at least as adequate as levels in bloater chub and lake herring, whereas levels in smelt may be less than adequate. Superficially, alewives, on the basis of muscle thiamine concentrations, appear to be a better source of thiamine for predators such as lake trout than either native coregonids or the exotic smelt. However, this was not reflected in the egg thiamine content of lake trout that fed on alewives (Fitzsimons and Brown 1998). Nearshore Lake Superior lake trout have a diet of 58% lake herring and 24% smelt, so it would be expected, on the basis of prey thiamine content, that their egg concentrations would be intermediate between those of lake trout that fed exclusively on alewives and those of lake trout that feed on smelt that exhibited the highest and lowest thiamine concentrations. On the contrary, thiamine concentrations in the eggs of nearshore Lake Superior lake trout were 4.7–8.8 times higher than those in the eggs of lake trout from Lakes Michigan and Ontario, where lake trout fed almost exclusively on alewives. Similarly, compared with concentrations in Lakes Huron and Erie, where lake trout fed almost exclusively on smelt, egg thiamine concentrations in nearshore Lake Superior lake trout were 4.4–7.3 times higher. Fitzsimons and Brown (1998) found that egg thiamine concentrations in Lakes Ontario and Michigan lake trout did not differ from those in lake trout from Lakes Huron and Erie.

The fact that thiamine levels in lake trout that fed almost exclusively on smelt or alewives were low implicates the high but similar thiaminase content of these two species (Ji and Adelman 1998) as a possible determining factor. Ji and Adelman (1998) and others (Krampitz and Wooley 1944; Melnick et al. 1945) reported the almost complete destruction of large quantities of naturally occurring and supplementary thiamine in periods as short as 30 min. This is well within the gut passage times for most fish species (Karpevitch and Bokoff 1937). The coldwater habitat of the lake trout is unlikely to significantly reduce the activity of thiaminase, based on the fact that Krampitz and Wooley (1944) found only a 50% difference in the amount of thiamine destroyed in a given time at temperatures of 0 and 37°C. In addition, the low end of the pH range for thiaminase activity (pH 3–7; Deolalkar and Sohonie 1954; Anglesea and Jackson 1985) is similar to that of the teleost stomach (Vonk and Mennega 1938; Vonk 1939), indicating that thiaminase would be active in the gut. Consumption of either smelt or alewives could also affect thiamine assimilation from other species, even if their thiaminase content is low. Bloater chub and alewives can at certain times of the year occur at the same water depth, so that they could also occur in the gut of a predator at the same time (M. Holey, U.S. Fish and Wildlife Service, personal communication). Hence, the thiaminase content of an ingested alewife, in addition to affecting the availability of its thiamine content to a predator, could also affect the thiamine availability from a bloater chub ingested at the same time.

Based on Lakes Ontario and Michigan, there is no evidence of between lake, within species, or within genus variation in mean thiamine concentrations for alewives, coregonids, and smelt. Whether this represents similarities in the diets, the physiological requirements for thiamine, or a combination of these two factors is not known. Diets of alewives and smelt in Lakes Ontario and Michigan are quite similar (see Figures 1 and 2; Foltz and Norden 1977; Janssen and Brandt 1980; Kiriluk et al. 1995). Given the similarity across lakes and within genera, it seems unlikely that the five- to eightfold higher thiamine levels in lake trout eggs from Lake Superior compared with the other Great Lakes (Fitzsimons and Brown 1998) are the result of anomalously high thiamine levels in the lake herring of Lake Superior, a major part of the diet of lake trout in this lake.

Differences in mean thiamine concentrations among species, which are unrelated to size, also appeared to be independent of the thiamine concentration in their diets, even though thiamine is an essential nutrient (Halver 1989). In Lake Ontario, alewives are largely planktivorous (Kiriluk et al. 1995; see Figures 1 and 2), whereas lake herring, based on data from Lake Superior, would likely feed on *Mysis* and *Diporeia* (Dryer and Beil 1964). Small smelt feed on *Mysis* and *Diporeia* (Scott and Crossman 1973), whereas larger smelt appear to become increasingly piscivorous, feeding on slimy sculpin in Lake Ontario (Brandt and Madon 1986; Kiriluk et al. 1995). The two- to sixfold difference in thiamine concentrations among these three fish in Lake Ontario, however, is not reflected in the levels in zooplankton, *Mysis*, and *Diporeia*. Moreover, the transition to piscivory in older smelt should tend to increase thiamine concentrations because, in Lake Michigan, sculpin had the highest thiamine concentrations after alewives, and so a diet of sculpin should increase thiamine levels in a predator. Similarly, in Lake Michigan, the order of thiamine concentrations in fish (alewives, slimy sculpin > bloater chub > smelt) also does not correspond to the thiamine concentrations in their major dietary items; alewives feed on zooplankton (Janssen and Brandt 1980), slimy sculpin feed on *Diporeia* (Kraft and Kitchell 1986), and bloater chub feed on *Mysis* and *Diporeia* (Wells and Beeton 1963). Smelt in Lake Michigan also feed on *Mysis* and *Diporeia* while young but become increasingly piscivorous when their length exceeds 180 mm, at which point their consumption of young-of-the-year alewives is three times that of smaller smelt (Foltz and Norden 1977). Given that the average length of smelt in this study was 130 mm, it would be expected that their thiamine levels would be intermediate to those of bloater chub and alewives. Instead, average thiamine levels were less than in either species, possibly indicating, because of the high thiaminase content of alewives (Ji and Adelman 1998), a negative effect of alewife consumption on thiamine levels in Lake Michigan smelt. The twofold higher thiamine concentrations in sculpin compared with bloater chub from Lake Michigan also cannot be explained on the basis of diet. One would expect that the diversification of the diet from one wholly dependent on *Diporeia*, as is the case for sculpin, to one constituted of *Diporeia* and *Mysis*, which is characteristic of bloater chub, would increase thiamine concentration. Average thiamine concentrations in *Mysis* were 1.5 times higher than in *Diporeia*.

We conclude that thiamine levels in prey fish should be adequate to prevent effects on growth, whereas the adequacy of these levels to support normal reproductive processes is unknown. Although we documented species differences in amounts of thiamine, the patterns observed differed from published lake trout egg thiamine levels and corresponding diets, leading us to hypothesize that thiaminase content, rather than thiamine content, may be an important factor in determining the thiamine content of a predator's eggs. It follows then that variation in the thiaminase content of prey could be as important as variation in the thiamine content in explaining variability in the occurrence of thiamine-responsive EMS. Although Niimi et al. (1997) provided some preliminary data on thiamine levels in Lake Ontario food chains, the data presented here provide the first comprehensive analysis of thiamine levels in Great Lakes prey fish and invertebrates using modern analytical methods. For this reason, it is not possible to determine if levels have changed over time. Consequently, the involvement of thiamine in the previously reported epizootics of early mortality syndromes remains unknown. Our results will provide valuable baseline data against which to assess any future changes.

Acknowledgments

We thank Rick Kiriluk, Mike Whittle, Mike Keir, Dawn Walsh, Ralph Stedman, Chuck Bronte, Gary Cholwek, and Floyd Cornelius, who contributed samples for this study. We also thank Mike Hornung, Arthur Niimi, and an anonymous reviewer, who reviewed the manuscript and provided valuable comments.

References

Anglesea, J. D., and A. J. Jackson. 1985. Thiaminase activity in fish silage and moist fish feed. Animal Feed Science and Technology 13:39–46.

Blom, J. H., and K. Dabrowski. 1995. Reproductive success of female rainbow trout (*Oncorhynchus mykiss*) in response to graded dietary ascorbyl monophosphate levels. Biology of Reproduction 52:1073–1080.

Borgmann, U., and D. M. Whittle. 1983. Particle-size conversion efficiency and contaminant concentrations in Lake Ontario biota. Canadian Journal of Fisheries and Aquatic Sciences 40:328–336.

Borgmann, U., and D. M. Whittle. 1994. Particle-size-conversion efficiency, invertebrate production, and potential fish production in Lake Ontario. Canadian Journal of Fisheries and Aquatic Sciences 51:693–700.

Brandt, S. B., and S. P. Madon. 1986. Rainbow smelt (*Osmerus mordax*) predation on slimy sculpin (*Cottus cognatus*) in Lake Ontario. Journal of Great Lakes Research 12:322–325.

Brown , S. B., J. D. Fitzsimons, V. P. Palace, and L. Vandenbyllaardt. 1998a. Thiamine and early mortality syndrome in lake trout. Pages 18–25 *in* McDonald et al. (1998).

Brown, S. B., D. C. Honeyfield, and L. Vandenbyllaardt. 1998b. Thiamine analysis in fish tissues. Pages 73–81 *in* McDonald et al. (1998).

Cornelius, F. C., K. M. Muth, and R. Kenyon. 1995. Lake trout rehabilitation in Lake Erie: a case history. Journal of Great Lakes Research 21(Supplement 1):65–82.

Deolalkar, S. T., and K. Sohonie. 1954. Thiaminase from fresh-water, brackish-water and salt-water fish. Nature 4402:489–490.

Deutsch, H. F., and A. D. Hasler. 1943. Distribution of a vitamin B_1 destructive enzyme in fish. Proceedings of the Society for Experimental Biology and Medicine 53:63–65.

Dryer, W. R., and J. Beil. 1964. Life history of the lake herring in Lake Superior. U.S. Fish and Wildlife Service Fishery Bulletin 63:493–530.

Fisher, J. P., J. D. Fitzsimons, G. F. Combs, Jr., and J. M. Spitsbergen. 1996. Naturally occurring thiamine deficiency causing reproductive failure in Finger Lakes Atlantic salmon and Great Lakes lake trout. Transactions of the American Fisheries Society 125:167–178.

Fisher, S. J., and B. L. Swanson. 1996. Diets of siscowet lake trout from the Apostle Islands region of Lake Superior, 1993. Journal of Great Lakes Research 22 (Supplement 2):463–468.

Fitzsimons, J. D. 1995. The effect of B-vitamins on a swim-up syndrome in Lake Ontario lake trout. Journal of Great Lakes Research 21 (Supplement 1):286–289.

Fitzsimons, J. D., and S. B. Brown. 1998. Reduced egg thiamine levels in inland and Great Lakes lake trout and their relationship with diet. Pages 160–171 *in* McDonald et al. (1998).

Fitzsimons, J. D., S. Huestis, and B. Williston. 1995. Occurrence of a swim-up syndrome in Lake Ontario lake trout in relation to contaminants and cultural practices. Journal of Great Lakes Research 21(Supplement 1):277–285.

Foltz, J. W., and C. R. Norden. 1977. Food habits and feeding chronology of rainbow smelt , *Osmerus mordax*, in Lake Michigan. U.S. National Marine Fisheries Service Fishery Bulletin 75:637–640.

Gnaedinger, R. H. 1964. Thiaminase activity in fish: an improved assay method. Fishery Industrial Research 2:55–59.

Gnaedinger, R. H., and R. A. Krzeczkowski. 1966. Heat inactivation of thiaminase in whole fish. Commercial Fisheries Review 28(8):11–14.

Halver, J. E. 1989. The vitamins. Pages 37–43 *in* Fish nutrition, second edition. Academic Press, Toronto

Hornung, M. W., L. Miller, R. E. Peterson, S. Marcquenski, and S. B. Brown. 1998. Efficacy of thiamine, astaxanthin, β-carotene, and thyroxine treatments in reducing early mortality syndrome in Lake Michigan salmonid embryos. Pages 124–134 *in* McDonald et al. (1998).

Janssen, J., and S. B. Brandt. 1980. Feeding ecology and vertical migration of adult alewives (*Alosa pseudoharengus*) in Lake Michigan. Canadian Journal of Fisheries and Aquatic Sciences 37:177–184.

Ji, Y. Q., and I. R. Adelman. 1998. Thiaminase activity in alewives and smelt in Lakes Huron, Michigan, and Superior. Pages 154–159 *in* McDonald et al. (1998).

Ji, Y. Q., J. J. Warthesen, and I. R. Adelman. 1998. Thiamine nutrition, synthesis, and retention in relation to lake trout reproduction in the Great Lakes. Pages 99–111 *in* McDonald et al. (1998).

Jude, D. J., F. J. Tesar, S. F. Deboe, and T. J. Miller. 1987. Diet and selection of major prey species by Lake Michigan salmonines, 1973–1982. Transactions of the American Fisheries Society 116:677–691.

Karpevitch, A., and E. Bokoff. 1937. The rate of digestion in marine fishes. Zoologicheskii Zhurnal 16:28–44. (Russian; English summary.)

Kiriluk, R. M., M. R. Servos, D. M. Whittle, G. Cabana, and J. Rasmussen. 1995. Using ratios of stable nitrogen and carbon isotopes to characterize the biomagnification of DDE, mirex, and PCB in a Lake Ontario pelagic food web. Canadian Journal of Fisheries and Aquatic Sciences 52:2660–2674.

Kraft, C. E., and J. F. Kitchell. 1986. Partitioning of food resources by sculpins in Lake Michigan. Environmental Biology of Fishes 16:309–316.

Krampitz, L. O., and D. W. Wooley. 1944. The manner of inactivation of thiamine by fish tissue. Journal of Biological Chemistry 152:9–17.

Mac, M. J., and C. C. Edsall. 1991. Environmental contaminants and the reproductive success of lake trout in the Great Lakes: an epidemiological approach. Journal of Toxicology and Environmental Health 33:375–394.

Madenjian, C. P., T. J. DeSourcie, and R. M. Stedman. 1998. Ontogenetic and spatial patterns in diet and growth of lake trout in Lake Michigan. Transactions of the American Fisheries Society 127:236–252.

Marcquenski, S. V., and S. B. Brown 1997. Early mortality syndromes in the Great Lakes. Pages 135–152 *in* R. M. Rolland, M. Gilbertson, and R. E. Peterson, editors. Chemically induced alterations in functional development and reproduction in fishes. SETAC (Society of Environmental Toxicology and Chemistry), Pensacola, Florida.

McDonald, G., J. D. Fitzsimons, and D. C. Honeyfield, editors. 1998. Early life stage mortality syndrome in fishes of the Great Lakes and Baltic Sea. American Fisheries Society, Symposium 21, Bethesda, Maryland.

Melnick, D., M. Hochberg, and B. L. Oser. 1945. Physiological availability of the vitamins. II. The effect of dietary thiaminase in fish products. Journal of Nutrition 30:81–88.

Morito, C. L. H., D. H. Conrad, and J. W. Hilton. 1986. The thiamine deficiency signs and requirement of rainbow trout (*Salmo gairdneri*, Richardson). Fish Physiology and Biochemistry 1:93–104.

Nielands, J. B. 1947. Thiaminase in aquatic animals of Nova Scotia. Journal of the Fisheries Research Board of Canada 7:94–99.

Niimi, A. J., C. C. Jackson, and J. D. Fitzsimons. 1997. Thiamine dynamics in aquatic ecosystems and its biological implications. Internationale Revue der gesamten Hydrobiologie 1:47–56.

Phillips, A. M., Jr., and seven coauthors. 1945. The nutrition of the trout. Fishery Research Bulletin 7, New York State Conservation Department, Albany.

Rand, P. S., and D. J. Stewart. In press. Dynamics of salmonine diets and foraging in Lake Ontario 1983–1993: a test of a bioenergetic model prediction. Canadian Journal of Fisheries and Aquatic Sciences.

Scott, W. B., and E. J. Crossman. 1973. Freshwater fishes of Canada. Bulletin of the Fisheries Research Board of Canada 184.

Snedecor, G. W., and W. G. Cochran. 1967. Statistical methods. Iowa State University Press, Ames.

Symula, J., and six coauthors. 1989. Blue-sac disease in Lake Ontario lake trout. Journal of Great Lakes Research 16:41–52.

Vonk, H. J. 1939. Die biologische bedeutung des pH-optimums der verdauungsenzyme bei den vertebraten. Ergebnisse der Enzymforschung 8:55–56.

Vonk, H. J., and A. M. W. Mennega. 1938. Das pH-optimum des pepsins und der pH des magenin-haltes. Acta Brevia Neerlander Physiology and Pharmacology 8:27–28.

Wells, L., and A. M. Beeton. 1963. Food of the bloater, *Coregonus hoyi*, in Lake Michigan. Transactions of the American Fisheries Society 92:245–255.

American Fisheries Society Symposium 21:99–111, 1998

Thiamine Nutrition, Synthesis, and Retention in Relation to Lake Trout Reproduction in the Great Lakes

YING Q. JI[1]
Department of Fisheries and Wildlife, University of Minnesota
1980 Folwell Avenue
St. Paul, Minnesota 55108-6124, USA

JOSEPH J. WARTHESEN
Department of Food Science and Nutrition, University of Minnesota

IRA R. ADELMAN[2]
Department of Fisheries and Wildlife, University of Minnesota

Abstract.—Juvenile and adult lake trout *Salvelinus namaycush* that were fed semipurified, thiamine-deficient diets or alewives *Alosa pseudoharengus* containing thiaminase, a thiamine-destroying enzyme, showed no overt symptoms of thiamine deficiency. Growth rates and ovulation rates were similar among all treatments. However, liver thiamine pyrophosphate (TPP), a biochemical indicator of impending thiamine deficiency, in juvenile lake trout fed thiamine-deficient diets was reduced to 35 pmol/g compared with 59 pmol/g in control groups. Blood TPP in adult female lake trout fed alewives was one-third of that in controls fed a commercial diet. Adult lake trout from Lake Michigan had blood TPP levels similar to those of fish fed the alewife diet in the laboratory. Lake Superior lake trout had TPP levels similar to those of fish fed the control diet in the laboratory. Thiamine synthesis occurred in the intestine of lake trout. At least 81% of thiamine in the posterior intestine was synthesized, presumably by bacteria, when a ^{14}C-labeled thiamine diet was force-fed to lake trout. Thiamine had a long retention time in the lake trout: at 27 weeks after fish were injected with radioactive thiamine, blood cells retained 11% of the radioactivity that was present at 2 d and liver tissue retained 34% of the 2-d level. Lack of self-sustaining lake trout reproduction by Lake Michigan fish may be related to their lower blood thiamine levels. Thiamine deficiency may cause early mortality syndrome, which is common in Lake Michigan but not Lake Superior fish with higher blood thiamine levels.

Forty years after their demise throughout the Great Lakes, self-sustaining lake trout *Salvelinus namaycush* populations have been restored only in Lake Superior. This is in spite of massive stocking of lake trout and control of the sea lamprey *Petromyzon marinus* (Eshenroder et al. 1995; Hansen et al. 1995; Holey et al. 1995). Also during the past 40–50 years, the primary forage species of lake trout in the Great Lakes has shifted from lake herring *Coregonus artedi* and other coregonids to alewives *Alosa pseudoharengus* and smelt *Osmerus mordax* (Berst and Spangler 1972; Lawrie and Rahrer 1972; Wells and McLain 1972). Smelt and alewives have become important components of lake trout diets in the upper Great Lakes (Jude et al. 1987; Diana 1990; Miller and Holey 1992; Conner et al. 1993).

Because smelt and alewives contain thiaminase, a thiamine-destroying enzyme (Gnaedinger and Krzeczkowski 1966), lake trout that consume those species may develop a thiamine deficiency. Such a nutritional deficiency may result in subnormal reproductive success because thiamine is an essential vitamin for fish (Halver 1989). When raw fish containing thiaminase were fed to fish, symptoms of thiamine deficiency were found (Wolf 1942; Harrington 1954). If lake trout in the Great Lakes are suffering from a thiamine deficiency caused by consumption of smelt or alewives, their reproductive success might be impaired. That impairment might manifest itself as early mortality syndrome (EMS) of lake trout larvae (Fitzsimons 1995; Fisher et al. 1996).

Thiamine, a water-soluble vitamin, has a high turnover rate, and deficiency symptoms are rapid and severe in mammals (Gubler 1991). In contrast, the development time for overt symptoms in fish is relatively long (Halver 1957; Coble 1965; Morito et al. 1986; Masumoto et al. 1987; Morris and Davies 1995; Morris et al. 1995). Two possible causes for this prolonged time for development of deficiency symptoms may be that fish can obtain thiamine from a nondietary source or that thiamine is retained by fish for a long period of time.

[1] Present address: Minnesota Department of Agriculture, 90 West Plato Boulevard, St. Paul, Minnesota 55107, USA.
[2] To whom reprint requests should be addressed.

The objectives of this study were to (1) determine the effect of thiamine-deficient and thiaminase-containing diets on lake trout reproduction, (2) assess the thiamine nutritional status of adult lake trout in Lakes Superior and Michigan, (3) determine if thiamine is synthesized in the gastrointestinal tract of lake trout, and (4) determine the relative retention time of thiamine in lake trout.

Methods

Feeding Experiments

Three laboratory feeding experiments were conducted. In experiments 1 and 2, adult and juvenile lake trout, respectively, were fed semipurified diets containing different levels of thiamine. In experiment 3, adult lake trout were fed alewives containing thiaminase or a commercial trout diet.

Fish in experiments 1 and 3 were held in circular tanks, 1.8 m in diameter and 90 cm deep, with a volume of about 2,250 L. The tanks were continuously supplied with aerated well water at a constant temperature of 11°C. Water flow of approximately 20 L/min per tank maintained dissolved oxygen concentrations at approximately 8 mg/L. A 60-W fluorescent tube and a 40-W incandescent bulb were suspended above a 50 × 50 cm screened opening in the plywood cover of each tank. Photoperiod was synchronized weekly with the local photoperiod at 45° N latitude. Sunrise and sunsets of 0.5 h were simulated by lighting the incandescent bulb only.

Fish in experiment 2 were held in six covered rectangular tanks, 60 × 50 × 50 cm deep, holding approximately 150 L of water. The flow rate of the 11°C water was approximately 5 L/min. A hole of approximately 10 cm in diameter allowed feeding and limited light penetration; the photoperiod was adjusted weekly to local conditions.

In experiment 1, 60 adult (6 years old) female lake trout broodstock that had previously spawned once in the hatchery were obtained in January 1987 from the Crystal Springs Hatchery, Minnesota Department of Natural Resources. Fish were about 60 cm long and weight averaged 2.1 kg. Ten fish were randomly assigned to each of the six circular tanks. All fish were fed a commercial trout grow-out diet (Glencoe Mills, Glencoe, Minnesota) for 3 months. During that time, food consumption returned from a much reduced rate to the rate at the hatchery before transportation, approximately 0.5% of body weight per day. Semipurified diets containing approximately 0, 1, and 40 mg/kg thiamine were then randomly assigned, two tanks for each diet. Fish were fed to satiation twice daily on weekdays and once daily on weekends. Experiment 1 was conducted for 16 months, from April 1987 to August 1988.

Three attempts were made from mid-November to early December 1987 to manually strip eggs from all fish that had ovulated. Each time a fish ovulated, blood was taken for determination of thiamine nutritional status by measurement of thiamine pyrophosphate (TPP). Length and weight were measured on all fish on the third attempt at stripping on 3 December 1987. On 10 August 1988, an accident occurred in the water supply system that killed about two-thirds of the experimental fish, equally distributed among treatments. Length, weight, and weight of ovaries of the fish that died were measured and liver samples were taken. Ovary weight was used to compute gonadosomatic index as an indicator of reproductive development.

In experiment 2, 90 juvenile lake trout, with an average weight of 387 g, were obtained from the St. Paul Metro Hatchery, Minnesota Department of Natural Resources, and were randomly assigned to the six experimental tanks. All fish were individually tagged and fed the commercial trout diet for 2 weeks and then the semipurified 40 mg/kg thiamine diet for about 1 week. The same semipurified diets used in experiment 1 were then randomly assigned to the tanks. Feeding procedures were the same as in experiment 1.

The experiment ended after approximately 5.5 months when the accident in the water supply system caused the death of all of the fish. Food consumption rate was measured each day during the experimental period. Liver samples were taken from the dead fish at the termination of the experiment.

In experiment 3, Lake Michigan alewives or a commercial trout diet were fed to adult female lake trout. Frozen alewives, purchased from Schilling Fisheries (Ocono, Wisconsin), contained no detectable thiamine. Thiaminase activity, expressed as the amount of thiamine destroyed per gram of fish per minute, was approximately 118 pmol $\cdot$ g^{-1} $\cdot$ min^{-1}.

Thirty-two adult female lake trout, average weight 3.2 kg, from the same source as in experiment 1 were randomly distributed into four experimental tanks in January 1989. They were fed the commercial trout diet for 3 weeks during acclimation to the laboratory. These fish had previously spawned twice at the hatchery.

The experiment was begun on 8 February 1989, when fish in two tanks were fed thawed alewives and fish in the other two tanks continued to receive the commercial diet. All fish were fed to satiation twice daily on weekdays and once daily on week-

TABLE 1.—Composition of the semipurified diets used in feeding experiments 1 and 2. Thiamine was added at the rate of 0, 1, or 40 mg/kg to create the three experimental diets.

Ingredient	Amount (% by weight)
Vitamin-free casein	42
Dextrin	10
Dextrose	7
α-Cellulose	10
Bernhart-Tomarelli Salt mix	5
Herring oil	12
Gelatin	10
Choline Cl	1
Vitamin pre-mix without thiamine[a]	3
Thiamine	0, 0.0001, 0.004
DL-Methionine	0.5
Arginine (free base)	1
L-Tryptophan	0.04

[a] The vitamin premix provided the following vitamin content in 1 kg of feed: vitamin A palmitate, 10,000 IU; vitamin D3, 4,000 IU; vitamin E acetate, 200 IU; vitamin K, 50 mg; riboflavin, 50 mg; biotin, 0.5 mg; folic acid, 20 mg; vitamin B12 crystal, 0.2 mg; niacin, 300 mg; pyridoxine HCl, 40 mg; inositol, 500 mg; ascorbic acid, 500 mg; D-calcium pantothenate, 100 g.

ends. The experiment was conducted for about 21 months, from 8 February 1989 to 12 November 1990. Length and weight were determined and blood samples were taken at the beginning of the experiment and after 5, 10, 14, 18, and 21 months.

A "thiamine-free," casein-based, semipurified diet was made in the laboratory (Table 1). This formulation is that of Poston (1976) with minor modifications by Masumoto et al. (1987) and Morito et al. (1986). Thiamine was added to produce diets with three different thiamine (dry weight) levels: 0, 1, and 40 mg/kg. Because "thiamine-free" ingredients contained trace amounts of thiamine, the actual thiamine contents of the three diets were 0.17, 1.3, and 40 mg/kg. The 1 mg/kg thiamine diet is the recommended minimum needed by salmonids to avoid deficiency symptoms (NRC 1981; Morito et al. 1986). The 40 mg/kg level was chosen because commercial grow-out diets usually contain 20 mg/kg thiamine and manufacturers sometimes double the grow-out vitamin content in broodstock feeds.

All ingredients were purchased from the United States Biochemicals Corp. (Cleveland, Ohio) except herring oil, which was supplied by Glencoe Mills. Animal gelatin, dissolved in hot water, was used as a binder to provide a diet with a soft, rubbery texture with 50% water content. The feed was frozen at −20°C until use.

Thiamine Nutritional Status of Wild Lake Trout

Adult lake trout blood samples for determination of TPP were taken in the vicinity of Saugatuck, Michigan, for Lake Michigan and Bayfield, Wisconsin, for Lake Superior. Reproduction of lake trout in the Saugatuck area was thought to be nonexistent, whereas naturally reproduced lake trout were common in the Bayfield area (Hansen et al. 1995; Holey et al. 1995).

Fish were collected on five dates spanning approximately 14 months. Actual sampling dates for Lake Michigan were 27 September 1987 (prespawning), 2 November 1987 (spawning), 19 May 1988 (spring), 11 September 1988 (prespawning), and 3 November 1988 (spawning). For Lake Superior, sampling dates were 20 September 1987 (prespawning), 22 October 1987 (spawning), 9 May 1988 (spring), 15 September 1988 (prespawning), and 16 October 1988 (spawning).

Fish were captured in gill nets from the Saugatuck area by the U.S. Fish and Wildlife Service. For the spring sampling in 1988, fish were captured by angling. Samples obtained from the Bayfield area were gillnetted by the Red Cliff Band of Lake Superior Chippewa Indians of Wisconsin or the Wisconsin Department of Natural Resources.

Only fish still alive when pulled from the water were used for blood collection. However, because of the multitude of activities on the research vessels, blood could not always be drawn from fish immediately upon capture. A comparison of the stability of TPP levels in blood taken at 0, 20, 40, and 60 min after death indicated no significant differences. Thus, blood samples taken within 1 h of a fish's death adequately represented the TPP levels at the time of death. Blood samples were immediately placed on dry ice for transportation to the laboratory.

Thiamine Synthesis Experiment

Radioactive thiamine as a percentage of total thiamine was used in this experiment to determine the presence or absence of thiamine synthesis in the gastrointestinal tract of lake trout. This approach was based on the principle that a radioactive isotope behaves in the same manner as its nonradioactive counterpart. When radioactive thiamine was fed to fish, ^{14}C thiamine should behave identically to ^{12}C thiamine in the gastrointestinal tract. Radioactive thiamine as a percentage of total thiamine would remain constant as feed passed through the gastrointestinal tract. The percentage would decrease if a nondietary source of thiamine, such as thiamine synthesis, was present. Thus, the ratios of radioactive thiamine to total thiamine in the contents of the stomach and the anterior and posterior intestine were used to confirm the presence or absence of a nondietary source of thiamine in the gastrointestinal tract.

To conduct this experiment, a feed containing radioactive thiamine was prepared. Thiazole-2-^{14}C-labeled thiamine hydrochloride, in units of 50 μCi and with a specific activity of 24.2 mCi/mmol, was purchased from Amersham Corp. (Arlington Heights, Illinois). A stock solution was prepared by dissolving one 50-μCi unit into 5 mL of 0.1 N HCl. Approximately 1.0 mL of the stock solution was mixed with 1 kg (dry weight) of thiamine-free ingredients to make about 2 kg of moist gelatin feed as described above for the feeding experiments.

The amount of radioactive thiamine (micrograms per kilogram) in the feed and gastrointestinal contents was calculated as:

$$^{14}\text{C thiamine} = [(\text{sample CPM} - \text{blank CPM}) \times \text{MW} \times 1{,}000]/[\text{SW} \times \text{QC efficiency} \times 62.4 \times 2.22 \times 10^6)$$

where CPM is counts per minute, MW is molecular weight, SW is sample weight, QC efficiency is quenching and counting efficiency (95.4%), 62.4 is the theoretical maximum specific radioactivity, and 2.22×10^6 represents disintegrations per minute (dpm) per microcurie. Theoretical maximum specific radioactivity was used to calculate the thiamine content that is 100% radioactive with ^{14}C atoms at the 2-position of the thiazole ring. The radioactive thiamine used contained only 38.78% radioactive thiamine. Quenching and counting efficiency was determined by using a toluene standard spike combined with a factory-sealed ^{14}C standard.

The radioactivity in the feed was confirmed in random samples as 11,799 (SE = 549) dpm/g of feed. This is equivalent to a thiamine supplement of 74.2 (SE = 3.5) μg/kg total thiamine, of which 28.8 μg/kg was ^{14}C thiamine. The trace amount of thiamine that existed in the thiamine-deficient diet was 170 μg/kg (dry weight) and the feed from which radioactivity was measured had a 50% water content; thus, the total thiamine in the feed was approximately 160 μg/kg (wet weight), with ^{14}C thiamine being 18% of the total thiamine. Supplemental thiamine was intentionally low so that the feed would be classified as thiamine-deficient (NRC 1981) yet have sufficient thiamine to be measurable. Wet weight was used because the total thiamine content and radioactive thiamine were analyzed on a wet weight basis.

The fish used in this experiment were from the control groups in feeding experiment 3. The fish were held in a circular tank as described above for feeding experiments 1 and 3, except that a screen was placed about 15 cm from the bottom to minimize the potential for coprophagy by the fish. Before the experiment, fish were fed the thiamine-deficient, semipurified diet for 3 months.

After acclimation to the semipurified diet, 12 fish were starved for 3 d, then anesthetized with tricaine methanesulfate (MS-222), and force-fed approximately 20 g of the radioactive diet per fish with a caulk gun. After 24 h, all fish were killed with an overdose of the anesthetic and dissected. The gastrointestinal tract was removed and separated into three parts: the stomach, the anterior half of the intestine, and the posterior half of the intestine. Approximately 2 g of stomach contents and all of the anterior and posterior intestinal contents were taken. These samples were then divided into two parts: about 0.2 g from each gastrointestinal tract section was placed in tared liquid scintillation vials for radioactive analysis, and the remaining contents were analyzed for total thiamine by column exchange.

To determine the presence and amount of nondietary thiamine, the following equations were used:

$$T_1 = (1 - R_a/R_s) \times 100$$

$$T_2 = (1 - R_p/R_s) \times 100$$

where T_1 and T_2 are the percentages of nondietary thiamine in the anterior and posterior intestine, respectively; R_a is the ratio of radioactive thiamine to total thiamine in the contents of the anterior intestine; R_s is the ratio of radioactive thiamine to total thiamine in the stomach contents (diet); and R_p is the ratio of radioactive thiamine to total thiamine in the contents of the posterior intestine. To distinguish the percentage of nondietary thiamine in the posterior intestine that originated in the anterior intestine, the following formulas were used:

$$T_3 = (1 - R_p/R_a) \times 100$$

$$T_4 = (R_p/R_a - R_p/R_s) \times 100$$

where T_3 is the percentage of nondietary thiamine of posterior origin and T_4 is the percentage of nondietary thiamine of nonposterior origin.

To determine tissue uptake of radioactive thiamine from the fish that were force-fed the ^{14}C-labeled thiamine, approximately 0.2 g of liver, stomach, pyloric ceca, and anterior and posterior intestine were washed and placed in tared liquid scintillation vials. The tissues were then digested with 1.5 mL of Soluene (Packard Instruments Co., Meriden, Connecticut) for 48 h in a 55°C water bath. Scintillation fluid (15 mL of Ecocint A, National Diagnostics, Manville, New Jersey) was added and radioactivity was measured with a Beckman LS-1000 liquid scintillation spectrometer (Beckman Instruments, Inc., Schaumburg, Illinois).

Thiamine Retention Experiment

Fish from the same source and holding conditions as in the thiamine synthesis experiment were used to determine the length of time that thiamine was retained in various fish tissues. Fish were fed the semipurified, thiamine-deficient diet for 3 months before and for the 26-week experimental period.

Units of thiazole-2-^{14}C thiamine were dissolved in a 0.9% NaCl solution. A dose of approximately 1 μCi/kg of fish was injected into the caudal artery after the fish were anesthetized with MS-222. Blood samples were taken from the caudal artery 48 h after injection with a 10-mL heparinized Vacutainer tube. The blood was then centrifuged at 6,500 g for 10 min. The supernatant was discarded and 200 μL of packed cells was pipetted into a scintillation vial. The elapsed time of 48 h ensured that the injected thiamine had sufficient time to be taken into blood cells. This was confirmed by samples of plasma taken 48 h after injection in which radioactivity was only slightly above background and negligible compared with that in blood cells.

Liver biopsy samples were taken with a 14-gauge, 11.4-cm Monoject Actuated Biopsy Cutting Needle (Sherwood Medical, St. Louis, Missouri). After a fish was anesthetized, a 4-mm incision in the integument was made posterior to the base of the pelvic fins. About 20–50 mg of liver was obtained from each fish and placed in a tared liquid scintillation vial. Multiple biopsy sections were needed to obtain the desired amount of sample material. Occasionally, inadequate amounts were obtained so that data were not available from all fish at all sampling dates. Oxytetracycline was injected into each fish to prevent possible infection of the incision. The sampling of packed cells and liver tissue was repeated at 42, 109, and 171 d after injection.

On day 42 after the injection, two fish were killed to determine the distribution of radioactivity in various organs. On day 189, the experiment was terminated. Radioactivity was determined in about 0.2 g of the muscle, liver, stomach, heart, kidney, spleen, intestine, and ovarian tissue of the eight remaining fish.

Blood Sampling Procedures and Chemical Analysis

Except as noted otherwise, blood samples were drawn in the following manner in the laboratory and field. Fish were first anesthetized with MS-222. Blood (2–3 mL) was drawn from the caudal artery into a 10-mL heparinized Vacutainer tube with a 22-gauge needle. The blood samples were placed on ice before transfer to a freezer and then stored at −20°C until analysis.

Blood and liver TPP, the active coenzyme form of thiamine, was used as an indicator of thiamine nutritional status. TPP levels were determined by high-pressure liquid chromatography (HPLC). The procedures of Baines (1985) were followed except that whole blood was used instead of erythrocytes. The preparation of liver tissue was according to Masumoto et al. (1987) except that TPP was extracted into methanol instead of trichloroacetic acid, and then Baines' (1985) method was followed.

A recovery experiment with a pooled lake trout blood sample was conducted to measure the percentage of standard TPP extracted and measured by the HPLC procedure. After the first centrifugation for removal of debris, the pooled sample was divided into three tubes of 1.8 mL each. One tube received no TPP spike, one was spiked with 0.2 mL of 1 pmol/mL TPP standard solution to achieve an increase in TPP content of 100 pmol/mL, and one was spiked with 0.2 mL of 4 pmol/mL TPP standard solution to achieve an increase in TPP content of 400 pmol/mL. The recovery rates were approximately 92 and 94% for the 100 and 400 pmol/mL spikes, respectively.

The stability of TPP during storage was tested. Approximately 60 mL of blood was taken from a group of juvenile lake trout. The pooled blood was then divided into four groups. One group was analyzed for TPP immediately and the others were analyzed after 1, 2, or 4 weeks of storage at −20°C. No significant difference in TPP was found among the four groups.

Because blood could not always be frozen immediately, a comparison was made of the effects on TPP content of different times elapsed before freezing. The TPP content of blood frozen 3 h after drawing was 96% of that of blood frozen immediately

TABLE 2.—Mean weight, number of ovulated lake trout, and blood thiamine pyrophosphate (TPP) levels for lake trout fed for 8 months on semipurified diets containing three different thiamine levels in experiment 1. Values shown in parentheses are SEs.

Dietary thiamine (mg/kg)	Number of fish	Number ovulated	Initial weight (kg)	Weight gained (kg)	Blood TPP (pmol/mL)
0	20	11	2.2 (0.13)	0.25	63 (6)
1	20	10	2.0 (0.11)	0.22	57 (7)
40	17	9	2.1 (0.14)	0.31	73 (7)

after drawing. These differences were not statistically significant. All analyses for total thiamine were conducted by Medallion Laboratories, General Mills, Inc. (Minneapolis, Minnesota).

Statistical Analysis

A randomized block design with multiple group comparisons was used to analyze for differences in blood or liver TPP contents in feeding experiments 1 and 2. A t-test was used in experiment 3 to compare blood TPP levels between lake trout fed alewives and those fed the commercial diet at different times. Also, t-tests were used in the field surveys to compare blood TPP levels between Lake Michigan and Lake Superior fish.

Paired comparison t-tests were used to compare percentages of radioactive thiamine in anterior and posterior intestinal contents with those of stomach contents in the same fish. Samples with total thiamine concentrations below the minimum detectable limit (50 μg/g) were excluded from the statistical analysis. As a result, sample sizes were reduced to six for anterior and five for posterior intestinal contents.

Regression analysis was used to determine the relationship between radioactivity in packed blood cells or in liver and days after thiamine injection. Two-factor analysis of variance was used to compare radioactivity in different organs at different times in the thiamine retention experiment. Unless noted otherwise, significant differences were those with P-values < 0.05.

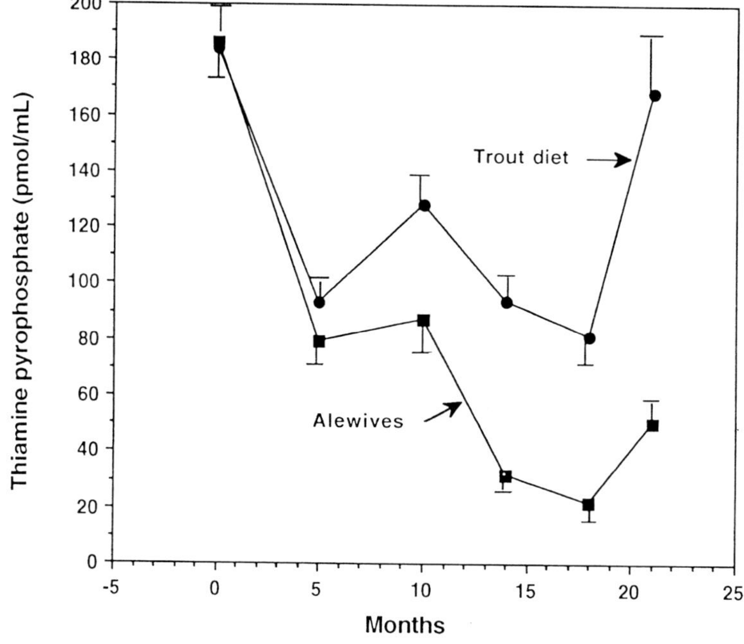

FIGURE 1.—Thiamine pyrophosphate levels in blood of lake trout fed a commercial trout diet or alewives containing thiaminase at various times after the start of experiment 3. Bars shown above or below the mean are SEs.

TABLE 3.—Mean weight, liver thiamine pyrophosphate (TPP) levels, and gonadosomatic index (grams of ovaries per gram of fish × 100) for lake trout fed for 16 months on the semipurified diets in experiment 1. Values shown in parentheses are SEs.

Dietary thiamine (mg/kg)	Number of fish	Weight (kg)	Liver TPP (pmol/g)	Gonadosomatic index
0	14	2.8 (0.29)	204 (22)	5.5 (0.94)
1	14	2.3 (0.27)	150 (24)	4.9 (1.24)
40	12	2.9 (0.28)	191 (33)	5.4 (0.95)

Results

Feeding Experiments

In experiment 1, growth rates were not significantly different among adult lake trout receiving 0, 1, or 40 mg/kg thiamine. Fish in all tanks fully consumed the 0.5% daily ration. However, fish gained little weight during the experiment (Table 2). Three fish that received the 0 mg/kg thiamine diet died from unknown causes.

Many fish ovulated during the spawning season, approximately 8 months after the start of the experiment. The percentage of fish that ovulated was similar among the three diet treatments: 55% for fish fed the 0 mg/kg thiamine diet, 50% for fish fed the 1 mg/kg thiamine diet, and 53% for fish fed the 40 mg/kg thiamine diet (Table 2). The TPP levels in blood at the time of ovulation were not significantly different among fish fed the three diets.

About 70% of the experimental fish died 16 months after the start of the experiment after an accident in the water supply system. At that time, neither weight, gonadosomatic index, nor liver TPP levels differed significantly as a result of diet (Table 3).

In experiment 2, the juvenile lake trout fed diets containing the three different levels of thiamine had similar food consumption and growth rates after 5.5 months (Table 4). Liver TPP levels were significantly different among the experimental groups ($P < 0.001$). Fish fed the 0 mg/kg thiamine diet had the lowest level of liver TPP, whereas those fed the 1 mg/kg thiamine diet had the highest liver TPP concentration.

In experiment 3, essentially all energy consumed went to the production of eggs, because after eggs were stripped at 9 and 21 months, somatic growth ranged from slightly negative to slightly positive with no significant difference among treatments (Table 5). During the 1989 spawning season, 87% of the fish ovulated, and during 1990, 86% ovulated, with no significant difference between fish fed the commercial diet and the alewives.

Fish fed either alewives or the commercial diet had similar blood TPP levels (approximately 185 pmol/mL) at the start of the experiment (Figure 1). After 5 months, blood TPP contents of fish fed alewives began to differ from those of fish fed the commercial diet. These differences became statistically significant ($P < 0.001$) by the 10th month and remained so thereafter.

Thiamine Synthesis Experiment

Mean total and radioactive thiamine concentrations declined between the stomach contents and the contents of the two intestinal segments (Table 6). The thiamine concentration measured in the stomachs of force-fed lake trout was 153 μg/kg, with 20.2% radioactive; this approximated the level that we estimated for the feed, 160 μg/kg, with 18% radioactive. Radioactive thiamine as a percentage of total thiamine declined progressively as food passed

TABLE 4.—Mean gain in weight, food consumption rate, and liver thiamine pyrophosphate (TPP) levels of juvenile lake trout fed semipurified diets for 5.5 months in experiment 2. Values shown in parentheses are SEs.

Dietary thiamine (mg/kg)	Initial weight (g)	Weight gain (g)	Food consumption (grams of fish per week)	TPP levels (pmol/g)
0	389 (23)	160 (16)	49.3 (2.2)	35 (2.8)
1	373 (15)	151 (24)	47.1 (0.9)	72 (6.1)
40	397 (17)	160 (10)	48.6 (1.0)	59 (5.2)

TABLE 5.—Mean weight (kg) and number of ovulated lake trout in experiment 3. Fish were fed either a commercial pelleted trout diet or alewives containing thiaminase, over 21 months, including two spawning cycles. Values shown in parentheses are SEs.

Months after start	Diet type	Number of fish	Number ovulated	Initial weight	Weight after egg stripping
10	Alewives	16	14	2.61 (0.17)	2.68 (0.28)
	Commercial	15	13	2.95 (0.20)	2.79 (0.22)
21	Alewives	14	12	2.83 (0.26)	3.07 (0.28)
	Commercial	14	12	2.80 (0.21)	2.89 (0.20)

from the stomach to the anterior intestine to the posterior intestine, with both anterior and posterior intestinal contents statistically different from the stomach content ($P < 0.001$) but not different from each other (Table 6). The percentages of nondietary thiamine were calculated as 72.8% in the anterior intestine and 81.2% in the posterior intestine, with 30.9% of the latter of posterior origin and 50.3% of nonposterior origin.

Radioactive thiamine was absorbed into the various tissues of the gastrointestinal tract and the liver. Tissue radioactivity in increasing order (on a wet tissue basis) was: stomach, 299 dpm/100 mg (SE = 32.7); posterior intestine, 300 dpm/100 mg (SE = 34.5); anterior intestine, 400 dpm/100 mg (SE = 38.0); pyloric ceca, 524 dpm/100 mg (SE = 32.7); liver, 660 dpm/100 mg (SE = 69.4).

Thiamine Retention Experiment

Radioactive thiamine had a relatively long retention time in both packed cells and liver tissue of lake trout. At 27 weeks, packed blood cells still retained 11% of the radioactivity present at 2 d and liver retained 34% of the 2-d level (Figure 2).

The radioactivity in different tissues changed between samples taken at 6 and 27 weeks, although the data from 6 weeks are somewhat uncertain because of the small sample size (only two fish; Table 7). At 6 weeks, the highest level of radioactivity was in heart tissue, followed by liver, kidney, and ovaries. At 27 weeks, heart tissue continued to have the highest radioactivity, but liver tissue had lower levels than ovarian and kidney tissue. There was a significant difference in radioactivity among tissues at the different times and also a significant interaction

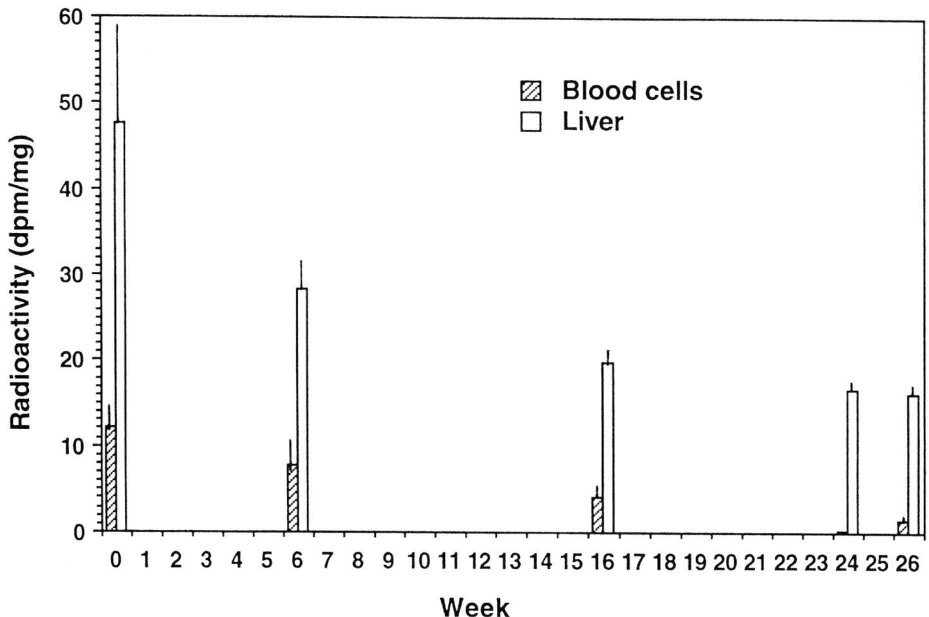

FIGURE 2.—Radioactivity (disintegrations per minute; dpm) in packed blood cells and liver tissue of lake trout at various times after injection of ^{14}C-labeled thiamine. Bars indicate SE values.

TABLE 6.—Total thiamine, radioactive thiamine, and the percentage of radioactive thiamine in the contents of the stomach, anterior intestine, and posterior intestine of lake trout. Fish were force-fed a diet containing ^{14}C-labeled thiamine and samples were taken 24 h later. Values shown in parentheses are SEs.

Contents site	Number of samples	Total thiamine (μg/kg)	Radioactive thiamine (μg/kg)	Percentage radioactive thiamine
Stomach	12	153 (16)	30.0 (4.0)	20.2 (1.8)
Anterior intestine	6	91 (11)	4.8 (0.8)	5.5 (0.9)
Posterior intestine	5	108 (16)	3.7 (0.6)	3.8 (0.7)

between tissue radioactivity and time ($P < 0.01$). Thus, radioactivity was not moving into different tissues uniformly: while radioactivity in some tissues declined, it increased in others.

Thiamine Nutritional Status of Wild Lake Trout

Throughout the 14 months of sampling in the Bayfield area for Lake Superior lake trout and in the Saugatuck area for Lake Michigan lake trout, blood TPP levels were significantly lower ($P < 0.01$) in the Lake Michigan fish (Figure 3). TPP levels of Lake Superior fish were usually at least two times those of Lake Michigan fish.

Discussion

Feeding Experiments

Thiamine, a water-soluble vitamin, generally has a high turnover rate and is not thought to be stored in large amounts or for any substantial period of time in any tissue, at least in mammals (Gubler 1991). Insufficient intake of thiamine results in rapid development of clinical symptoms of deficiency (Gubler 1991). This deficiency has been reported to cause beriberi disease in humans (Shimozono and Katsura 1965), Chastek's paralysis in foxes (Green and Evans 1940), bracken staggers in horses (Evans 1975), and cerebrocortical necrosis in cattle and sheep (Edwin et al. 1979).

In fish, a dietary thiamine requirement has been demonstrated in many species, and typical symptoms of deficiency include anorexia, muscle atrophy, convulsions, loss of equilibrium, edema, hyperexcitability, and poor growth (NRC 1983; Halver 1989). In contrast to mammals, overt thiamine deficiency symptoms in fish take a relatively long time to develop. Various studies have reported development times ranging from 8 to 14 weeks for smaller fish (Halver 1957; Morito et al. 1986; Morris and Davies 1995; Morris et al. 1995) and up to 30 weeks with no symptoms for larger fish (Coble 1965).

In the present study, we observed none of the overt symptoms of thiamine deficiency described above. Juvenile and adult fish fed thiamine-deficient or thiaminase-containing diets for 5.5, 16, or 21 months in three experiments showed no differences in behavior, food consumption rate, growth, or ovulation rate. However, biochemical indicators of thiamine deficiency were detected in two experiments. Juvenile fish in experiment 2 had reduced liver TPP levels after 5.5 months of consuming a semipurified, thiamine-deficient diet of 0.17 mg/kg thiamine. In experiment 3, adult fish fed a thiaminase-containing diet of alewives had lower blood TPP concentrations by 10 months into the experiment than fish fed a commercial diet. Blood and liver TPP is reported to be a sensitive indicator of the potential onset of thiamine deficiency in trout (Masumoto et al. 1987), yet overt symptoms were not observed.

It is uncertain why the adult lake trout did not exhibit overt symptoms of thiamine deficiency. In experiment 1, fish fed a semipurified, thiamine-deficient diet did not even show reduced blood TPP after 8 months or reduced liver TPP after 16 months. As indicated by our thiamine synthesis and thiamine retention experiments, a nondietary source of thiamine and a long retention time of thiamine in fish tissues may be two factors that contributed to this prolonged time for development of symptoms of thiamine deficiency.

TABLE 7.—Radioactivity (disintegrations per minute per milligram) in different tissues of lake trout at 6 and 27 weeks after injection of ^{14}C-labeled thiamine. Values shown in parentheses are SEs.

Tissue	Week 6	Week 27
Heart	62 (5.1)	36 (5.0)
Liver	36 (6.2)	16 (1.3)
Kidney	21 (10.6)	22 (2.8)
Ovaries	20 (6.2)	25 (6.8)
Spleen		20 (2.0)
Stomach	20 (0.5)	9 (1.2)
Intestine	18 (1.2)	11 (1.1)
Packed cells	8 (1.9)	1 (0.5)
Muscle	5 (0.5)	5 (0.8)

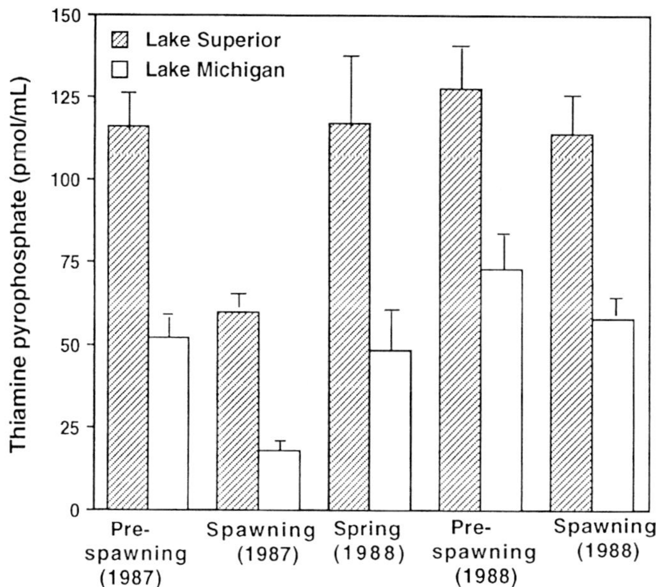

FIGURE 3.—Mean thiamine pyrophosphate levels in blood of lake trout from Lakes Michigan and Superior. See text for actual sampling dates. Bars indicate SE values.

Thiamine Synthesis Experiment

The significant decrease in percentage of radioactive thiamine from stomach contents, anterior intestinal contents, and posterior intestinal contents indicated a significant nondietary source of thiamine that increased the percentage of nonradioactive thiamine in the intestine of lake trout.

Thiamine is not known to be synthesized by animals, only by bacteria, yeast, and higher plants (Gubler 1991). Among mammals, substantial thiamine synthesis occurs in ruminants, but that synthesis is of microbial origin (Breves et al. 1980, 1981). In ruminants, absorption of thiamine occurs in the small intestine (Miller et al. 1986a, 1986b) through a carrier-mediated process (Hoyumpa 1982). In nonruminant mammals, significant synthesis of thiamine may occur in the gastrointestinal tract (Shibata 1950; Wostmann et al. 1962), but that thiamine is generally believed to be unavailable to the host animal without coprophagy (Gubler 1991). Without coprophagy by lake trout, intestinal absorption would have to occur for synthesis to make a contribution to thiamine nutrition. Although we occasionally observed lake trout ingesting feces in feeding experiments 1 and 3, they invariably ejected it immediately, and the screened tank bottom largely prevented consumption of feces in the thiamine synthesis experiment.

Synthesis of thiamine in the lake trout intestines seems plausible because synthesis of vitamin B or vitamin B-producing bacteria has been found in other fish species. Trepsiene et al. (1977) isolated thiamine-producing bacteria in carp *Cyprinus carpio* intestines. Sugita et al. (1991) isolated vitamin B_{12}-producing bacteria from six freshwater fishes. Limsuwan and Lovell (1981) and Lovell and Limsuwan (1982) reported intestinal synthesis and absorption of vitamin B_{12} in channel catfish *Ictalurus punctatus* and *Tilapia*.

The actual level of thiamine in the anterior intestine of the lake trout in our synthesis study was very low (0.0048 mg/kg) compared with the minimum requirement in feed (1 mg/kg) recommended by the National Research Council (NRC 1981). However, we do not know if synthesized thiamine may have been absorbed rapidly by the intestine and thus may have contributed significantly to thiamine nutrition, despite its low concentration in the intestinal contents. With nondietary thiamine content in the posterior intestine as high as 81% of total thiamine, the contribution to thiamine nutrition of thiamine synthesized in the gastrointestinal tract may be quite significant.

To our knowledge, our method for determining thiamine synthesis has not previously been used. Measurement of nutrient absorption in the intestine was complicated by a potential new source of thiamine, microbial synthesis. The ratio of radioactive thiamine to total thiamine enables detection of the addition of nondietary thiamine; however, our method cannot measure absorption rate. When synthesis is present, use of a nondigestible marker such as chromic oxide still would not permit determination of absorption because of the addition of nondietary thiamine. The combination of the radioactivity and chromic oxide would reveal the absorption rate of the dietary thiamine alone by measuring radioactive thiamine against the indigestible marker. However, it would not address the absorption rate of nondietary thiamine because the total quantity of nondietary thiamine remains unknown.

Our measurement of radioactive thiamine in contents of the gastrointestinal tract assumed that all measured radioactivity resulted from intact ^{14}C-labeled thiamine, but in reality, measured radioactivity could also have resulted from degraded thiamine. Radioactive and nonradioactive thiamine degrade at the same rate. Measurement of radioactivity in degraded thiamine would give the appearance of a higher percentage of radioactive thiamine in the intestinal contents and lead to the conclusion that a smaller increase in nondietary thiamine had occurred than was the case. Thus, our measurement is conservative.

Although thiamine synthesis seemed to occur in the gastrointestinal tract of the lake trout, it is difficult to ascertain what role that synthesis might play in preventing thiamine deficiency in field situations. If a thiamine deficiency in female spawners causes a deficiency in eggs that results in EMS, then thiamine synthesis is not sufficient to overcome that deficiency. However, if the deficiency is caused by the consumption of thiaminase-containing prey, as is assumed, the thiaminase may remain active in the intestine and thus negate any synthesis that might occur. In feeding experiment 1, no evidence of thiamine deficiency was found in lake trout fed a thiamine-deficient diet for 16 months, but in experiment 3, fish had reduced blood TPP levels after 10 months of feeding on thiaminase-containing alewives. This suggests that the presence of thiaminase had a greater effect on the development of thiamine deficiency than the absence of thiamine in the diet.

Thiamine Retention Experiment

The long retention time of thiamine by lake trout may also contribute to the prolonged time for development of thiamine deficiency symptoms in fish in the feeding experiments. At 27 weeks after injection, radioactivity in blood cells was still 16% of radioactivity at 2 d and radioactivity in liver was 34% of the 2-d levels. However, while those tissues were losing thiamine, it was increasing in other tissues, particularly kidney and ovaries.

Very few thiamine turnover or thiamine retention studies have been done with mammals, and we are aware of none with fish. Trebukhina et al. (1985) injected ^{14}C thiamine into mice fed a thiamine-deficient diet and reported the rate at which thiamine was incorporated into various tissues. The tissues with high turnover rates were liver, kidney, heart, stomach, spleen, and brain. In the present study, we measured the retention rate, or the rate at which radioactive thiamine was depleted, as opposed to the rate at which radioactive thiamine was incorporated. We found high radioactivity in the same tissues in which Trebukhina et al. (1985) found it in mice.

Thiamine Nutritional Status of Wild Lake Trout

The thiamine nutritional status of fish collected from Lake Michigan resembled that of lake trout fed the alewife diet for 10 months in feeding experiment 3. Blood TPP levels of fish from Lake Michigan ranged from 18 to 73 pmol/mL for samples taken over 14 months (Figure 3). The TPP levels in lake trout fed the thiaminase-containing diet ranged from 22 to 87 pmol/mL for the period between 10 months, when TPP levels first differentiated from controls, and 21 months, when the experiment was terminated (Figure 1). The blood TPP levels in Lake Superior lake trout, which ranged from 60 to 128 pmol/mL, were similar to those of control fish in experiment 3, which ranged from 81 to 168 pmol/mL.

The difference in blood TPP levels between lake trout from Lakes Michigan and Superior may be caused by a combination of diets composed of thiaminase-containing species and the amount of thiaminase activity in those prey species. In the vicinity of Bayfield, Lake Superior, thiaminase-containing smelt accounted for 66% of lake trout diets in 1987 (Conner et al. 1993). In Lake Michigan, the diet of nearshore lake trout during 1984–1988 consisted of 81% thiaminase-containing alewives (Miller and Holey 1992). In lake trout sampled in 1986 from Saugatuck, Lake Michigan, alewives constituted 82% and smelt constituted 2% of lake trout stomach contents (R. F. Elliot, U.S. Fish and Wildlife Service, unpublished data). The remaining 16% of the diet consisted of bloaters *Coregonus hoyi* and yellow perch *Perca flavescens*, which are not known to contain thiaminase. Whether the higher percentage of thiaminase-containing forage fish consumed by Lake Michigan lake trout was sufficient to cause their lower thiamine nutritional status is uncertain. Also, it is difficult to assess whether differences in thiaminase activity between alewives and smelt caused the differences in blood TPP levels between lake trout from the two lakes. Ji and Adelman (1998, this volume) found that thiaminase activities of these two species were highly variable depending on species, sampling location, and time, with a significant interaction among these variables.

The lower TPP levels in Lake Michigan lake trout compared with Lake Superior fish suggest a possible link between thiamine nutritional status and reproductive success, including the occurrence of EMS (Fitzsimons 1995; Fisher et al. 1996). Self-sustaining populations of lake trout have been reestablished in most of Lake Superior (Hansen et al. 1995), whereas self-sustaining reproduction of lake trout in Lake Michigan has been nonexistent (Holey et al. 1995). Furthermore, EMS has been observed in lake trout from Lake Michigan but not Lake Superior (Fitzsimons 1995). However, the level of TPP activity in blood below which females produce larvae having EMS remains to be established.

At the time the present study was undertaken, thiamine deficiency had not been implicated in EMS of lake trout sac fry (Fitzsimons 1995; Fisher et al. 1996). From our laboratory experiments and field observations, it appears that adult lake trout can ovulate and spawn successfully when consuming thiamine-deficient or thiaminase-containing diets. However, sufficient thiamine for ovulation and spawning may not be enough to prevent EMS in sac fry, particularly because lake trout in Lake Michigan feed on thiaminase-containing species for most of their lives.

Acknowledgments

This work is the result of research sponsored by the Minnesota Sea Grant Program, which is supported by the National Oceanic and Atmospheric Administration Office of Sea Grant, United States Department of Commerce, under grant R/F-23. This paper is journal reprint number JR 434 of the Minnesota Sea Grant College Program. We are indebted to personnel from the Red Cliff Band of Lake Superior Chippewa Indians of Wisconsin, the U.S. Fish and Wildlife Service, and the Wisconsin Department of Natural Resources for assistance in collecting fish; the Minnesota Department of Natural Resources for providing experimental fish; George R. Spangler for providing the intellectual impetus to conduct this research; and two anonymous reviewers for suggestions for revision of the original manuscript.

References

Baines, M. 1985. Improved high performance liquid chromatographic determination of thiamin diphosphate in erythrocytes. Clinica Chimica Acta 153:43–48.

Berst, A. H., and G. R. Spangler. 1972. Lake Huron: effects of exploitation, introductions, and eutrophication on the salmonid community. Journal of the Fisheries Research Board of Canada 29:877–887.

Breves, G., M. Brandt, H. Hoeller, and K. Rohr. 1981. Flow of thiamin in the duodenum in dairy cows fed different rations. Journal of Agricultural Science 96:587–591.

Breves, G., H. Hoeller, J. Harmeyer, and H. Martens. 1980. Thiamin balance in the gastrointestinal tract of sheep. Journal of Animal Science 51:1177–1181.

Coble, D. D. 1965. Effect of raw smelt on lake trout. Canadian Fish Culturist 36:27–34.

Conner, D. J., C. R. Bronte, J. H. Selgeby, and H. L. Collins. 1993. Food of salmonine predators in Lake Superior, 1981–87. Great Lakes Fishery Commission Technical Report 59.

Diana, J. S. 1990. Food habits of angler-caught salmonines in western Lake Huron. Journal of Great Lakes Research 16:271–278.

Edwin, E. E., L. M. Markson, J. Shreeve, R. Jackman, and P. J. Carroll. 1979. Diagnostic aspects of cerebrocortical necrosis. Veterinary Record 104:4–8.

Eshenroder, R. L., N. R. Payne, J. E. Johnson, C. Bowen, II, and M. P. Ebener. 1995. Lake trout rehabilitation in Lake Huron. Journal of Great Lakes Research 21(Supplement 1):108–127.

Evans, W. C. 1975. Thiaminases and their effects on animals. Vitamins and Hormones 33:467–504.

Fisher, J. P., J. D. Fitzsimons, G. F. Combs, Jr., and J. M. Spitsbergen. 1996. Naturally occurring thiamine deficiency causing reproductive failure in Finger Lakes Atlantic salmon and Great Lakes lake trout. Transactions of the American Fisheries Society 125:167–178.

Fitzsimons, J. D. 1995. The effect of B-vitamins on a swim-up syndrome in Lake Ontario lake trout. Journal of Great Lakes Research 21(Supplement 1):286–289.

Gnaedinger, R. H., and R. A. Krzeczkowski. 1966. Heat inactivation of thiaminase in whole fish. Commercial Fisheries Review 28:11–14.

Green, R. G., and C. A. Evans. 1940. A deficiency disease of foxes. Science 92:154–155.

Gubler, C. J. 1991. Thiamin. Pages 233–281 *in* L. J. Machlin, editor. Handbook of vitamins: nutritional, biochemical, and clinical aspects. Marcel Dekker, Inc. New York.

Halver, J. E. 1957. Nutrition of salmonid fishes. III. Water soluble vitamin requirements of chinook salmon. Journal of Nutrition 62:225–243.

Halver, J. E. 1989. The vitamins. Pages 32–109 *in* J. E. Halver, editor. Fish nutrition. Academic Press, San Diego, California.

Hansen, M. J., and 11 coauthors. 1995. Lake trout (*Salvelinus namaycush*) populations in Lake Superior and their restoration in 1959–1993. Journal of Great Lakes Research 21 (Supplement 1):152–175.

Harrington, R., Jr. 1954. Contrasting susceptibilities of two fish species to a diet destructive to vitamin B-1. Journal of the Fisheries Research Board of Canada 11:529–534.

Holey, M. E., and eight coauthors. 1995. Progress toward lake trout restoration in Lake Michigan. Journal of Great Lakes Research 21(Supplement 1):128–151.

Hoyumpa, A. M. 1982. Characterization of normal intestinal thiamin transport in animals and man. Annals of the New York Academy of Sciences 378:337–343.

Ji, Y. Q., and I. R. Adelman. 1998. Thiaminase activity in alewives and smelt in Lakes Huron, Michigan, and Superior. Pages 154–159 *in* G. McDonald, J. D. Fitzsimons, and D. C. Honeyfield, editors. Early life stage mortality syndrome in fishes of the Great Lakes and Baltic Sea. American Fisheries Society, Symposium 21, Bethesda, Maryland.

Jude, D. J., F. J. Tesar, S. F. Deboe, and T. J. Miller. 1987. Diet and selection of major prey species by Lake Michigan salmonines 1973–1982. Transactions of the American Fisheries Society 116:677–691.

Lawrie, A. H., and J. F. Rahrer. 1972. Lake Superior: effects of exploitation and introductions on the salmonid community. Journal of the Fisheries Research Board of Canada 29:287–295.

Limsuwan T., and R. T. Lovell. 1981. Intestinal synthesis and absorption of vitamin B-12 in channel catfish. Journal of Nutrition 111:2125–2132.

Lovell, R. T., and T. Limsuwan. 1982. Intestinal synthesis and dietary nonessentiality of vitamin B12 for *Tilapia nilotica*. Transactions of the American Fisheries Society 111:485–490.

Masumoto, T., R. W. Hardy, and E. Casillas. 1987. Comparison of transketolase activity and thiamin pyrophosphate levels in erythrocytes and liver of rainbow trout (*Salmo gairdneri*) as indicators of thiamin status. Journal of Nutrition 117:1422–1426.

Miller, B. L., J. C. Meiske, and R. D. Goodrich. 1986a. Effects of dietary additives on B-vitamin production and absorption in steers. Journal of Animal Science 62:484–496.

Miller, B. L., J. C. Meiske, and R. D. Goodrich. 1986b. Effects of grain source and concentrate level on B-vitamin production and absorption in steers. Journal of Animal Science 62:473–483.

Miller, M. A., and M. E. Holey. 1992. Diets of lake trout inhabiting nearshore and offshore Lake Michigan environments. Journal of Great Lakes Research 18:51–60.

Morito, C. L. H., D. H. Conrad, and J. W. Hilton. 1986. The thiamin deficiency signs and requirement of rainbow trout (*Salmo gairdneri*, Richardson). Fish Physiology and Biochemistry 1:93–104.

Morris, P. C., and S. J. Davies. 1995. Thiamin supplementation of diets containing varied lipid:carbohydrate ratios given to gilthead seabream (*Sparus aurata* L.). Animal Science 61:597–603.

Morris, P. C., S. J. Davies, and D. M. Lowe. 1995. Qualitative requirement for B vitamins in diets for the gilthead seabream (*Sparus aurata* L.). Animal Science 61:419–426.

NRC (National Research Council). 1981. Nutrient requirements of coldwater fishes. National Academy Press, Washington, DC.

NRC (National Research Council). 1983. Nutrient requirements of warmwater fishes and shellfishes. National Academy Press, Washington, DC.

Poston, H. A. 1976. Optimum level of dietary biotin for growth, feed utilization, and swimming stamina of fingerling lake trout (*Salvelinus namaycush*). Journal of the Fisheries Research Board of Canada 33:1803–1806.

Shibata, N. 1950. Thiamine contents of various organs in the adult rats. Vitamins 3:23–29.

Shimozono, N., and E. Katsura, editors. 1965. Review of Japanese literature on beriberi and thiamin. Kyoto University, Japan.

Sugita, H., C. Miyajima, and Y. Deguchi. 1991. The vitamin B12 producing ability of the intestinal microflora of freshwater fish. Aquaculture 92:267–276.

Trebukhina, R. V., Y. M. Ostrovsky, V. S. Shapot, G. N. Mikhaltsevich, and V. N. Tumanov. 1985. Turnover of ^{14}C thiamin and activities of thiamin pyrophosphate-dependent enzymes in tissues of mice with Ehrlich ascites carcinoma. Nutrition and Cancer 6:260–273.

Trepsiene, O., K. Jankevicius, and V. Lubianskiene. 1977. Synthesis of B vitamin complex by intestinal bacteria of carps fed on artificial food. Trudy Akadamii Nauk Litovskoi SSR Seriya C3(70):71–78.

Wells, L., and A. L. McLain. 1972. Lake Michigan: effects of exploitation, introduction and eutrophication on the salmonid community. Journal of the Fisheries Research Board of Canada 29:889–898.

Wolf, L. E. 1942. Fish diet disease of trout. Fisheries Research Bulletin 2, New York State Conservation Department, Albany.

Wostmann, B. S., P. L. Knight, and D. F. Kan. 1962. Thiamine in germfree and conventional animals: effect of the intestinal microflora on thiamine metabolism of the rat. Annals of the New York Academy of Sciences 98:516–527.

American Fisheries Society Symposium 21:112–123, 1998

Interspecies Comparisons of Blood Thiamine in Salmonids from the Finger Lakes, and Effect of Maternal Size on Blood and Egg Thiamine in Atlantic Salmon with and without Cayuga Syndrome

JEFFREY P. FISHER[1]
Department of Avian and Aquatic Animal Medicine, College of Veterinary Medicine Cornell University, Ithaca, New York 14853, USA

SCOTT B. BROWN[2]
Department of Fisheries and Oceans, Freshwater Institute Winnipeg, Manitoba R3T 2N6, Canada

STEPHEN CONNELLY
Environmental Conservation-Horticulture Department, Finger Lakes Community College 4355 Lake Shore Drive, Canandaigua, New York 14424-8395, USA

THOMAS CHIOTTI
New York State Department of Environmental Conservation, Region 7 Headquarters 1285 Fisher Avenue, Cortland, New York 13045, USA

CHARLES C. KRUEGER
Department of Natural Resources, Cornell University

Abstract.—A lethal thiamine deficiency afflicting larval landlocked Atlantic salmon *Salmo salar* in several of New York's Finger Lakes has been linked to a maternal diet of the exotic, thiaminase-rich alewife *Alosa pseudoharengus*. To evaluate why trout and char species in the Finger Lakes are apparently not affected by this "Cayuga syndrome," levels of thiamine in the whole blood of syndrome-positive and syndrome-negative stocks of Atlantic salmon were compared with levels in lake trout *Salvelinus namaycush*, brown trout *Salmo trutta*, and rainbow trout *Oncorhynchus mykiss* from Cayuga and/or Seneca lakes. Thiamine levels did not differ between sexes within any species or stock. Consistent with the hypothesis that thermal habitat partitioning may predispose the salmon to more dietary thiaminase than other Finger Lakes salmonids, thiamine levels in the salmon that produced syndrome-positive sac fry were significantly lower than levels measured in Finger Lakes brown trout and rainbow trout. In contrast, there was no difference between the syndrome-positive salmon and Finger Lakes lake trout, possibly because the male char were in starved (postspawned) condition. Regressions of maternal blood or egg thiamine versus maternal weight and length were not significant for salmon that produced syndrome-positive sac fry; yet, a significant inverse relationship was detected for the syndrome-negative salmon from the Adirondack progenitor stock. These findings may reflect the transition of these reference control salmon from a thiaminase-poor invertebrate diet to a piscivorous diet of thiaminase-active smelt *Osmerus mordax*.

Reproduction is impaired in salmonid populations that grow to maturity in the Finger Lakes of New York State (Fisher et al. 1995a), the lower Great Lakes of Canada and the United States (Mac et al. 1985; Skea et al. 1985; Mac and Edsall 1991; Fitzsimons et al. 1995), and the Baltic Sea (Norrgren et al. 1993). In each of these regions, reproductive impairment is observed as "early mortality syndromes" in sac fry (i.e., alevins) or first-feeding fry. In the Finger Lakes (FL), the Cayuga syndrome has afflicted sac fry of landlocked Atlantic salmon *Salmo salar* since at least 1974, when it was first observed (Fisher and Spitsbergen 1990; Fisher et al. 1995a). Affected salmon populations previously identified include those in Cayuga Lake (CL), Seneca Lake (SL), and Keuka Lake (KL). Recent studies have also documented the condition in Atlantic salmon from Green Pond (GP) in the Adirondack Mountains and Otsego Lake (OL), the headwaters of the Susquehanna River (Fisher et al. 1996a).

Every adult female Atlantic salmon captured from CL, SL, and KL produced sac fry with the Cayuga syndrome, and mortality in these sac fry nearly

[1] Present address: Pentec Environmental, Inc., 120 Third Avenue South, Suite 110, Edmonds, Washington 98020, USA.

[2] Present address: Environment Canada, Canada Centre for Inland Waters, 867 Lakeshore Road, Box 5050, Burlington, Ontario L7R 4A6, Canada.

always reached 100% (Fisher et al. 1995a). Nutrition was implicated as a possible mediator of the disease because only populations with diets that included the nonnative, thiaminase-rich alewife *Alosa pseudoharengus* produced sac fry that exhibited syndrome-related mortality (Fisher and Spitsbergen 1990; Fisher et al. 1995a). Evaluations of gross lesions and neurological signs in sac fry with Cayuga syndrome (Fisher et al. 1995b), reduction of mortality after thiamine treatment in lake trout *Salvelinus namaycush* swim-up fry (Fitzsimons 1995) and syndrome-positive Atlantic salmon sac fry (Fisher et al. 1996b), and depressed thiamine concentrations in syndrome-positive offspring of both species (Fisher et al. 1996b) gave strong support to the role of thiamine in these early mortality syndromes.

Multiple salmonid species suffer syndrome-related mortalities in the Great Lakes (Marcquenski and Brown 1997) and Baltic Sea (Norrgren et al. 1998, this volume). In contrast, Cayuga syndrome has been observed in landlocked Atlantic salmon only within the affected FL (Fisher et al. 1995a). For example, the New York State Department of Environmental Conservation (NYSDEC) routinely spawns lake trout from SL for stocking programs and has not previously documented the early mortality syndromes seen in Great Lakes lake trout (Fitzsimons et al. 1995). Likewise, viability investigations of CL rainbow trout *Oncorhynchus mykiss* (Skea et al. 1985) and brown trout *Salmo trutta* (Fisher 1995; Fisher et al. 1995a) did not reveal syndrome-related mortality.

The apparent sensitivity of FL Atlantic salmon to Cayuga syndrome has been a source of confusion and contention. Fisher et al. (1996b) suggested that the Atlantic salmon consumed more thiaminase-rich alewife than other salmonid species because of the preference of both the salmon and the alewife for epilimnetic waters before the salmons' fall spawning season (Lackey 1969, 1970; Brandt et al. 1980; Haynes 1995). Under this hypothesis, the salmon would be exposed to higher concentrations of dietary thiaminase than the more metalimnetic and hypolimnetic brown trout and lake trout (Jude et al. 1987; Haynes 1995). Consequently, the transovarian deposition of thiamine in the salmon would be relatively reduced.

A valid criticism of the "alewife connection" to the Cayuga syndrome is that it ignores other means of inducing thiamine deficiency. For example, the exotic rainbow smelt *Osmerus mordax* is also abundant in the FL and also exhibits thiaminase activity (Deutsch and Ott 1942; Gnaedinger 1964; Ji and Adelman 1998, this volume). Fisher et al. (1995a) considered it unlikely that smelt were responsible for the thiamine deficiency in FL salmon because smelt were the principal diet of salmon in Little Clear Pond (LC), the FL progenitor stock, and no syndrome-related mortality had been seen in the LC sac fry. Thiaminase activity in smelt was also reported to be roughly one-third that in alewife (Gnaedinger 1964). Furthermore, in waters where smelt and alewife coexisted, smelt were confined to the colder, hypolimnetic and metalimnetic waters (Brandt et al. 1980; Jude et al. 1987; Haynes 1995). Thus, there would be fewer opportunities for FL salmon to consume smelt during the summer months. Finally, lake trout and brown trout feed on smelt to at least some extent during the spring, summer, and fall, yet no syndrome-like reproductive problems have been recorded in FL populations of these species.

To address questions raised by the hypothesized dietary association of Cayuga syndrome, we compared blood levels of each thiamine moiety between FL trout and char stocks and landlocked Atlantic salmon that were or were not thiamine-deficient (i.e., syndrome-positive, SYN[+], or syndrome-negative, SYN[−]). These data provide the first evaluation of thiamine blood profiles from multiple salmonid species within the same systems. Because predator size also influences prey preference (Brandt 1986; Jude et al. 1987), we also sought to establish how thiamine levels in the blood and eggs of the landlocked salmon varied with maternal size and whether a difference existed between populations that produced SYN[+] sac fry and those that did not. This latter question was especially important with respect to earlier investigations of the LC sac fry, whose thiamine levels, although severalfold higher than those of SYN[+] sac fry, were comparable with those of lower Great Lakes stocks of lake trout that exhibited variable levels of swim-up mortality (Fisher et al. 1996b).

Materials and Methods

Source of Fish

All Atlantic salmon sampled were captured by electroshocking tributaries or setting trap nets during the fall 1994 spawning migrations or egg harvests (Table 1). The reference control salmon stock for these studies (i.e., LC) is the progenitor source for all lakes stocked with landlocked salmon in New

TABLE 1.—Source and sex of salmon and trout sampled for these studies.

Species sampled	Source of salmon and trout[a]	Male (*N*)	Female (*N*)	UK[b] (*N*)	Date bled
Atlantic salmon	Little Clear Pond	2	10	0	9 November 1994
Salmo salar	Little Clear Pond Hatchery	0	5	0	9 November 1994
	Green Pond	0	1	0	9 November 1994
	Cayuga Lake	3	3	0	21 November 1994
	Otsego Lake	7	11	0	16 November 1994
	Seneca Lake	2[c]	0	0	14 and 17 November 1994
Lake trout	Cayuga Lake	1[d]	0	0	22 May 1994
Salvelinus namaycush	Seneca Lake	4	0	0	17 November 1994
Brown trout	Cayuga Lake	1[d]	0	0	21 May 1994
Salmo trutta	Cayuga Lake	2	5	4	14 and 15 November 1994
	Seneca Lake	2	0	0	17 November 1994
Rainbow trout	Seneca Lake	3	6	4	14 November 1994
Oncorhynchus mykiss	Seneca Lake	0	0	2	15 November 1994
	Seneca Lake	1	4	2	17 November 1994

[a] Salmon, brown trout, and lake trout were sexually mature (i.e., expressed either eggs or milt) at time of sampling, unless otherwise noted.

[b] Sex not recorded.

[c] Immature yearling salmon, no milt expressed.

[d] Sampled from angler catches during annual spring fishing derby; no milt expressed.

York State; this stock subsists naturally on a diet of invertebrates and smelt (Fisher et al. 1995a). The four experimental stocks came from systems with alewife forage (i.e., CL, SL, OL, and GP), and salmon from these systems produce sac fry that die from the Cayuga syndrome (Fisher et al. 1995a, 1996a). Alewives were introduced unintentionally into CL and SL through the building of the Erie Canal in the late 1800s. Alewives were introduced into OL without permission during the late 1980s. Alewives were introduced intentionally into GP in 1957 and 1959 to provide forage for splake *Salvelinus fontinalis* × *S. namaycush*. Three of these systems also have smelt populations (CL, SL, and OL). The hatchery stock (LCH) also originated from LC brood and were fed New York Diet #4, a broodstock diet that is fortified with 2,863 mg/kg thiamine mononitrate. Because smelt also express thiaminase (Gnaedinger 1964; Ji and Adelman 1998), the LCH stock provided a dietary control for this study. Additional stock and watershed characteristics are described elsewhere (Oglesby 1978; Fisher et al. 1995a).

All salmon were ripe at the time of blood sampling except those from CL, one female each from OL and LCH that had already spawned, and the two salmon from SL, which were immature male yearlings. Salmon from CL were transported to the Resource Ecology and Management Facility at Cornell University, where they were held for 2 weeks until ripe in a 2.6-m (diameter) tank with flow-through, dechlorinated CL water. Salmon from CL and GP were killed immediately before sampling with a blow to the head. Salmon from LC, LCH, and OL were briefly anesthetized in tricaine methanesulfonate (MS-222, Sigma Chemical Co., St. Louis, Missouri) before sampling on site and released.

Trout and char (i.e., rainbow trout, brown trout, and lake trout) were collected during efforts to capture salmon on Cayuga and Seneca lakes, with the exception of one brown trout and one lake trout that were donated (live) by anglers during a spring 1994 fishing derby on CL (Table 1). All brown trout caught in the fall were ripe or nearly ripe. Seneca Lake lake trout spawn from late September to mid-October; hence, although the four males captured from SL still expressed milt, they were gaunt and in poor condition, having spawned probably a month or more earlier. Rainbow trout from SL were captured near the mouth of Katherine Creek at the beginning of their spawning run. Spawning of SL rainbow trout occurs in early March in the headwaters of Katherine Creek; thus, they were not ripe at the time of sampling. All trout were sampled in the field and released or transported back to Cornell University and held for a maximum of 4 d in a tank identical to that used to ripen CL salmon.

Blood and Egg Collection

Blood samples were taken from the caudal vein of all salmon, trout, and char captured. Blood was drawn using 22-gauge needles and Vacutainer™ collection ampules, and samples were frozen directly on dry ice. Twenty eggs from each landlocked Atlantic salmon spawned were also frozen to determine thiamine status. Survival of the sac fry progeny from each of the salmon spawned was evaluated in a related study (Fisher et al. 1996a); these survival results were used in the present report only to identify blood samples from salmon that produced SYN[+] offspring. Survival of the progeny from the FL trout and char was not examined because previous studies have indicated that they were not affected by the Cayuga syndrome (Skea et al. 1985; Fisher 1995) and because limited laboratory facilities precluded the monitoring of offspring survival in all the salmonid species captured.

Thiamine Analyses

Gradient reversed phase high-performance liquid chromatography was used to detect and quantify free thiamine, thiamine monophosphate (TMP), and thiamine pyrophosphate (TPP) in the whole blood of all salmonids sampled and in the egg samples of all salmon spawned. The method is described in detail by Brown et al. (1998, this volume). Product recovery in samples spiked with free thiamine ranged from 85 to 90%; recovery in samples spiked with TPP ranged from 80 to 90%. Assay detection limits were 0.002, 0.004, and 0.005 nmol/g for free thiamine, TPP, and TMP, respectively. The coefficient of variation for an egg sample analyzed 6 times was 7.47%; the coefficient of variation for a blood sample analyzed 10 times was 5.96%.

Statistical Analyses

Blood thiamine comparisons.—Differences in mean levels of thiamine in the whole blood were evaluated for significance using one-way analysis of variance (ANOVA) techniques (Zar 1974). Thiamine levels were log-transformed to adjust for heterogeneous variance. Mean levels of thiamine were compared among (1) stock, species, and sex, and (2) sexes within stocks. Findings of significance ($\alpha \leq 0.05$) were followed with the Bonferroni multiple-comparison test.

If the Bonferroni multiple-comparison test did not reveal differences between stocks or between sexes within stocks, then stocks were pooled by species (e.g., blood data from male and female CL and SL brown trout were pooled into "FL brown trout"). The pooling of blood data from salmon stocks was modified slightly from that of trout and char stocks in that it was specifically performed to examine differences between SYN[+] and SYN[−] salmon. For female salmon, syndrome status was determined based on the survival of their sac fry progeny, as discussed above (Fisher et al. 1996a). Because no correlate of thiamine status to male salmon viability has been specifically identified, the syndrome status of male salmon was assigned according to whether their blood levels differed significantly from those of the females of the same stock, unless maturity levels of the salmon would have prevented their consideration as SYN[+]. Thus, the SYN[−] Atlantic salmon group (N = 17) consisted of all male and female salmon from LC, the three female salmon from OL whose progeny did not die from the Cayuga syndrome (Fisher et al. 1996a), and the two immature SL salmon; the LCH salmon were excluded from the SYN[−] group because of their artificial, thiamine-fortified diet. The SYN[+] group (N = 22) consisted of all salmon from CL, GP, and OL, except for the three OL females just described.

Thiamine levels versus maternal size.—Regression analyses were performed to determine whether maternal length or weight of landlocked Atlantic salmon related to the thiamine levels in their blood or eggs. Initially, data from all female salmon were pooled, and regression analyses were performed for each of the thiamine moieties. These graphic analyses suggested clustering of the data that closely corresponded to the SYN[−] and SYN[+] groups (i.e., including both sexes) described in the preceding section. Subsequent regressions were performed to examine whether the effect of maternal size on blood and egg thiamine was different among (1) reference control LC salmon, (2) SYN[−] salmon, and (3) salmon that produced SYN[+] sac fry (H_o, $\beta = 0$; H_a, $\beta \neq 0$). The SYN[−] group included the control LC females, and the three OL females that produced normal sac fry (Fisher et al. 1996a). The SYN[+] group included the three female CL salmon and the seven female OL salmon whose sac fry died from Cayuga syndrome in the associated study (Fisher et al. 1996a). No weight or length data were available for the GP (SYN[+]) female. Likewise, the LCH salmon were excluded from the SYN[−] group because of their artificial diet. All statistical calculations were assisted by Data Desk version 4.1 (Data Description, Inc., Ithaca, New York).

Results

Interspecies and Stock Comparisons of Blood Thiamine

The principal form of thiamine detected in the whole blood of all species and stocks was the pyrophosphate moiety, constituting from 70.7 (SL rainbow trout) to 90% (SL brown trout) of the total thiamine in the systemic circulation (Figure 1). Concentrations of TMP and free thiamine were more variable between stocks and species than TPP or total thiamine levels (Figure 2). Thiamine monophosphate ranged from 3.5 to 20% of total thiamine in the blood, whereas free thiamine ranged from 2.9 to 14.9% of the total.

Thiamine levels did not differ between sexes within stocks, so data from both sexes were pooled by stock and ANOVAs were computed again. Levels of each thiamine moiety differed between stocks and species ($F_{\text{log TMP}}$ = 9.065, df – 11, 78; $F_{\text{log TPP}}$ = 8.365; $F_{\text{log free thiamine}}$ = 8.0783; $F_{\text{log total thiamine}}$ = 11.426). Reflective of their diet fortified with free thiamine, the LCH stock had the highest levels of systemic thiamine for nearly every moiety (Figures 1 and 2); however, the levels did not differ significantly from those found in the SYN[−] LC salmon. Thiamine levels in the blood of the naturally fortified SL rainbow trout were also exceptionally high and did not differ from those of the LC control stock. Despite

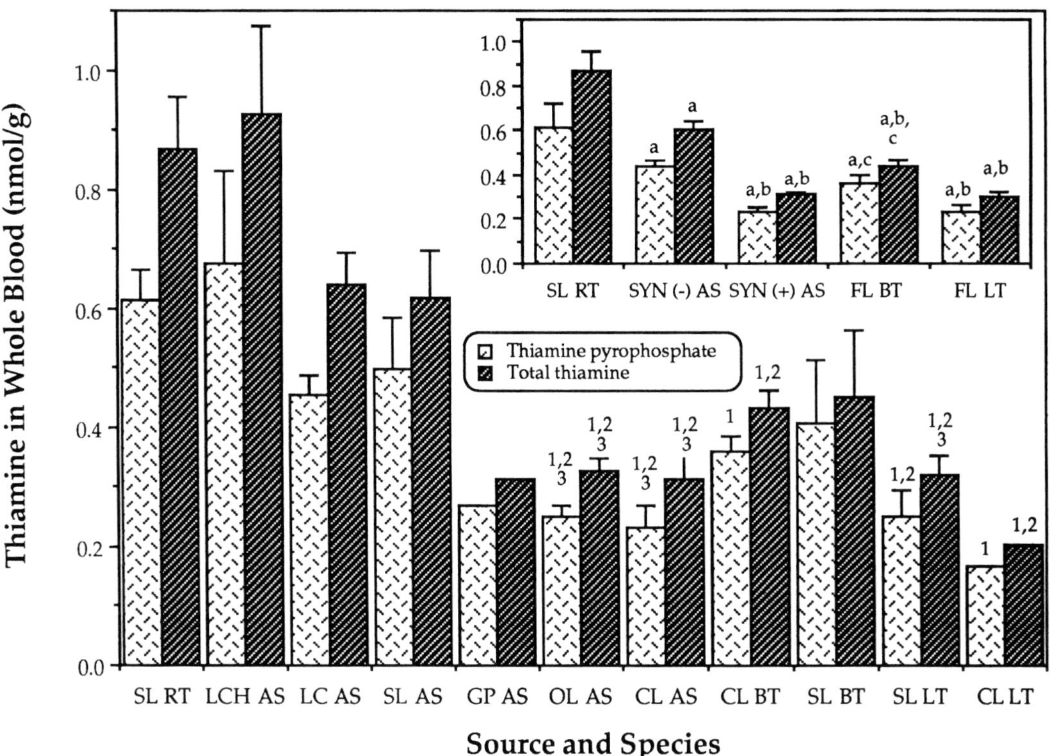

FIGURE 1.—Thiamine pyrophosphate and total thiamine concentrations in the whole blood of salmon, trout, and char populations from lakes with syndrome-positive (SYN[+]) and syndrome-negative (SYN[−]) Atlantic salmon stocks. Codes, from left to right, depict the following stocks and species: Seneca Lake rainbow trout (SL RT, N = 22), Little Clear Hatchery Atlantic salmon (LCH AS, N = 5), Little Clear Pond Atlantic salmon (LC AS, N = 12), Seneca Lake Atlantic salmon (SL AS, N = 2), Green Pond Atlantic salmon (GP AS, N = 1), Otsego Lake Atlantic salmon (OL AS, N = 18), Cayuga Lake Atlantic salmon (CL AS, N = 6), Cayuga Lake brown trout (CL BT, N = 17), Seneca Lake brown trout (SL BT, N = 2), Seneca Lake lake trout (SL LT, N = 4), and Cayuga Lake lake trout (CL LT, N = 1). Significance of multiple comparisons are depicted as: 1 = different from SL RT, 2 = different from LCH AS, and 3 = different from LC AS ($P \leq 0.05$). The inset depicts the pooled species or stock data as described in the text. Categories from left to right are: SL RT (N = 22), SYN[−] Atlantic salmon (N = 17); SYN[+] Atlantic salmon (N = 22), Finger Lakes (FL) brown trout (N = 5), and FL lake trout (N = 4). Significance of multiple comparisons depicted in the inset are as follows: a = different from SL RT, b = different from SYN[−] AS, and c = different from SYN[+] AS ($P \leq 0.05$).

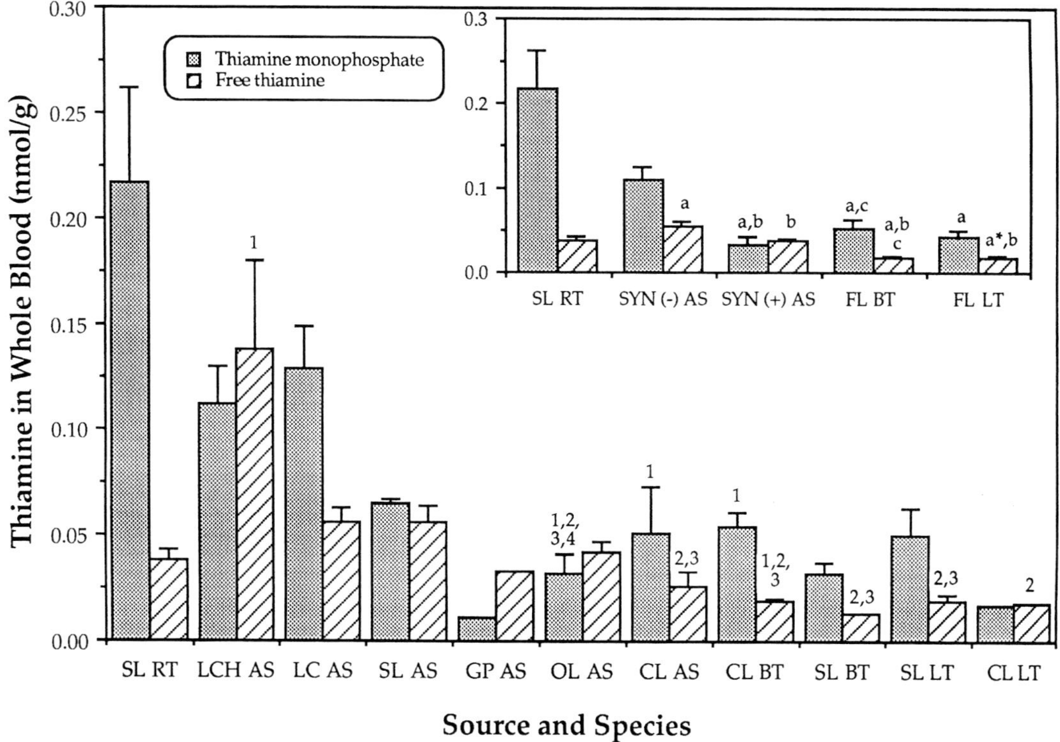

FIGURE 2.—Thiamine monophosphate and free thiamine concentrations in the whole blood of salmon, trout, and char populations from lakes with syndrome-positive (SYN[+]) and syndrome-negative (SYN [−]) Atlantic salmon stocks. Codes, from left to right, depict the following stocks and species: Seneca Lake rainbow trout (SL RT, N = 22), Little Clear Hatchery Atlantic salmon (LCH AS, N = 5), Little Clear Pond Atlantic salmon (LC AS, N = 12), Seneca Lake Atlantic salmon (SL AS, N = 2), Green Pond Atlantic salmon (GP AS, N = 1), Otsego Lake Atlantic salmon (OL AS, N = 18), Cayuga Lake Atlantic salmon (CL AS, N = 6), Cayuga Lake brown trout (CL BT, N = 17), Seneca Lake brown trout (SL BT, N = 2), Seneca Lake lake trout (SL LT, N = 4), and Cayuga Lake lake trout (CL LT, N = 1). Significance of multiple comparisons are depicted as: 1 = different from SL RT, 2 = different from LCH AS, 3 = different from LC AS, and 4 = different from CL BT ($P \leq 0.05$). The inset depicts the pooled species or stock data as described in the text. Categories from left to right include: SL RT (N = 22), SYN[−] Atlantic salmon (N = 17), SYN[+] Atlantic salmon (N = 22), Finger Lakes (FL) brown trout (N = 5), and FL lake trout (N = 5). Significance of multiple comparisons depicted in the inset are as follows: a = different from SL RT, b = different from SYN[−] AS, and c = different from SYN[+] AS ($P \leq 0.05$, $^*P \leq 0.01$).

previous documentation of Cayuga syndrome in sac fry offspring from female SL salmon, blood levels of thiamine in the immature male SL Atlantic salmon were not different from those of the SYN[−] LC control stocks. Further multiple comparisons revealed that syndrome-afflicted CL, OL, and GP stocks generally had the lowest levels of circulating thiamine, usually significantly lower than those measured in the LCH Atlantic salmon, LC Atlantic salmon, and SL rainbow trout (Figures 1 and 2). Thiamine levels in the blood of brown trout and lake trout from CL and SL were also significantly lower than those from LC (SYN[−]) salmon and SL rainbow trout stocks (Figures 1 and 2). Thiamine concentrations in the blood of lake trout from CL and SL were not different from those in SYN[+] Atlantic salmon stocks.

Thiamine Comparisons between Species and Stocks: Pooled Data

If Bonferroni multiple comparisons did not reveal significant differences between stocks of the same species, data were pooled by species and ANOVAs were recomputed, thereby increasing the power of the test. Thus, whole blood data were pooled for each trout and char species, and their thiamine

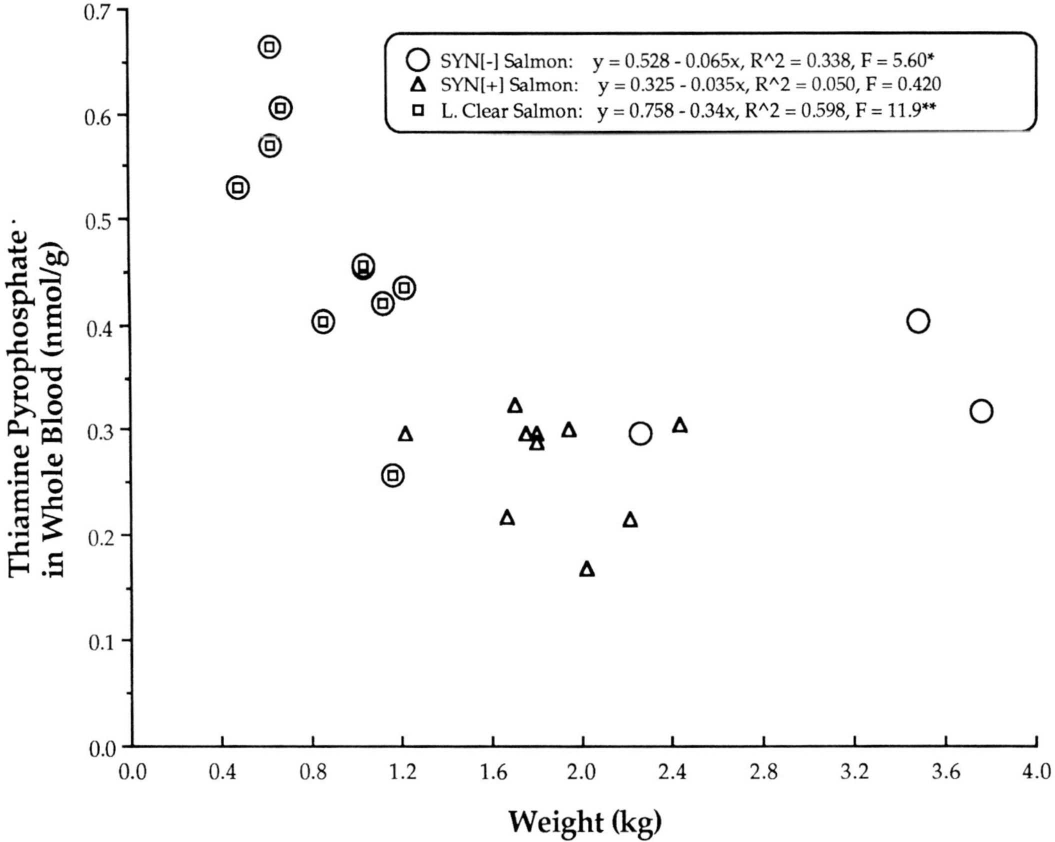

FIGURE 3.—Scatterplots and regressions of whole blood thiamine pyrophosphate versus weight in mature female Atlantic salmon. Little Clear Pond reference control salmon and syndrome-negative Otsego Lake salmon = SYN[−]. Cayuga Lake and syndrome-positive Otsego Lake salmon ($*P \leq 0.05$, $**P \leq 0.01$) = SYN[+].

levels were compared with those found in landlocked salmon that produced either SYN[+] or SYN[−] offspring (Figures 1 and 2, insets).

The ANOVA of the pooled stock data revealed significant differences ($P \leq 0.0001$) between stocks for mean levels of each thiamine moiety ($F_{\text{log TMP}} = 19.387$, df = 4, 80; $F_{\text{log TPP}} = 24.177$; $F_{\text{log free thiamine}} = 13.751$; $F_{\text{log total thiamine}} = 29.068$). The SYN[−] Atlantic salmon had significantly more TPP and total thiamine in their blood than the SYN[+] Atlantic salmon and the FL brown trout and lake trout. The SYN[−] Atlantic salmon also had more TMP than the SYN[+] Atlantic salmon and more free thiamine than all of the other stocks (Figures 1 and 2, insets). Thiamine concentrations in SL rainbow trout exceeded those found in SYN[−] Atlantic salmon for all moieties except free thiamine.

Multiple comparisons of thiamine levels were also performed to isolate differences in thiamine levels between SYN[+] salmon and FL trout and char. Seneca Lake rainbow trout had between twofold and threefold more TMP, TPP, and total thiamine than SYN[+] Atlantic salmon, FL brown trout, and FL lake trout (Figures 1 and 2, insets). Similarly, FL brown trout blood had significantly higher concentrations of TMP, TPP, and total thiamine than the blood from Atlantic salmon with SYN[+] offspring. In contrast, thiamine levels in the blood of FL lake trout and SYN[+] Atlantic salmon did not differ.

Blood and Egg Thiamine versus Maternal Size

Maternal length and weight of the landlocked salmon were inversely related to the blood and egg concentrations of each thiamine moiety. Because TPP was the most concentrated moiety in blood and free thia-

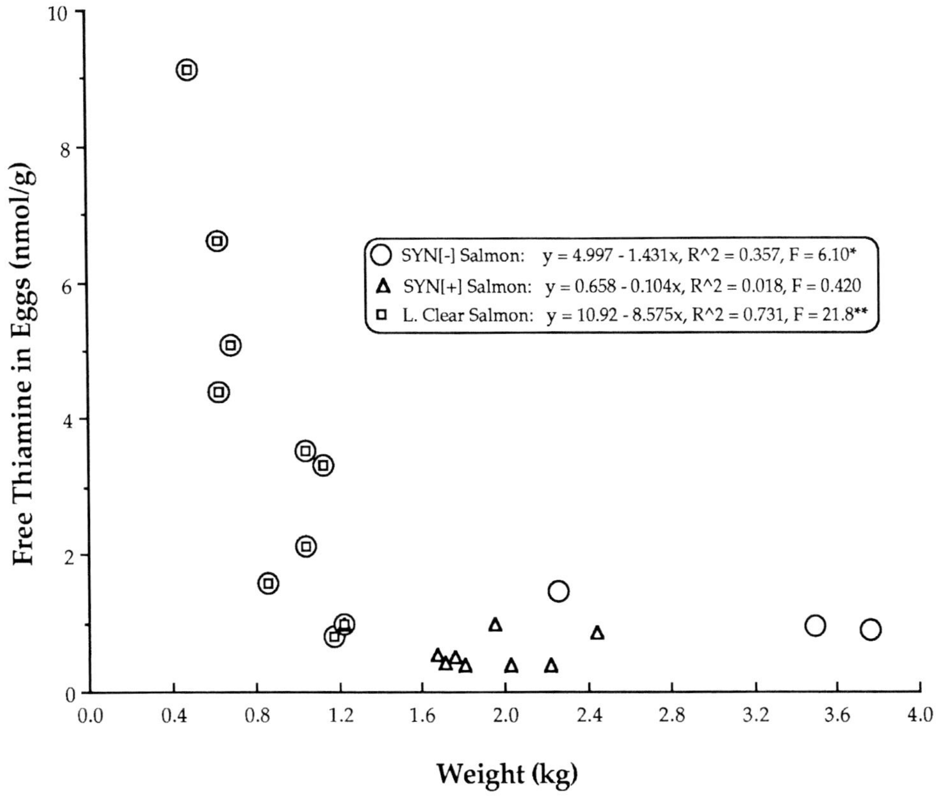

FIGURE 4.—Scatterplots and regressions of egg free thiamine versus weight in mature female Atlantic salmon. Little Clear Pond reference control salmon and syndrome-negative Otsego Lake salmon = SYN[−]. Cayuga Lake and syndrome-positive Otsego Lake salmon ($*P \leq 0.05$, $**P \leq 0.01$) = SYN[+].

mine was the most concentrated moiety in eggs, only these regression analyses are presented. Similarly, weight was a slightly better predictor of thiamine status than length; thus, only weight data are shown. The graphic relationships identified were somewhat curvilinear, roughly corresponding to the natural groupings of SYN[−] LC salmon (i.e., with or without the three SYN[−] OL salmon) and SYN[+] salmon. For the blood, regressions of TPP versus length and weight were highly significant for salmon with SYN[−] sac fry but insignificant for salmon with SYN[+] sac fry (Figure 3). For the eggs, regressions of free thiamine versus length and weight were highly significant for salmon with SYN[−] sac fry but again insignificant for salmon with SYN[+] sac fry (Figure 4).

Discussion

The current results reveal that whole blood measurements are sufficiently robust to detect substantial interspecies and intraspecies differences in thiamine status of salmonids that feed to varying degrees on forage species that express thiaminase. Hematocrit and washed packed cell volume were not essential to assess the relationship between blood and egg thiamine profiles in this field-based study. Finger Lakes rainbow trout and brown trout and mature Atlantic salmon that produced SYN[−] sac fry had thiamine levels significantly higher than Atlantic salmon that produced SYN[+] sac fry. Thiamine levels in the blood of SL rainbow trout exceeded those in all other stocks. It was not possible in the current study to monitor the viability of the SL rainbow trout eggs and sac fry. However, total thiamine concentrations in the blood of SL rainbow trout were more than twofold higher than the maternal blood threshold in Atlantic salmon (i.e., 0.44 nmol/g) that prevented syndrome-related mortality in their sac fry progeny (J. P. Fisher, unpublished observations). Given the high levels of thiamine in the SL rainbow trout, the previous demonstration of high viability in CL rainbow trout (Skea et al. 1985), and the great physical and chemical similarities between SL and CL (Oglesby 1978), it is unlikely that SL rainbow trout suffer mortality akin to the Cayuga or swim-up syndromes.

The current study revealed that TPP was the principal form of thiamine in the blood of all salmonid species investigated, which is in agreement with similar findings in mammals (Combs 1992). Indeed, the relative proportion of the thiamine moieties differed little between the SYN[−] Atlantic salmon, trout, and char species. Given the roles of TPP in bioenergetics (e.g., TPP serves as a critical cofactor in the metabolism of pyruvate and α-ketoglutaric acid), it is understandable that this thiamine moiety predominated in the blood. In SYN[+] salmon, TPP levels were depressed out of proportion with regard to the other moieties. These results indicate that TPP represents the most sensitive indicator of thiamine status in blood and suggest that the quantification of other thiamine moieties may not be necessary for the general screening of thiamine status in the field.

In the current study, evidence that alewife consumption is the cause of depressed thiamine levels was consistent with that presented previously (Fisher et al. 1995a). Salmon from two systems with alewife and marginal (OL) or nonexistent (GP) smelt populations had significantly reduced thiamine levels in their blood. In contrast, the ability of smelt to depress thiamine levels was also suggested by (1) the insignificant difference in thiamine levels in the blood of syndrome-afflicted landlocked salmon (presumed alewife consumption before spawning) and FL lake trout (presumed smelt and alewife consumption), and (2) the significant inverse relationship between growth and thiamine levels in the blood of reference control LC salmon, which presumably increase their consumption of smelt (there is no alewife in LC) as their size increases.

The high levels of thiamine in the blood of SL rainbow trout may reflect the consumption of zooplankton and benthic invertebrates (Jude et al. 1987; N. D. McBride and K. Sanford, NYSDEC, unpublished data, 1996). Such forage species have not been demonstrated to express high thiaminase activity. In turn, predation on thermally partitioned prey reflects the wide temperature tolerance of this species (Haynes et al. 1986). On the basis of Halver's (1989) dietary recommendations for salmonid thiamine requirements (i.e., 33–55 nmol/g), Fitzsimons et al. (1998, this volume) found that Great Lakes invertebrate resources such as *Mysis relicta* and *Diporeia* species have enough thiamine to prevent deficiencies. It remains to be seen whether these invertebrates, which are also significant forage species for SL rainbow trout, also express thiaminase. Given the high levels of thiamine in the SL rainbow trout and the observations that blood thiamine is rapidly reduced in salmonids fed alewife (Ji et al. 1998, this volume) or the thiamine antagonist amprolium (Fynn-Aikins et al., in press), it is unlikely that the invertebrate prey of salmonids in the FL pose any risk to thiamine nutrition.

The current data showing that brown trout have higher levels of circulating thiamine than Atlantic salmon are also consistent with the hypothesis that brown trout may be eating less thiaminase-rich alewife because of their preference for colder waters within the thermocline (and for the more diversified diet found therein; Jude et al. 1987; Haynes 1995). These data support previous observations of high viability of this species' sac fry in CL and SL (Fisher 1995; Fisher et al. 1995a). Thiamine levels in brown trout from the pooled FL stocks (i.e., FL brown trout in insets to Figures 1 and 2) are, nonetheless, near the survival threshold for maternal blood thiamine in landlocked salmon. Furthermore, despite their elevated levels relative to those of the SYN[+] salmon, they are significantly depressed relative to levels in the SL rainbow trout and the SYN[−] stocks of Atlantic salmon. These data strongly suggest that the FL brown trout are consuming enough thiaminase (probably from a variety of both alewife and smelt) to depress their thiamine levels, but not to a critical level for this species. It is also possible that the brown trout are less sensitive to the effects of thiaminase than the Atlantic salmon.

One of the most surprising findings in the present study was the very low level of thiamine detected in the blood of male SL and CL lake trout. The SL lake trout stock has been captured and cultured routinely for years without documentation of syndrome-related mortality, and the viability of the CL stock was confirmed during earlier studies of the Cayuga syndrome (Fisher 1995). However, in this volume Fitzsimons et al. (1998) report levels of thiamine in SL lake trout eggs of approximately 1.5 nmol/g, less than half the proposed threshold for survival of lake trout swim-up fry from Lake Ontario. Apparently, about 5% swim-up mortality was also seen in the fry from these eggs (K. Osika, NYSDEC, Bath Hatchery, unpublished data). The low levels of thiamine in the blood of male lake trout described here are consistent with the depressed levels seen in the eggs from the subsequent 1995 year-class examined by Fitzsimons et al. (1998).

Several scenarios may explain the low levels of thiamine in SL lake trout blood relative to those found in lower Great Lakes stocks (Fisher et al. 1996b; Fitzsimons et al. 1998). First, the lake trout and/or alewife may be less thermally restricted in SL than they are in Lakes Michigan (Wells 1968; Brandt et al. 1980) and Ontario (Haynes 1995). Thus, they may be eating more alewife than was suggested previously (Fisher et al. 1996b). Second, the lake trout may increase their consumption of smelt in the summer, as shown in Lakes Michigan (Jude et al. 1987) and Ontario (Elrod 1983), but the activity of the smelt thiaminase may be comparable with that of alewife (Ji and Adelman 1998) rather than lower, as demonstrated previously (Gnaedinger 1964). Third, thiamine levels recorded in male lake trout may be erroneously low as a result of their starved, postspawned condition. Finally, factors in the diets of salmonids from the lower Great Lakes, such as contaminants that induce lipid peroxidation (Palace et al. 1998, this volume), may accelerate thiamine metabolism (Lychko et al. 1987) and possibly lead to a higher requirement for the vitamin (Fisher et al. 1995b).

Given the results of numerous studies indicating that smelt are displaced to deeper, colder waters when they are in competition with alewife (Wells 1968; Brandt et al. 1980; Hartman 1988), it seems unlikely that the lake trout in Seneca and Cayuga lakes are consuming only alewife during the critical summer and fall months of oogenesis. In the FL (Youngs and Oglesby 1972), OL (McBride and Sanford, unpublished data), and GP (R. Preall, NYSDEC, region 5, personal communication), salmonid species appear to be vertically stratified only during the summer and fall, when the thermocline is established and stable. Hence, it is conceivable that during periods of thermal stratification, gut content analyses would reveal an increased proportion of smelt and deepwater coregonids in lake trout, a "mixed bag" of smelt, alewife, and midwater invertebrates (e.g., *Mysis* species) in brown trout, and a nearly exclusive diet of alewife in the epilimnetic Atlantic salmon. With this schema, one would also expect little to no interspecies differences in forage items from gut contents of salmonids taken in the winter and spring.

As a preliminary test of this hypothesis, we acquired gut contents from lake trout (N = 11), brown trout (N = 4), landlocked Atlantic salmon (N = 3), and rainbow trout (N = 2) from the spring fishing derby on CL mentioned above. Both smelt and alewife were found in the stomachs of each species except rainbow trout (the stomachs of which were empty or the contents unidentifiable), and the smelt was always more digested than the alewife. These early results lend support for the lack of thermal partitioning during the spring. Similar results were obtained by NYSDEC personnel during an April 1990 investigation: both smelt and alewife were found in the stomachs of lake trout, rainbow trout, brown trout, and landlocked salmon. In contrast, only alewife was identified in the stomachs of nine adult (i.e., piscivorous) lake trout ($\geq$500 mm) collected in August 1990 (T. Chiotti, NYSDEC, unpublished data), a clear departure from what might be expected from thermal habitat partitioning. More gut content samples are needed from each season to determine whether thermal habitat partitioning can account for the apparent species sensitivity for thiamine deficiency among salmonids in the FL.

Although thiaminase activity has been demonstrated in rainbow smelt (Deutsch and Ott 1942; Deutsch and Hasler 1943; Nielands 1947; Gnaedinger 1964; Ji and Adelman 1998), the ability of smelt diets to produce thiamine deficiency in salmonids under controlled conditions has been equivocal (Wolf 1942; Coble 1965; Ji et al. 1998). The stability of the enzyme in smelt and its ability (or inability) to induce thiamine deficiency in lake trout and other salmonids may be affected, in part, by its digestibility relative to that of alewife and other thiaminase-containing forage species (e.g., buckeye shiner *Notropis atherinoides*; Wolf 1942). Thus, thiaminase activity measured in smelt may be similar to that of alewife, as found by Ji and Adelman (1998), but its functionality in vivo may not account for the thiamine deficiency in lake trout. It could be reasoned that a deficiency contributed by smelt is more the result of the lower levels of thiamine in its tissues (Fitzsimons et al. 1998) than of the thiaminase present in its gut.

Perhaps the data that most support a diet–thiaminase connection to reproductive failure in salmonids (be it caused by alewife, smelt, or a combination thereof) comes, surprisingly enough, from the present study, in which blood and egg thiamine levels in the SYN[−] LC Atlantic salmon were regressed against maternal growth indices (Figures 3 and 4). The LC stock lacks an alewife forage, does not show evidence of reproductive impairment (Fisher et al. 1995a, 1995b), and has significantly more blood and egg thiamine than the syndrome-afflicted FL, OL, and GP stocks (Fisher et al. 1996a, 1996b). Yet, larger LC salmon had substantially less thiamine than smaller LC salmon (Figures 3 and 4). Levels of total thiamine in the sac fry of the LC stock averaged 3.06 nmol/g in the 1994 year-class (Fisher et al. 1996a) and 1.86 nmol/g in the 1993 year-class (Fisher et al. 1996b), both below the threshold of 3.3 nmol/g proposed for lake trout survival (Fitzsimons and Brown 1998). Although smelt are considered the primary forage species of LC Atlantic salmon, populations of golden shiner *Notemigonus crysoleucas*, pumpkinseed sunfish *Lepomis gibbosus*, white sucker *Catostomus commersoni*, and brook trout *Salvelinus fontinalis* are also present (R. Foster, NYSDEC, Adirondack Hatchery, personal communication). Data depicted in Figures 3 and 4 suggest that LC salmon shift their diet as they grow from prey items with low or nonexistent thiaminase to the thiaminase-active (and larger) rainbow smelt. This switch to piscivory thus gradually reduces thiamine levels over time; however, reproduction is not impaired in the LC salmon because either they have not targeted smelt for a long enough period to reduce their thiamine intake to a critical level or the smelt diet is not capable of reducing thiamine levels to a great enough degree to cause reproductive impairment, for whatever reason (e.g., digestibility, thiaminase activity, etc.). Similarly, regressions of blood thiamine versus weight or length of SYN[+] salmon were not significant because maternal blood levels were already below the critical threshold necessary for thiamine deposition to occur in the eggs.

Acknowledgments

This work was supported by National Oceanic and Atmospheric Administration award NA 46RG0090 to the Research Foundation of the State University of New York for the New York Sea Grant Institute. Unpublished information on alewife and other fish populations in Otsego Lake, Green Pond, and Little Clear Pond was provided by R. Fieldhouse, R. Preall, and R. Foster (NYSDEC, Albany, New York), respectively. Assistance with study execution was also provided by P. R. Bowser and G. Wooster (Cornell University, Aquatic Animal Health Program, College of Veterinary Medicine, Ithaca, New York).

References

Brown, S. B., D. C. Honeyfield, and L. Vandenbyllaardt. 1998. Thiamine analysis in fish tissues. Pages 73–81 *in* McDonald et al. (1998).

Brandt, S. B. 1986. Food of trout and salmon in Lake Ontario. Journal of Great Lakes Research 12:200–205.

Brandt, S. B., J. J. Magnuson, and L. B. Crowder. 1980. Thermal habitat partitioning by fishes in Lake Michigan. Canadian Journal of Fisheries and Aquatic Sciences 37:1557–1564.

Coble, D. D. 1965. Effects of a diet of raw smelt on lake trout. Canadian Fish Culturist 36:27–34.

Combs, G. F., Jr. 1992. The vitamins. Academic Press, San Diego, California.

Deutsch, H. F., and A. D. Hasler. 1943. Distribution of a vitamin B-1 destructive enzyme in fish. Proceedings of the Society for Experimental Biology and Medicine 53:63–65.

Deutsch, H. F., and G. L. Ott. 1942. Mechanism of vitamin B-1 destruction by a factor in raw smelt. Proceedings of the Society for Experimental Biology and Medicine 51:119–122.

Elrod, J. H. 1983. Seasonal food of juvenile lake trout in U.S. waters of Lake Ontario. Journal of Great Lakes Research 9:396–402.

Fisher, J. P. 1995. Early life stage mortality of Atlantic salmon, *Salmo salar*, epizootiology of the 'Cayuga syndrome.' Doctoral dissertation. Cornell University, Ithaca, New York.

Fisher, J. P., S. Brown, P. R. Browser, G. A. Wooster, and T. Chiotti. 1996a. Continued investigations into the role of thiamine and thiaminese-rich forage in the Cayuga syndrome of New York's landlocked Atlantic salmon. Pages 79–81 *in* B.-E. Bengtsson, C. Hill, and S. Nellbring, editors. Report from the second workshop on reproduction disturbances in fish. Swedish Environmental Protection Agency Report 4534, Stockholm.

Fisher, J. P., J. D. Fitzsimons, G. F. Combs, Jr., and J. M. Spitsbergen. 1996b. Naturally occurring thiamine deficiency causing reproductive failure in Finger Lakes Atlantic salmon and Great Lakes lake trout. Transactions of the American Fisheries Society 125:167–178.

Fisher, J. P., and six coauthors. 1995a. Reproductive failure in landlocked Atlantic salmon from New York's Finger Lakes: investigations into the etiology and epidemiology of the "Cayuga syndrome." Journal of Aquatic Animal Health 7:81–94.

Fisher, J. P., and J. M. Spitsbergen. 1990. Investigations into the Cayuga Lake Atlantic salmon *Salmo salar* syndrome. Pages 16–19 *in* M. Gilbertson, editor. Proceedings of the roundtable on contaminant-caused reproductive problems in salmonids. International Joint Commission, Windsor, Ontario.

Fisher, J. P., J. M. Spitsbergen, T. Iamonte, E. E. Little, and A. DeLonay. 1995b. Pathological and behavioral manifestations of the "Cayuga syndrome," a thiamine deficiency in larval landlocked Atlantic salmon. Journal of Aquatic Animal Health 7:269–283.

Fitzsimons, J. D. 1995. The effect of B-vitamins on a swim-up syndrome in Lake Ontario lake trout. Journal of Great Lakes Research 21 (Supplement 1):286–289.

Fitzsimons, J. D., and S. B. Brown. 1998. Reduced egg thiamine levels in inland and Great Lakes lake trout and their relationship with diet. Pages 160–171 *in* McDonald et al. (1998).

Fitzsimons, J. D., S. B. Brown, and L. Vandenbyllaardt. 1998. Thiamine levels in food chains of the Great Lakes. Pages 90–98 *in* McDonald et al. (1998).

Fitzsimons, J. D., S. Huestis, and B. Williston. 1995. Occurrence of a swim-up syndrome in Lake Ontario lake trout and the effects of cultural practices. Journal of Great Lakes Research 21 (Supplement 1): 227–285.

Fynn-Aikins, K., P. R. Bowser, D. C. Honeyfield, J. D. Fitzsimons, and H. G. Ketola. In press. Effect of dietary amprolium on tissue thiamin and Cayuga syndrome in Atlantic salmon. Transactions of the American Fisheries Society.

Gnaedinger, R. H. 1964. Thiaminase activity in fish: an improved assay method. Fishery Industrial Research 2:55–59.

Halver, J. E. 1989. Fish nutrition, second edition. Academic Press, Toronto.

Hartman, W. L. 1988. Historical changes in the major fish resources of the Great Lakes. Pages 103–131 *in* M. S. Evans, editor. Toxic contaminants and ecosystem health: a Great Lakes focus. Wiley, New York.

Haynes, J. M. 1995. Thermal ecology of salmonids in lake Ontario. Great Lakes Research Review 2:17–22.

Haynes, J. M., and five coauthors. 1986. Movements of rainbow steelhead trout (*Salmo gairdneri*) in Lake Ontario and a hypothesis for the influence of spring thermal structure. Journal of Great Lakes Research 12:304–313.

Honeyfield, D. C., J. G. Hnath, J. Copeland, K. Dabrowski, and J. H. Blom. 1998. Correlation of nutrients and environmental contaminants in Lake Michigan coho salmon with incidence of early mortality syndrome. Pages 135–145 *in* McDonald et al. (1998).

Ji, Y. Q., and I. R. Adelman. 1998. Thiaminase activity in alewives and smelt in Lakes Huron, Michigan, and Superior. Pages 154–159 *in* McDonald et al. (1998).

Ji, Y. Q., J. J. Warthesen, and I. R. Adelman. 1998. Thiamine nutrition, synthesis, and retention in relation to lake trout reproduction in the Great Lakes. Pages 99–111 *in* McDonald et al. (1998).

Jude, D. J., F. J. Tesar, S. F. Deboe, and T. J. Miller. 1987. Diet and selection of major prey species by Lake Michigan salmonines, 1973–1982. Transactions of the American Fisheries Society 116:677–691.

Lackey, R. T. 1969. Food interrelationships of salmon, trout alewives and smelt in a Maine lake. Transactions of the American Fisheries Society 98:641–646.

Lackey, R. T. 1970. Seasonal depth distribution of landlocked Atlantic salmon, brook trout, landlocked alewives, and American smelt in a small lake. Journal of the Fisheries Research Board of Canada 27:1656–1661.

Lychko, A. P., A. A. Pentiuk, and N. B. Lutsiuk. 1987. Effect of various thiamine supplies of the body on the enzyme activity in the metabolism of xenobiotics and lipid peroxidation in rat liver microsomes. Ukrainskii Biokhimicheskii Zhurnal 59:44–49.

Mac, M. J., and C. C. Edsall. 1991. Environmental contaminants and the reproductive success of lake trout in the Great Lakes: an epidemiological approach. Journal of Toxicology and Environmental Health 33:375–394.

Mac, M. J., C. C. Edsall, and J. G. Seelye. 1985. Survival of lake trout eggs and fry reared in water from the upper Great Lakes. Journal of Great Lakes Research 11:520–529.

Marcquenski, S. V., and S. B. Brown. 1997. Early mortality syndrome (EMS) in salmonid fishes from the Great Lakes. Pages 135–152 *in* R. M. Rolland, M. Gilbertson, and R. E. Peterson, editors. Chemically induced alterations in functional development and reproduction of fishes. SETAC (Society of Environmental Toxicology and Chemistry), Pensacola, Florida.

McDonald, G., J. D. Fitzsimons, and D. C. Honeyfield, editors. 1998. Early life stage mortality syndrome in fishes of the Great Lakes and Baltic Sea. American Fisheries Society, Symposium 21, Bethesda, Maryland.

Nielands, J. B. 1947. Thiaminase in aquatic animals of Nova Scotia. Journal of the Fisheries Research Board of Canada 7:94–99.

Norrgren, L., P. Amcoff, H. Börjeson, and P.-O. Larsson. 1998. Reproductive disturbances in Baltic fish: a review. Pages 8–17 *in* McDonald et al. (1998).

Norrgren, L., T. Andersson, P. A. Bergqvist, and I. Bjorklund. 1993. Chemical physiological and morphological studies of feral Baltic salmon (*Salmo salar*) suffering from abnormal fry mortality. Environmental Toxicology and Chemistry 12:2065–2076.

Oglesby, R. T. 1978. The limnology of Cayuga Lake. Pages 2–120 *in* J. A. Bloomfield, editor. Lakes of New York state. Academic Press, New York.

Palace, V. P., S. B. Brown, C. L. Baron, J. D. Fitzsimons, and J. F. Klaverkamp. 1998. Relationship between induction of the phase I enzyme system and oxidative stress: relevance for lake trout from Lake Ontario and early mortality syndrome of their offspring. Pages 146–153 *in* McDonald et al. (1998).

Skea, J. C., J. Symula, and J. Miccoli. 1985. Separating starvation losses from other early feeding fry mortality in steelhead trout *Salmo gairdneri*, chinook salmon *Oncorhynchus tshawytscha*, and lake trout *Salvelinus namaycush*. Bulletin of Environmental Contamination and Toxicology 35:82–91.

Wells, L. 1968. Seasonal depth distribution of fish in southeastern Lake Michigan. U.S. Fish and Wildlife Service Fishery Bulletin 67:1–15.

Wolf, L. E. 1942. Fish diet disease of trout. Fisheries Research Bulletin 2, New York State Conservation Department, Albany.

Youngs, W. D., and R. T. Oglesby. 1972. Cayuga Lake: effects of exploitation and introductions on the salmonid community. Journal of the Fisheries Research Board of Canada 29:787–794.

Zar, J. H. 1974. Biostatistical analysis. Prentice-Hall, Englewood Cliffs, New Jersey.

American Fisheries Society Symposium 21:124–134, 1998

Efficacy of Thiamine, Astaxanthin, β-Carotene, and Thyroxine Treatments in Reducing Early Mortality Syndrome in Lake Michigan Salmonid Embryos[1]

MICHAEL W. HORNUNG
Environmental Toxicology Center, University of Wisconsin, Madison, Wisconsin 53706, USA

LEAH MILLER
School of Pharmacy, University of Wisconsin

RICHARD E. PETERSON[2]
Environmental Toxicology Center and School of Pharmacy, University of Wisconsin

SUSAN MARCQUENSKI
Bureau of Fish Management, Wisconsin Department of Natural Resources Madison, Wisconsin 53707, USA

SCOTT B. BROWN
Environment Canada, Canada Center for Inland Waters Burlington, Ontario L7R 4A6, Canada

Abstract.—Lake Michigan Skamania strain steelhead *Oncorhynchus mykiss* and coho salmon *O. kisutch* fry exhibit an early mortality syndrome (EMS) in which death is preceded by loss of equilibrium, inability or lack of feeding, and general lethargy. It was hypothesized that decreased egg concentrations of carotenoid pigments, thyroxine, or thiamine contributed to this syndrome. Thiamine analyses of Lake Michigan coho salmon eggs from individual family groups exhibited 16–97% EMS if egg total thiamine concentrations were less than 0.9 nmol/g or egg free thiamine concentrations were less than 0.3 nmol/g. In eggs with total or free thiamine concentrations greater than 0.9 or 0.3 nmol/g, respectively, the range of EMS in fry was 5–12%. Immersion of steelhead and coho salmon eggs in 1.4 mM or greater thiamine hydrochloride significantly decreased EMS compared with controls. Immersion of coho salmon eggs in 2.8 mM thiamine increased the mean concentration of free thiamine in the eggs to 1.0 nmol/g, compared with 0.26 nmol/g in controls. Injection of either β-carotene or astaxanthin (0.86 or 8.6 μg/g, respectively) in steelhead eggs did not significantly reduce the occurrence of EMS. Early mortality syndrome was not decreased in steelhead after immersion of eggs in 2 mg/L thyroxine, but it was significantly decreased in steelhead sac fry immersed in 2 mg/L thyroxine. These results suggest that low egg thiamine is a predisposing factor for EMS; however, other factors that are variable among individual coho salmon females may influence the occurrence of EMS-related mortality. Whether the addition of exogenous thiamine corrects a thiamine deficiency or protects fry from developing EMS through some other mechanism is currently unknown.

Coho salmon *Oncorhynchus kisutch*, chinook salmon *O. tshawytscha*, and steelhead *O. mykiss* constitute a significant portion of the Great Lakes multimillion dollar sportfishing industry. Because these species do not sustain their populations through natural reproduction, U.S. states and Canadian provinces bordering the Great Lakes collect returning adult fish and spawn them at hatcheries where the eggs are incubated before release back into the Great Lakes as fingerlings or yearlings. Thus, the production of hatchery-reared salmonids is essential to maintain the populations of these fish in the Great Lakes.

Recent increased mortality of Lake Michigan coho salmon, chinook salmon, and steelhead sac fry and swim-up fry reared in these hatcheries has raised concerns about the ability of the hatcheries to meet their stocking goals. This salmonid mortality, which characteristically occurs at the end of the sac fry stage or early in the alevin stage (after absorption of the yolk) and is preceded by loss of equilibrium, inability or lack of feeding, and general lethargy, is referred to as early mortality syndrome (EMS). The magnitude of the problem may be increasing: EMS-related mortality has increased from 33% in 1988 to 50% for some stocks of steelhead from Wisconsin (Marcquenski 1991).

[1] Portions of this publication were presented at the Second Workshop on Reproductive Disturbances in Fish, Stockholm, Sweden (1995).

[2] To whom correspondence should be addressed at School of Pharmacy, 425 North Charter Street, Madison, Wisconsin 53706, USA.

Possible causes of this mortality syndrome in Lake Michigan were hypothesized based on the occurrence of early life stage mortality syndromes in other salmonid stocks, egg nutriture, and the efficacy of different treatments in reducing mortality resulting from EMS. These included the role of thiamine in early mortality syndromes in lake trout *Salvelinus namaycush* from Lake Ontario (Fitzsimons 1995) and Atlantic salmon *Salmo salar* from New York State (Fisher et al. 1995b, 1996) and the Baltic Sea (Bylund and Lerche 1995). In addition, an association has been observed between concentrations of carotenoid pigments, specifically astaxanthin, in the eggs of Atlantic salmon from the Baltic Sea and a form of early life stage mortality the signs of which are similar to those associated with EMS (Norrgren et al. 1993; Lignell 1994). The documented alteration of thyroid hormone homeostasis in the salmon introduced into the Great Lakes (reviewed by Leatherland 1993) suggested that it too may be a factor involved in EMS.

To evaluate the potential role of thiamine, carotenoids, and thyroid hormone on EMS, several experiments were conducted. The endogenous levels of free thiamine, thiamine monophosphate, and thiamine pyrophosphate in Lake Michigan coho salmon eggs were determined. Newly fertilized steelhead and coho salmon eggs were immersed in water containing graded concentrations of thiamine to determine the concentration required to effectively reduce EMS. The corresponding concentration of thiamine in the eggs was determined after immersion. Additionally, steelhead eggs were microinjected with the carotenoid pigments astaxanthin or β-carotene to determine whether increasing the egg carotenoid concentrations would reduce EMS. Finally, steelhead eggs and newly hatched embryos were treated with thyroxine in an attempt to reduce EMS in the fry.

Methods

Egg Thiamine and EMS Levels in Lake Michigan Coho Salmon

In 1993 and 1994, coho salmon eggs were collected from gravid females (N = 10 in 1993, N = 8 in 1994) from Lake Michigan and fertilized with milt pooled from several males. An average of 700 eggs from each female were incubated in a 38-L aquarium that received a constant flow of 11 ± 1.5°C dechlorinated tap water (pH 7.6; dissolved oxygen = 9.8 ppm, hardness = 306 ppm $CaCO_3$, alkalinity = 308 ppm). Two days after fertilization, 10 eggs from each group of eggs from an individual female were sampled and flash frozen in liquid N_2. Eggs were shipped on dry ice to the Department of Fisheries and Oceans, Winnipeg, Manitoba, Canada, for thiamine analysis. Homogenates of three eggs from each female were measured by reverse phase high-performance liquid chromatography after conversion of thiamine and the thiamine phosphates to their respective thiochromes (Brown et al. 1998b, this volume).

Eggs were checked weekly for mortality and three times each week from hatch to 4 weeks after yolk absorption for signs of EMS. Signs included a loss of equilibrium as shown by fry swimming on their sides or in a corkscrew pattern, hyperexcitability to touch, lack of feeding, and lethargy (scored as fish lying on their sides on the bottom of the tank).

Immersion of Coho Salmon Eggs in Thiamine

In November 1994, eggs stripped from eight Lake Michigan coho salmon females were fertilized with 2 mL of milt pooled from eight male coho salmon. Immediately after fertilization, eggs were rinsed in water and four replicates of 50 eggs per treatment group were immersed for 2 h during the water-hardening stage in either well water or one of seven thiamine concentrations prepared with thiamine hydrochloride (Sigma Chemical Co., St. Louis, Missouri) as follows: 0.044, 0.089, 0.18, 0.36, 0.71, 1.4, and 2.8 mM (15, 30, 60, 120, 240, 480, and 960 mg/L, respectively). The pH of each solution was between 7.4 and 8.0 except for the 2.8 mM solution, which had a pH < 6.5 before being adjusted to 7.0–7.2 with 1 N NaOH. After immersion, eggs were rinsed three times with fresh well water and placed in 9.5-L aquariums that had a constant supply of 11°C dechlorinated tap water. Coho salmon were monitored for signs of EMS as described above. One day after immersion, five eggs from each replicate treatment group were collected and placed in liquid N_2 for subsequent determination of thiamine.

Immersion of Steelhead Eggs in Thiamine

In February 1995, eggs from six Lake Michigan Skamania strain steelhead were pooled and fertilized with milt from six male steelhead. Two replicates were water-hardened in well water at each thiamine concentration as described above for coho salmon except that no 0.044 or 0.089 mM treatment was used. Five eggs from each replicate treatment group were also sampled as described above for determination of thiamine in eggs. Groups of 60 eggs from these same females were also treated for 2 h in 1.4 mM thiamine hydrochloride at (1) water hardening, (2) hatch (300 cumulative centigrade degree-days after fertilization), (3) 1 week after hatch (375 degree-days), (4) 2 weeks after hatch (450 degree-days), (5) 3 weeks after hatch (525 degree-days), or (6) 4 weeks after hatch (600 degree-days). Additionally, groups of 60 eggs were immersed in 1.4 mM thiamine hydrochloride during water hardening and then individual groups were immersed a second time at one of the later times listed above.

Injection of Steelhead Eggs with Carotenoids

In March 1994, eggs were collected from six Lake Michigan Skamania strain steelhead, pooled, and fertilized for injection with the carotenoids astaxanthin or β-carotene. Astaxanthin (Hoffman-LaRoche, Inc., Nutley, New Jersey) or β-carotene (Sigma) was incorporated into phosphatidylcholine (PC; Avanti Polar Lipids, Alabaster, Alabama) liposomes as follows. Astaxanthin or β-carotene was dissolved in chloroform and quantitatively transferred to 5 mL of 10 mM PC in chloroform. Chloroform was evaporated under vacuum at room temperature, after which the carotenoid and PC were rehydrated with 0.9% sterile saline to give a final carotenoid concentration of 5 mg/mL in 50 mM PC. Astaxanthin or β-carotene in PC was diluted 1:10 with 50 mM PC to produce 0.5 mg/mL solutions. Argon gas was layered over the solutions before they were sonicated to produce unilamellar liposomes (Woodle and Papahadjopoulos 1989). Injection of 0.2 μL of the 5 or 0.5 mg/mL carotenoid stock solutions into the steelhead eggs using the methods of Walker et al. (1992) yielded nominal carotenoid concentrations of 0.86 or 8.6 μg/g, respectively. After injection, eggs within a treatment group were placed in a 400-mL beaker with a continuous flow of water (water quality as above). After hatch, steelhead sac fry were transferred from the beakers to 38-L aquariums to facilitate observation of the signs of EMS.

Immersion of Steelhead in Thyroxine Solutions

A subset of the steelhead eggs collected for the carotenoid injections were left untreated and were incubated to the eyed stage of development. These eyed embryos were immersed in either dechlorinated tap water or L-thyroxine (2 mg/L; L-thyroxine sodium, Sigma) for 1 h in a static water bath. Water temperature increased less than 1°C during this treatment period. After immersion, continuous flow conditions were resumed. This treatment protocol was repeated once the next day. This same 2-d treatment protocol was repeated within 2 d after 100% hatch with a second group of Skamania strain steelhead not previously treated. All fry were monitored for up to 4 weeks after yolk absorption for signs of EMS.

Statistical Analysis

Coho salmon thiamine dose response data were analyzed by Kruskal–Wallis nonparametric analysis of variance (ANOVA), and differences between groups were analyzed by the distribution-free multiple-comparison test with significance set at $P < 0.05$ (Gad and Weil 1991). Thiamine uptake by coho salmon eggs at each dose were compared by one-way ANOVA, and significant differences between groups were determined by t-test at $P < 0.05$. In coho salmon and steelhead, EMS-related mortality between treatment groups for all other treatments were determined by chi-square analysis with differences considered significant at $P < 0.05$. To determine whether there was a difference in the egg concentration of the three thiamine forms among family groups exhibiting low EMS and those exhibiting high EMS, the data were divided into two sets and compared by the Mann–Whitney U-test (Gad and Weil 1991). The two sets were considered significantly different at $P < 0.05$.

Results

Clinical Signs of EMS

Offspring from Lake Michigan coho salmon and steelhead broodstock exhibited loss of equilibrium, hyperexcitability to touch, lethargy, and lack of feeding before death during the late sac fry and early alevin stages. The percentage of EMS-related fry mortality varied considerably among females and ranged from 5 to 97% in family groups of coho salmon and from 5 to 83% in family groups of steelhead.

Relationship between Egg Thiamine Concentrations and EMS

Considerable variation was evident between egg thiamine concentrations and the corresponding occurrence of EMS (Figure 1). To determine whether there was a difference in egg thiamine concentrations between eggs that exhibited high EMS and those that exhibited low EMS, the coho salmon EMS mortality data were divided into two sets. One set included those family groups that exhibited less than

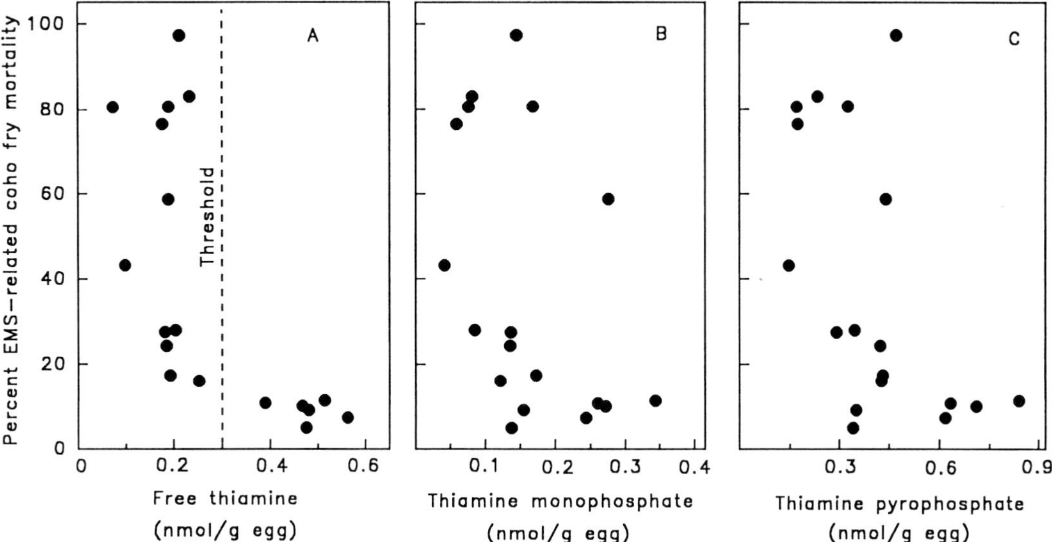

FIGURE 1.—Relationship between free thiamine (A), thiamine monophosphate (B), and thiamine pyrophosphate (C) concentrations in water-hardened eggs of 18 Lake Michigan coho salmon and percentage of EMS-related fry mortality. Each symbol represents the mean thiamine measurement of three eggs from one individual coho salmon female and the corresponding cumulative percentage of fry mortality in offspring from that female. The proposed egg thiamine threshold concentration (0.3 nmol/g), below which EMS-related mortality is highly variable and above which EMS-related mortality is consistently low, is indicated in panel A.

12% EMS (N = 6) and the other group included those family groups that exhibited greater than 16% EMS (N = 12). Coho salmon that exhibited less than 12% EMS had egg free thiamine concentrations (mean ± SE) of 0.48 ± 0.03 nmol/g, egg thiamine monophosphate concentrations of 0.24 ± 0.08 nmol/g, and egg thiamine pyrophosphate concentrations of 0.58 ± 0.20 nmol/g. Those that exhibited greater than 16% EMS had egg free thiamine, thiamine monophosphate, and thiamine pyrophosphate concentrations of 0.18 ± 0.05, 0.12 ± 0.06, and 0.32 ± 0.12 nmol/g, respectively. The egg concentrations of free thiamine, thiamine monophosphate, and thiamine pyrophosphate were significantly greater in the group with low EMS than in the group with high EMS (P = 0.0009, 0.017, and 0.022, respectively).

Effect of Thiamine

Thiamine treatment during water hardening reduced EMS-related fry mortality in both steelhead and coho salmon, but the effect was both species and dose dependent. Immersion of coho salmon eggs in 1.4 or 2.8 mM thiamine significantly reduced EMS mortality, from 29% in controls to 1.4 or 0.6%, respectively ($P < 0.05$; Figure 2). There was a significant increase in total thiamine and free thiamine but not in thiamine monophosphate or thiamine pyrophosphate concentrations in coho salmon eggs after immersion in 2.8 mM thiamine ($P < 0.05$; Figure 2). Immersion of coho salmon eggs in 2.8 mM thiamine increased mean concentration of free thiamine in the eggs to 1.0 nmol/g, compared with 0.26 nmol/g in controls. Immersion of steelhead eggs in 1.4 or 2.8 mM thiamine, but not lower concentrations, significantly reduced EMS mortality, from 72% in controls to 49 or 42%, respectively ($P <$ 0.05; Figure 3). The mean free thiamine in steelhead eggs based on two replicate treatments was 0.61 nmol/g in controls and 1.9 nmol/g in eggs treated with 2.8 mM thiamine.

Treatment of steelhead with 1.4 mM thiamine twice during development was more effective than a single treatment, although it did not completely eliminate EMS-related mortality. A single thiamine treatment significantly ($P < 0.05$) reduced EMS-related mortality, from 71% in controls to 40–48% in those groups treated at the six developmental stages, except at 375 centigrade degree-days (Table 1). When two treatments were used, once at water hardening and once again at either 525 or 600 centigrade degree-days, EMS-related mortality was significantly reduced compared with a single treatment at either of these times. This second treatment reduced EMS to 26 or 33%, compared with 40–48% for a single treatment.

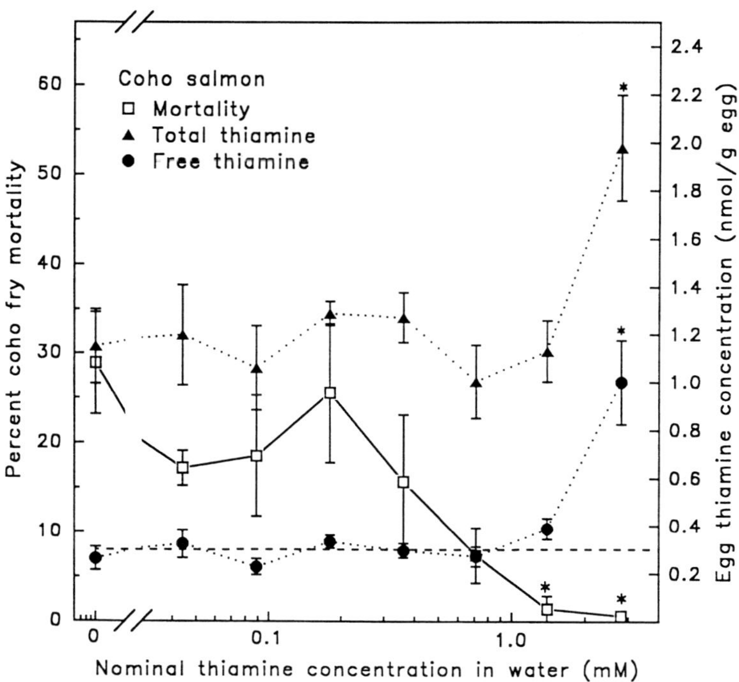

FIGURE 2.—Thiamine dose response curves for coho salmon (□) and uptake of total thiamine (▲) and free thiamine (●) in eggs after immersion in water containing graded concentrations of thiamine hydrochloride. Symbols represent the mean ± SE ($N = 4$). Asterisks indicate mortality significantly less than control or thiamine concentrations significantly greater than control ($P < 0.05$). The dashed line indicates the threshold level of egg free thiamine (0.3 nmol/g) for coho salmon suggested from the endogenous thiamine concentrations shown in Figure 1.

Effect of Carotenoid Treatment

Injection of newly fertilized Lake Michigan steelhead eggs (pooled from six females) with β-carotene or astaxanthin did not significantly reduce EMS mortality compared with controls. Control steelhead fry injected as eggs with PC alone exhibited 42% (10 of 24 fry) EMS. Eggs injected with astaxanthin at concentrations of 0.86 or 8.6 μg/g exhibited 35% (9 of 26 fry) or 22% (6 of 27 fry) EMS, respectively. Eggs injected with β-carotene at concentrations of 0.86 or 8.6 μg/g exhibited 37% (10 of 27 fry) or 21% (5 of 24 fry) EMS, respectively.

Effect of Thyroxine

Immersion in thyroxine affected EMS mortality, but this effect was stage dependent. The EMS mortality of 32% (14 of 44 fry) observed in steelhead eyed embryos immersed in thyroxine (2 mg/L) for 1 h on 2 successive days was not significantly different from the 46% (19 of 41 fry) mortality observed in controls. In contrast, immersion of newly hatched steelhead fry in thyroxine (2 mg/L) significantly reduced EMS to 16% (8 of 50 fry), compared with 38% (19 of 50 fry) in controls treated with water only ($P < 0.05$).

Discussion

Egg Thiamine Threshold Levels

The range of endogenous thiamine concentrations determined in Lake Michigan coho salmon eggs and the corresponding incidence of EMS suggests that a threshold concentration of thiamine exists in the eggs. Coho salmon fry with endogenous levels of free thiamine greater than 0.3 nmol/g exhibited low levels of EMS, as shown in Figure 1. Additionally, when free thiamine levels in coho salmon eggs were experimentally increased to more than 0.3 nmol/g, there was a significant reduction in EMS. The variability in incidence of EMS in Lake Michigan coho salmon with free thiamine levels less than the threshold level of 0.3 nmol/g suggests either a variability in responsiveness to thiamine or that other factors are also involved, including chemical and nonchemical stressors, genetic differences, or differences in diet. Although the present study suggests a

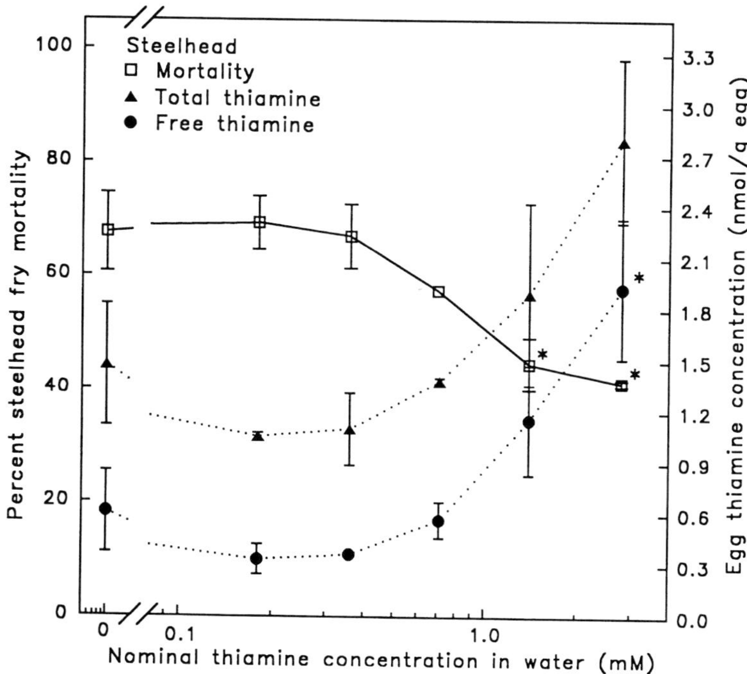

FIGURE 3.—Thiamine dose response curves for steelhead (□) and uptake of total thiamine (▲) and free thiamine (●) in eggs after immersion in water containing graded concentrations of thiamine hydrochloride. Symbols represent the mean and range of two replicates. Asterisks indicate mortality significantly less than control ($P < 0.05$).

threshold near 1 nmol/g for Lake Michigan steelhead (Figure 3), this needs to be verified by conducting thiamine dose response studies with eggs from individual steelhead family groups and comparing the results with endogenous levels of thiamine and the corresponding levels of EMS.

Other studies have also suggested that salmonid early life stage mortality is related to a threshold level of egg thiamine. Amcoff et al. (1998, this volume) reported a threshold level of thiamine between 0.1 and 0.2 μg/g in Baltic Sea Atlantic salmon, below which there was increased M74 syndrome. Based on free thiamine, this threshold level corresponds to 0.3–0.6 nmol/g and is similar to that found in the present study for coho salmon. Similarly, Fisher et al. (1996) suggested an egg thiamine threshold level between 0.124 and 0.234 μg/g for the occurrence of Cayuga syndrome in Atlantic salmon. This threshold level was based on the absence of the syndrome in lakes in which egg thiamine concentrations were greater than 0.234 μg/g and its presence in lakes in which egg thiamine concentrations were less than 0.124 μg/g. The egg thiamine threshold concentration of 1 μg/g reported by Brown et al. (1998a) was approximately 10 times higher than that for the salmon from the Baltic Sea or Cayuga Lake or for Lake Michigan coho salmon. Lake Ontario lake trout with egg thiamine concentrations less than 1 μg/g (3 nmol/g) exhibited swim-up mortality, whereas those with egg thiamine concentrations greater than 1 μg/g did not exhibit swim-up mortality.

Comparison of EMS with Other Salmonid Early Mortality

The clinical signs associated with EMS that were observed in this study, including disoriented swimming, hyperexcitability to touch, and lethargy, appear quite similar to those reported in lake trout during the same period from Lake Ontario. Fitzsimons et al. (1995) reported mean swim-up mortality of 33.5 ± 6% in 1990 and 1991 in Lake Ontario lake trout; this mortality could be reversed by immersing affected swim-up fry in a thiamine hydrochloride solution of 1 g/L and could be prevented by injection of 30 ng/mg thiamine hydrochloride solution into sac fry (Fitzsimons 1995). The signs associated with this mortality in Lake Ontario lake trout fry included loss of equilibrium, fry lying on their sides on the bottom of the tank, and hyperexcitability. The effect of thiamine on this condition

TABLE 1.—Steelhead EMS mortality in response to immersion in 1.4 mM thiamine once or twice during development. Asterisks indicate significant difference from control mortality by chi-square analysis ($P < 0.05$); daggers indicate significant difference from single treatment by chi-square analysis ($P < 0.05$).

	Single thiamine immersion[a]		Double thiamine immersion[b]	
Time of treatment	Number of fry with EMS per total number of fry	Percent EMS	Number of fry with EMS per total number of fry	Percent EMS
No immersion (control)	82 of 115	71		
Water hardening	53 of 113*	47		
300 degree-days	50 of 114*	44	37 of 99*	38
375 degree-days	71 of 119	60	58 of 132*†	44
450 degree-days	68 of 140*	49	50 of 125*	40
525 degree-days	56 of 137*	41	18 of 70*†	26
600 degree-days	63 of 132*	48	22 of 67*†	33

[a] Eggs or fry were immersed in 1.4 mM thiamine for 2 h once during development, either during water hardening or at 300, 375, 450, 525, or 600 centigrade degree-days. In these steelhead trout incubated at 10.5°C, hatching occurred at 300 centigrade degree-days and swim-up and the onset of exogenous feeding began at 600 centigrade degree-days.

[b] Eggs were immersed in 1.4 mM thiamine for 2 h during water hardening and again for 2 h at 300, 375, 450, 525, or 600 centigrade degree-days.

suggested that a thiamine deficiency resulting from the diet of the adult lake trout may be present (Fitzsimons 1995).

An association between salmonid early mortality in Atlantic salmon sac fry and the diet of the adults was also proposed by Fisher et al. (1996). These authors reported that Atlantic salmon in Cayuga Lake in New York State exhibit an early mortality syndrome called Cayuga syndrome that could be reversed or prevented by treatment of sac fry and alevins with 40 μg/g thiamine injected into the yolk sac or immersion of fry in 1% thiamine hydrochloride solution for 1 h. Cayuga syndrome was also postulated to be caused by a deficiency of thiamine induced by a dietary preference for alewife *Alosa pseudoharengus*, a species that contains thiaminase. Unlike EMS in steelhead and coho salmon from Lake Michigan, the signs associated with Cayuga syndrome included yolk sac opacities, edema, foreshortened maxillae, and occasional fin deformities (Fisher et al. 1995a). Cayuga syndrome in Atlantic salmon results in 100% mortality in all family groups, whereas EMS mortality in the present study was variable among family groups.

The signs associated with the early life stage mortality reported by Fisher et al. (1996) and Fitzsimons (1995) for salmonids in New York State and Lake Ontario, respectively, were completely eliminated by thiamine treatment. In the present study, EMS-related mortality was virtually eliminated in coho salmon fry immersed as eggs in 1.4 or 2.8 mM thiamine, whereas EMS-related mortality in steelhead fry was only reduced to 40% after eggs were immersed during water hardening in 2.8 mM thiamine, compared with 71% in controls. The background control mortality of 71% in eggs pooled from six female steelhead was greater than expected, based on the 35–40% mortality observed in steelhead fry the previous year. This increased mortality could be partially attributed to a 4°C increase in temperature caused by a pump failure that occurred after the eggs had hatched, although no increased mortality in the control or treatment groups was evident for several days after this event. The pooled sample of eggs could also constitute a greater proportion of severely affected family groups compared with those monitored the previous year. A second immersion in 1.4 mM thiamine during the time in which signs of EMS began to appear (525–600 degree-days) reduced EMS an additional 10%. Thiamine treatment did not eliminate all of the EMS-related mortality in the steelhead fry, which suggests that other stressors may be involved or that higher concentrations of thiamine are needed to completely eliminate EMS in steelhead.

The signs associated with salmonid early mortality described in the present study differ from those associated with salmonid early mortality reported elsewhere. Early mortality syndrome in Lake Michigan salmonids is different from the embryonic mortality reported by Smith et al. (1994) in Lake Ontario coho salmon and chinook salmon, in which mortality occurs before or during hatch; EMS mortality, on the other hand, occurs primarily near the time of swim-up. Mortality in these salmon embryos was also accompanied by pale egg color and small eyes. Pale egg color and low astaxanthin concentrations in eggs have been associated with M74, the early life stage mortality of Baltic Sea Atlantic salmon (Lignell 1994; Pettersson and Lignell 1996). Although small eyes and egg stage mortality have been observed in hatchery-incubated salmonids (S. Marcquenski, unpublished observations), neither of these signs was observed in steelhead or coho salmon eggs incubated in the laboratory in the present study. This suggests that cultural practices that stress the embryos during the egg stage of development could result in increased egg mortality that might be associated with EMS.

There has also been concern that EMS may be caused by persistent planar halogenated hydrocarbons such as 2,3,7,8-tetrachlorodibenzo-*p*-dioxin (TCDD) and related chemicals in Great Lakes salmonids. Rainbow trout (nonanadromous *Oncorhynchus mykiss*) fry exposed to sublethal concentrations of TCDD did not exhibit EMS-related signs but did exhibit an inability to maintain their vertical position in the water column while maintaining their lateral balance (M. W. Hornung, E. W. Zabel, and R. E. Peterson, University of Wisconsin, unpublished observation). These TCDD-exposed rainbow trout fry slowly sank to the bottom of the tank when they stopped swimming, which suggested an inability to maintain swim bladder inflation. A lack of swim bladder inflation has also been observed in early life stages of Japanese medaka *Oryzias latipes* (Harris et al. 1994) and zebrafish *Danio rerio* (Henry et al. 1997) exposed to TCDD. The characteristic signs of toxicity associated with lethal concentrations of TCDD and related chemicals in salmonid early life stages are identical to those of blue-sac disease (Wolf 1969) and include yolk sac and pericardial edema, multifocal hemorrhages, and a shortened snout (Spitsbergen et al. 1991; Walker and Peterson 1991). Based on these observations, TCDD is unlikely to be a causative agent of EMS in salmonids.

A direct causal link between persistent chlorinated hydrocarbons and salmonid early mortality similar to EMS does not seem likely, based on reports by other investigators. Fitzsimons et al. (1995) found no correlation between an extensive number of chlorinated and nonchlorinated aromatic hydrocarbons and heavy metals in lake trout eggs from Lake Ontario and the occurrence of mortality at swim-up. The Cayuga syndrome of Atlantic salmon does not appear to be linked to contaminants, as shown by low egg concentrations of PCBs, heavy metals, and TCDD equivalents (Fisher et al. 1995b). Additionally, these authors failed to produce mortality in control Atlantic salmon after injection of hexane extracts from Atlantic salmon eggs from Cayuga Lake. Mac et al. (1985) described fry mortality in Lake Michigan lake trout collected in 1980 that was associated with loss of equilibrium, erratic swimming, and lethargy, similar to the signs of EMS in the present study. These authors felt that PCBs or DDT were not the primary causative agents of this mortality because these signs were not observed in lake trout collected from 1972 to 1976, when the egg burden of these persistent chemicals was greater than in 1980. Also, fry survival in Lake Michigan lake trout increased to 65% in 1985 and remained between 65 and 95% through 1988, compared with less than 20% fry survival in 1980 and 1981 (Mac 1990). This vast improvement in survival over a very short time suggests that the mortality is caused by something other than persistent chemical contaminants.

Carotenoid Treatment

Lignell (1994) reported that egg concentrations of the carotenoid pigment astaxanthin were inversely related to the prevalence of M74 syndrome in Baltic salmon. This suggested that egg carotenoid levels might be involved in EMS in Lake Michigan salmonids. It was hypothesized that if EMS and M74 syndrome were caused by similar factors, injection of carotenoid pigments in Lake Michigan salmonids could reduce the level of EMS. Earlier observations of apparent differences in egg color between coho salmon from Lake Michigan and those from the Pacific Ocean, and the higher mortality in the Lake Michigan coho salmon, also suggested that carotenoids might be related to egg mortality (Degurse et al. 1973). Results from the current study, however, do not support the hypothesis that decreased carotenoid concentrations in eggs are the primary cause of EMS in Lake Michigan steelhead. The highest dose of β-carotene or astaxanthin injected into steelhead eggs (8.6 μg/g, or approximately 1.0 μg per egg if retained until the fry stage) was three times greater than the reported threshold level for M74 syndrome in Baltic salmon of 0.35 μg per fry (Lignell 1994).

Thyroxine Treatment

Treatment of Lake Michigan steelhead eggs was not effective at reducing EMS whereas treatment of sac fry may have been effective at reducing EMS due to the water-soluble thyroxine being more available to the newly hatched fry, with its large respiratory surface, than to the embryo inside the chorion. Previous studies in which significant effects on development and hatching were produced after eggs were immersed in thyroxine solutions (Dale and Hoar 1954; Reddy and Lam 1991) would suggest that the chorion is permeable to thyroxine. Thyroxine treatment of the eyed eggs in the present study is likely to have resulted in thyroxine uptake by the embryos, although it may have been insufficient to reduce EMS. Thyroxine levels have been shown to decline in some salmonids at hatch and then to increase as the last of the yolk is absorbed (Brown et al. 1987; Greenblatt et al. 1989). This decline and subsequent increase may represent utilization of maternally deposited reserves by the developing embryo and the onset of larval production of thyroid hormone (Greenblatt et al. 1989). Thus, immersion of newly hatched steelhead in the present study may have increased the thyroxine concentration in the sac fry during a period of development when these hormones are potentially at their lowest levels.

There are conflicting data on the relationship between the concentrations of thyroid hormones in early development and corresponding fry survival in various fish species. Although it has previously been reported that treatment of female striped bass *Morone saxatilis* with triiodothyronine (T_3) increased survival of the offspring (Brown et al. 1989), other authors have found no significant differences in early life stage mortality after treatments to alter egg thyroid concentrations by manipulation of maternal thyroid hormone levels (Tagawa and Hirano 1991; Ayson and Lam 1993). Leatherland et al. (1989) reported that egg thyroxine levels in coho salmon from Lake Erie were significantly lower than those in coho salmon from Lake Michigan or British Columbia, although there was no difference in egg or fry mortality among these three stocks. Unlike the eggs from Lake Michigan and British Columbia that showed a decline in egg thyroxine and an increase before complete resorption of their yolk, the Lake Erie stocks maintained constant low levels of thyroxine during these developmental stages. Also, treatment of larval striped bass with T_3 caused decreased survival at a concentration of 100 ng/mL of water (Huang et al. 1996).

The reduction of EMS in steelhead fry after thyroxine treatment in the present study should be considered in the context of the contradictory nature of the reports on the role of thyroid hormone in fish early survival. Further studies need to be conducted to determine whether the effect of thyroxine on EMS is stage-specific, to what extent EMS can be reduced by thyroxine treatment, and what effect thyroxine immersion has on normal functional development of the salmonid thyroid. Levels of thyroxine and thiamine should also be determined within family groups to determine whether a relationship exists that could explain the variability in EMS at low egg thiamine levels.

An interaction between thiamine and thyroxine could help to explain why low egg thiamine concentrations in coho salmon do not always lead to high EMS. If thyroxine has a role in regulating metabolism in developing fish, it may interact with thiamine pyrophosphate, a cofactor for several metabolic enzymes (Sebrell and Harris 1972). Coho salmon eggs with free thiamine levels less than 0.3 nmol/g exhibited a range of EMS from 16 to 97%. If coho salmon eggs had sufficient thyroxine to maintain normal development under conditions of low thiamine, they might exhibit higher survival than those with both low thiamine and low thyroxine. Under conditions of low egg thiamine and thyroxine, they might not maintain normal metabolic processes throughout early development and would die when the demand for thiamine or thyroxine is greater than that available to the developing fry. Whether this variability in mortality at low egg thiamine levels is related to thyroxine levels or some other factor that interacts with thiamine is unknown. There may be an underlying factor that can manifest its toxicity only under conditions of low thiamine. If egg thiamine concentrations are sufficiently high, the toxicity produced by this underlying factor may be prevented.

It is important to emphasize that although EMS is reversible and/or preventable by immersion of salmonid eggs or fry in thiamine, this is only an effective treatment; it does not establish that a thiamine deficiency is the primary cause of EMS. At present, hatcheries are successfully using thiamine treatments of eggs and/or fry to prevent EMS in Lake Michigan steelhead and coho salmon. Of potentially greater concern than the ability of hatcheries to produce healthy progeny and maintain stocking quotas are the physical, biological, or ecological conditions in the Great Lakes that may be affecting the adult broodstock and causing this reproductive failure. Furthermore, if there are basinwide changes that are affecting the reproductive potential of introduced salmonids in Lake Michigan, it raises the question of whether the reproductive health of native species is compromised as well.

Acknowledgments

This project was funded by Wisconsin Department of Natural Resources grants NMD 96363 and NME 91303. This is Environmental Toxicology Center, University of Wisconsin, Madison, Wisconsin, contribution #311. We thank Randy Link (Wisconsin Department of Natural Resources, Kettle Moraine Fish Hatchery, Adell) for providing steelhead eggs, Mark Opgenorth (Besadny Anadromous Fishery Facility, Kewaunee, Wisconsin) for providing coho salmon eggs, and Kristy Meyer, Matt Kotowski, and Mary Walker for technical assistance.

References

Amcoff, P., H. Börjeson, J. Lindeberg, and L. Norrgren. 1998. Thiamine concentrations in feral Baltic salmon exhibiting the M74 syndrome. Pages 82–89 *in* G. McDonald, J. D. Fitzsimons, and D. C. Honeyfield, editors. Early life stage mortality syndrome in fishes of the Great Lakes and Baltic Sea. American Fisheries Society, Symposium 21, Bethesda, Maryland.

Ayson, F. G., and T. J. Lam. 1993. Thyroxine injection of female rabbitfish (*Siganus guttatus*) broodstock: changes in thyroid hormone levels in plasma, eggs, and yolk-sac larvae, and its effect on larval growth and survival. Aquaculture 109:83–93.

Brown, C. L., C. V. Sullivan, H. A. Bern, and W. W. Dickhoff. 1987. Occurrence of thyroid hormones in early developmental stages of teleost fish. Pages 144–150 *in* R. D. Hoyt, editor. 10th annual larval fish conference. American Fisheries Society, Symposium 2, Bethesda, Maryland.

Brown, C. L., S. I. Doroshov, M. D. Cochran, and H. A. Bern. 1989. Enhanced survival in striped bass fingerlings after maternal triiodothyronine treatment. Fish Physiology and Biochemistry 7:295–299.

Brown, S. B., J. D. Fitzsimons, V. P. Palace, and L. Vandenbyllaardt. 1998a. Thiamine and early mortality syndrome in lake trout. Pages 18–25 *in* G. McDonald, J. D. Fitzsimons, and D. C. Honeyfield, editors. Early life stage mortality syndrome in fishes of the Great Lakes and Baltic Sea. American Fisheries Society, Symposium 21, Bethesda, Maryland.

Brown, S. B., D. C. Honeyfield, and L. Vandenbyllaardt. 1998b. Thiamine analysis in fish tissues. Pages 73–81 *in* G. McDonald, J. D. Fitzsimons, and D. C. Honeyfield, editors. Early life stage mortality syndrome in fishes of the Great Lakes and Baltic Sea. American Fisheries Society, Symposium 21, Bethesda, Maryland.

Bylund, G., and O. Lerche. 1995. Thiamine therapy of M74 affected fry of Atlantic salmon *Salmo salar*. Bulletin of the European Association of Fish Pathologists 15(3):93–97.

Dale, S., and W. S. Hoar. 1954. Effects of thyroxine and thiourea on the early development of chum salmon (*Oncorhynchus keta*). Canadian Journal of Zoology 32:244–251.

Degurse, P. E., D. Crochet, and H. R. Nielsen. 1973. Observations on Lake Michigan coho salmon (*Oncorhynchus kisutch*) propagation mortality in Wisconsin with an evaluation of the pesticide relationship. Wisconsin Department of Natural Resources Fisheries Management Report 62, Madison.

Fisher, J. P., J. D. Fitzsimons, G. E. Combs, Jr., and J. M. Spitsbergen. 1996. Naturally occurring thiamine deficiency causing reproductive failure in Finger Lakes Atlantic salmon and Great Lakes lake trout. Transactions of the American Fisheries Society 125:167–178.

Fisher, J. P., and six coauthors. 1995b. Reproductive failure of landlocked Atlantic salmon from New York's Finger Lakes: investigations into the etiology and epidemiology of the "Cayuga syndrome." Journal of Aquatic Animal Health 7:81–94.

Fisher, J. P., J. M. Spitsbergen, T. Iamonte, E. E. Little, and A. DeLonay. 1995a. Pathological and behavioral manifestations of the "Cayuga syndrome," a thiamine deficiency in larval landlocked Atlantic salmon. Journal of Aquatic Animal Health 7:269–283.

Fitzsimons, J. D. 1995. The effect of B-vitamins on a swim-up syndrome in Lake Ontario lake trout. Journal of Great Lakes Research 21(Supplement 1):286–289.

Fitzsimons, J. D., S. Huestis, and B. Williston. 1995. Occurrence of swim-up syndrome in Lake Ontario lake trout in relation to contaminants and cultural practices. Journal of Great Lakes Research 21(Supplement 1):277–285.

Gad, S., and C. S. Weil. 1991. Statistics and experimental design for toxicologists, 2nd edition. CRC Press, Boca Raton, Florida.

Greenblatt, M., C. L. Brown, M. Lee, S. Dauder, and H. A. Bern. 1989. Changes in thyroid hormone levels in eggs and larvae and in iodide uptake by eggs of coho and chinook salmon, *Oncorhynchus kisutch* and *O. tshawytscha*. Fish Physiology and Biochemistry 6:261–278.

Harris, G. E., Y. Kiparissis, and C. D. Metcalfe. 1994. Assessment of the toxic potential of PCB 81 (3,4,4',5-tetrachlorobiphenyl) to fish in relation to other non-ortho-substituted PCB congeners. Environmental Toxicology and Chemistry 13:1405–1413.

Henry, T. R., J. M. Spitsbergen, M. W. Hornung, C. C. Abnet, and R. E. Peterson. 1997. Early life stage toxicity of 2,3,7,8-tetrachlorodibenzo-*p*-dioxin in zebrafish *Danio rerio*. Toxicology and Applied Pharmacology 142:56–68.

Huang, L., J. L. Specker, and D. A. Bengtson. 1996. Effect of triiodothyronine on the growth and survival of larval striped bass (*Morone saxatilis*). Fish Physiology and Biochemistry 15:57–64.

Leatherland, J. F. 1993. Field observations on reproductive and developmental dysfunction in introduced and native salmonids from the Great Lakes. Journal of Great Lakes Research 19:737–751.

Leatherland, J. F., L. Lin, N. E. Down, and E. M. Donaldson. 1989. Thyroid hormone content of eggs and early developmental stages of three stocks of goitred coho salmon (*Oncorhynchus kisutch*) from the Great Lakes of North America, and a comparison with a stock from British Columbia. Canadian Journal of Fisheries and Aquatic Sciences 46:2146–2152.

Lignell, Å. 1994. Astaxanthin in yolk-sac fry from feral Baltic Salmon. Pages 94–95 *in* L. Norrgren, editor. Report from the Uppsala workshop in reproduction disturbances in fish. Swedish Environmental Protection Agency Report 4346, Uppsala.

Mac, M. J. 1990. Lake trout egg quality in lakes Michigan and Ontario. Pages 5–6 *in* M. Mac and M. Gilbertson, editors. Proceedings of the roundtable on contaminant-caused reproductive problems in salmonids. International Joint Commission and Great Lakes Fishery Commission, Windsor, Ontario.

Mac, M. J., C. C. Edsall, and J. G. Seelye. 1985. Survival of lake trout eggs and fry reared in water from the upper Great Lakes. Journal of Great Lakes Research 11:520–529.

Marcquenski, S. 1991. Drop-out syndrome in steelhead fry in Wisconsin. Pages 7–8 *in* M. Mac and M. Gilbertson, editors. Proceedings of the roundtable on contaminant-caused reproductive problems in salmonids. International Joint Commission and Great Lakes Fishery Commission, Windsor, Ontario.

Norrgren, L., T. Andersson, P.-A. Bergqvist, and I. Björklund. 1993. Chemical, physiological and morphological studies of feral Baltic salmon (*Salmo salar*) suffering from abnormal fry mortality. Environmental Toxicology and Chemistry 12:2065–2075.

Pettersson, A., and Å. Lignell. 1996. Decreased astaxanthin levels in the Baltic salmon and the M74 syndrome. Pages 28–29 *in* B.-E. Bengtsson, C. Hill, and S. Nellbring, editors. Report from the second workshop on reproductive disturbances in fish. Swedish Environmental Protection Agency Report 4534, Stockholm.

Reddy, P. K., and T. J. Lam. 1991. Effect of thyroid hormones on hatching in the tilapia, *Oreochromis mossambicus*. General and Comparative Endocrinology 81:484–491.

Sebrell, W. H., Jr., and R. S. Harris, editors. 1972. The vitamins, volume 5. Academic Press, New York.

Smith, I. R., B. Marchant, M. R. van den Heuvel, J. H. Clemons, and J. Frimeth. 1994. Embryonic mortality, bioassay derived 2,3,7,8-tetrachlorodibenzo-*p*-dioxin equivalents, and organochlorine contaminants in Pacific salmon from Lake Ontario. Journal of Great Lakes Research 20:497–509.

Spitsbergen, J. M., M. K. Walker, J. R. Olson, and R. E. Peterson. 1991. Pathologic alterations in early life stages of lake trout *Salvelinus namaycush*, exposed to 2,3,7,8-tetrachlorodibenzo-*p*-dioxin as fertilized eggs. Aquatic Toxicology 19:41–72.

Tagawa, M. and T. Hirano. 1991. Effects of thyroid hormone deficiency in eggs on early development of the Medaka, *Oryzias latipes*. Journal of Experimental Zoology 257:360–366.

Walker, M. K., L. C. Hufnagle, Jr., M. K. Clayton, and R. E. Peterson. 1992. An egg injection method for assessing early life stage mortality of polychlorinated dibenzo-p-dioxins, dibenzofurans, and biphenyls in rainbow trout (*Oncorhynchus mykiss*). Aquatic Toxicology 22:15–38.

Walker, M. K., and R. E. Peterson. 1991. Potencies of polychlorinated dibenzo-*p*-dioxin, dibenzofuran and biphenyl congeners, relative to 2,3,7,8-tetrachlorodibenzo-*p*-dioxin for producing early life stage mortality in rainbow trout (*Oncorhynchus mykiss*). Aquatic Toxicology 21:219–238.

Wolf, K. 1969. Blue-sac disease of fish. U.S. Fish and Wildlife Service Fish Disease Leaflet 15.

Woodle, M.C., and D. Papahadjopoulos. 1989. Liposome preparation and size characterization. Pages 193–217 *in* S. Fleisher and B. Fleisher, editors. Methods in enzymology, volume 171. Academic Press, San Diego, California.

American Fisheries Society Symposium 21:135–145, 1998

Correlation of Nutrients and Environmental Contaminants in Lake Michigan Coho Salmon with Incidence of Early Mortality Syndrome

DALE C. HONEYFIELD
Biological Resources Division, U.S. Geological Survey
Research and Development Laboratory
Wellsboro, Pennsylvania 16901, USA

JOHN G. HNATH AND JIM COPELAND
Michigan Department of Natural Resources, Fish Health Laboratory
Mattawan, Michigan 49071, USA

KONRAD DABROWSKI AND JOZEF H. BLOM
Ohio State University, School of Natural Resources
Columbus, Ohio 43210, USA

Abstract.—Muscle and egg samples from returning adult female Lake Michigan coho salmon *Oncorhynchus kisutch* were collected for thiamine analysis. Three groups of five females having low (2.5%), medium (42.4%), or high (92.6%) mean fry survival were selected for this study. Egg and muscle samples were collected at spawning and analyzed by high-performance liquid chromatography analysis for free thiamine, thiamine monophosphate (TP), and thiamine pyrophosphate (TPP). Egg concentrations of ascorbic acid, iron, zinc, magnesium, and potassium were measured. Twenty-five contaminants were also measured in muscle tissue of adult females. Total thiamine levels in eggs were similar between the medium and high survival groups but significantly lower in the low survival group. Eggs from the high and medium survival groups had higher levels of free thiamine and TP ($P < 0.01$) than eggs from the low survival group. There were no significant differences among the three groups in egg TPP. Muscle concentrations of TPP, TP, and total thiamine were similar among the three survival groups ($P > 0.10$). Correlations between fry survival and egg free thiamine ($r = 0.61$) and TP ($r = 0.52$) were observed. Fry survival was not correlated with adult muscle concentration of any form of thiamine or contaminant measured. Among the three groups, no differences in egg concentration were found for ascorbic acid, dehydroascorbic acid, iron, magnesium, zinc, and potassium. This research supports the hypothesis that low egg thiamine is an important factor in early mortality syndrome.

Recent reports of reproductive success in Lake Michigan salmonids show fry mortality of 70% for coho salmon *Oncorhynchus kisutch*, 60% for chinook salmon *O. tshawytscha*, 35% for steelhead trout *O. mykiss*, and 80% for Lake Ontario lake trout *Salvelinus namaycush* (Marcquenski 1996). In contrast, less than 30% mortality in these species was reported before 1990 (Simonin et al. 1990). These observations were reported from feral broodstocks spawned in hatcheries, but the problem is not caused by hatchery management of eggs or rearing of fry. Early mortality syndrome (EMS) is reported to be similar to M74 syndrome, which is observed in the Baltic region brown sea trout *Salmo trutta* and Atlantic salmon *Salmo salar* (Bengtsson et al. 1994; Norrgren 1994; Johansson et al. 1995), and Cayuga syndrome, which is observed in Atlantic salmon in the Finger Lakes region of New York State (Fisher et al. 1995). Thus, EMS has both national and international implications in the management of natural salmonid resources.

Fitzsimons (1995) first reported that sac fry survival was improved when fry were treated with thiamine. In the same study, no beneficial response was observed when sac fry were treated with nicotinic acid, riboflavin, folic acid, or pyridoxine. Furthermore, Bylund and Lerche (1995) reported that water hardening of eggs or treatment of sac fry in a 500-ppm thiamine bath significantly improved fish survival. Fisher et al. (1996) concluded that the decrease in salmonid fry survival from Cayuga Lake was directly linked to broodfish diets consisting only of alewife *Alosa pseudoharengus* and rainbow smelt *Osmerus mordax*. These two nonindigenous species, which are the dominant forage fish in Cayuga Lake, contain thiaminase, an enzyme that destroys thiamine (Fisher et al.

TABLE 1.—Mean (SE) thiamine concentration (nmol/g) in coho salmon captive broodstock eggs, muscle, and liver.

Tissue	TPP	TP	Free thiamine	Total thiamine
Eggs	1.12 (0.15)	1.06 (0.11)	27.64 (2.00)	29.82 (2.15)
Muscle	11.11 (0.61)	1.74 (0.12)	0.15 (0.03)	13.00 (0.72)
Liver	5.98 (3.09)	2.90 (0.95)	1.02 (0.12)	9.89 (4.06)

1995, 1996). The work by Fisher and coworkers strongly implicates thiaminase, which ultimately leads to reduction of thiamine in fish eggs taken from Cayuga Lake broodstock. Unlike the limited forage base in Cayuga Lake, the forage base in Lake Michigan is more diverse.

Studies with wild (Dabrowski 1991) and cultured salmonids (Blom and Dabrowski 1995) suggest that in mature fish the deposition of ascorbic acid in the ovaries greatly exceeds the deposition in other organs. The packing of ovaries with ascorbic acid during vitellogenesis and the subsequent use of this nutrient during embryogenesis and early exogenous feeding (Blom and Dabrowski 1996) indicate its importance to salmonid reproduction. In a recently reported study, ascorbic acid deficiency influenced production of steroids in female rainbow trout (nonanadromous *Oncorhynchus mykiss*), and in this manner it may affect the quality of eggs produced (Dabrowski et al. 1995). The saturation of ovarian ascorbic acid in rainbow trout resulted in maximum egg quantity and embryo survival (Blom and Dabrowski 1995). Therefore, it is hypothesized that

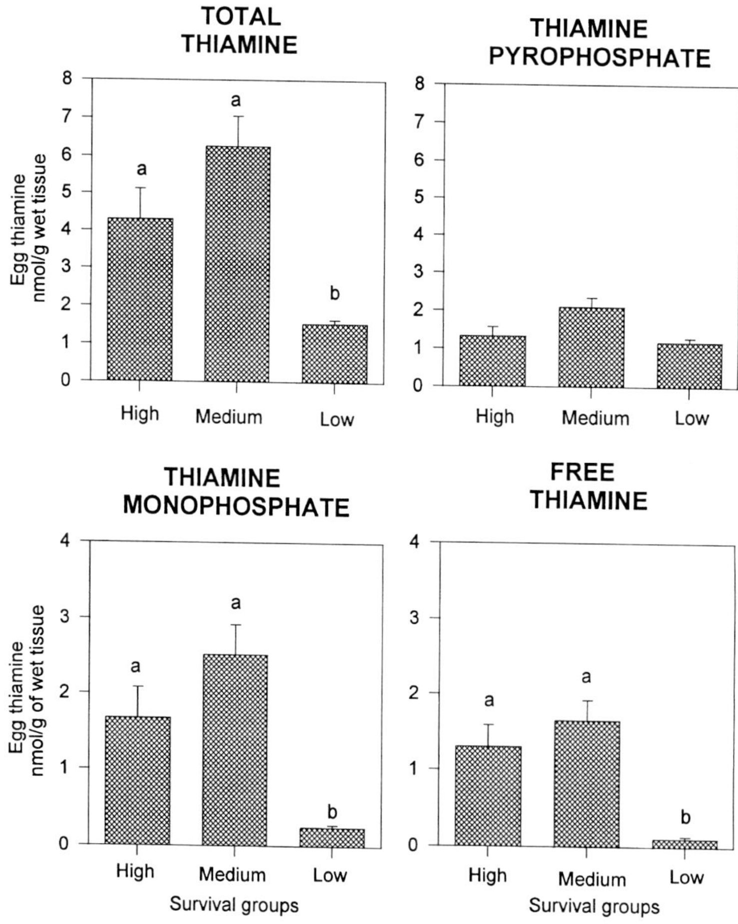

FIGURE 1.—Thiamine compounds in Lake Michigan coho salmon eggs based on fry survival: high (92.6%), medium (42.2%), and low (2.5%). Means with different letters within a panel are significantly different ($P < 0.05$).

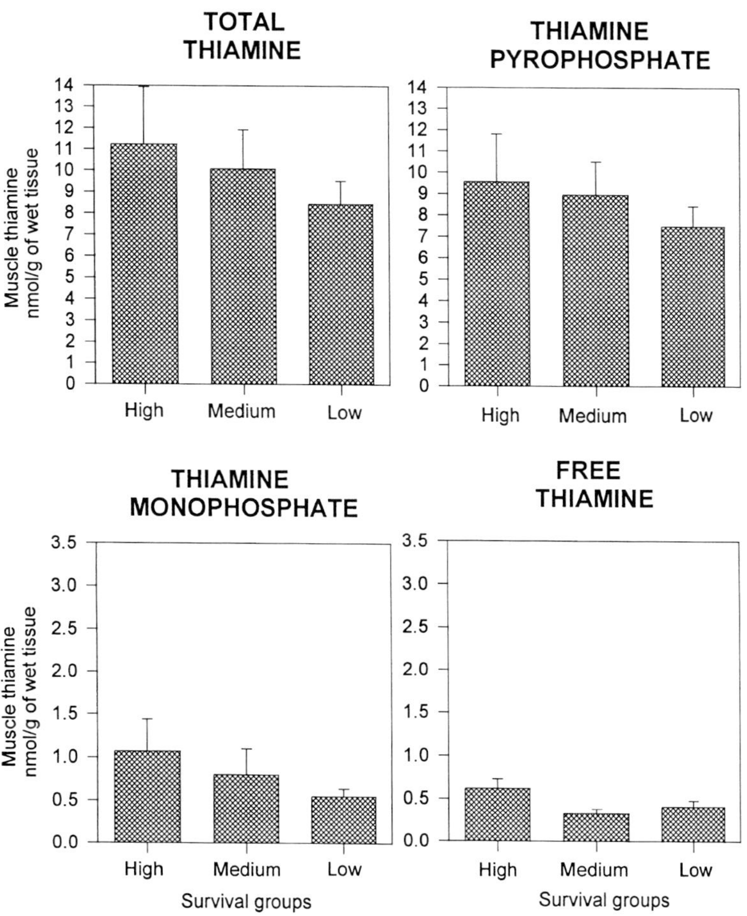

FIGURE 2.—Thiamine compounds in Lake Michigan female coho salmon muscle based on fry survival: high (92.6%), medium (42.2%), and low (2.5%).

transfer of ascorbic acid in aquatic food webs will change as a result of elongation of the food chain or type of prey consumed by piscivorous salmonids. Consequently, this may result in periodic deficiency of ascorbic acid in ovaries and increased mortality of fry before yolk absorption is completed.

Contaminants in Lake Michigan are also suspected of causing reproductive problems in salmonids (Miller 1994). To date, there is no convincing link between Lake Michigan contaminants and EMS (Fitzsimons et al. 1995). Stronger links, however, have been reported between contaminants and M74 in Baltic Sea fishes (Bengtsson et al. 1996). Thus, it appears that EMS and M74 may be related to thiamine deficiency, possibly to contaminants, or to other unknown factors. The objectives of the present study were to determine thiamine concentrations in eggs and muscle tissue of coho salmon from Lake Michigan, the concentrations of contaminants in muscle tissue of the adult females, and the concentrations of ascorbic acid and four minerals in eggs. Thereby, the relationship between nutrients and environmental contaminants and the incidence of EMS may be established.

Materials and Methods

Thirty female coho salmon were collected from Lake Michigan at the Platte River State Fish Hatchery in October 1994. Eggs from each fish were incubated separately. Fish were then assigned to one of three groups based on level of fry survival: high, medium, or low. Five fish from each group were randomly selected for laboratory analysis of eggs and muscle. The mean and range fry survival of the selected fish were: high (92.6%, 87–95%), medium (42.2%, 17–68%), and low (2.5%, 0–7%). Egg and muscle samples (fillets) were taken from each fish at spawning and stored frozen at −80°C until ana-

TABLE 2.—Mean (SE) egg concentration of ascorbic acid (μg/g of wet tissue) and minerals (μg/g of dry tissue) from the low (2.5%), medium (42.2%), and high (92.6%) survival groups of Lake Michigan coho salmon.

Variable	Survival group		
	Low	Medium	High
Ascorbic acid[a]	113.55 (7.89)	127.96 (6.81)	105.16 (4.17)
Dehydro-aa[b]	25.28 (1.25)	19.92 (1.57)	19.08 (1.32)
Iron	15.58 (1.49)	15.08 (0.44)	16.68 (0.37)
Zinc	49.14 (0.97)	51.04 (5.49)	47.14 (1.44)
Potassium	0.43 (0.05)	0.48 (0.06)	0.51 (0.01)
Magnesium	0.11 (0.01)	0.12 (0.01)	0.11 (0.01)

[a] The percentage of total ascorbic acid in the reduced form was: low, 77.4%; medium, 84.3%; high, 81.7%.

[b] Dehydroascorbic acid.

lyzed. Eggs, muscle, and liver tissue from a captive broodstock population with normal reproduction (no EMS) were also collected from a private hatchery in New York State. High-performance liquid chromatography was used to determine egg and muscle concentrations of thiamine, thiamine monophosphate (TP), and thiamine pyrophosphate (TPP; Brown et al. 1998, this volume). For ascorbic acid analysis, eggs were frozen and transported on dry ice and stored at −80°C. Duplicate subsamples of three eggs per female were analyzed for ascorbic acid and oxidized and reduced forms by a colorimetric method as described by Dabrowski and Hinterleitner (1989). For mineral analysis, eggs were freeze dried, pulverized, digested with a nitric acid–perchloric acid mixture, and analyzed by an inductively coupled plasma emission spectrometer (ICP, model ARL-3560, Applied Research Laboratory, Valencia, California).

Contaminants analysis was conducted at the Center for Environmental Health Sciences, Michigan Department of Public Health, Lansing, Michigan, as described by Price et al. (1986). Fillets with skin were analyzed for the following contaminants: mercury, aldrin, lindane, terphenyls (a group of polychlorinated triphenyl compounds such as Aroclor® 5432 and Aroclor® 5460), toxaphene, 4,4′-DDD 2,2Bis(4-chlorophenyl)-1,1 dichloroethane, 4,4′-DDE 2,2Bis(4-chlorophenyl)-1,1 dichloroethylene, 4,4′-DDT, total DDT, dieldrin, hexachlorobenzene, octachlorostyrene, PCB A-1254, α-chlordane, γ-chlordane, *cis*-nonachlordane, oxychlordane, total chlordane, heptachlor, mirex, pentachlorostyrene, hexachlorostyrene, heptachlorostyrene, Firemaster BP-6, and heptachlor epoxide.

Swim-up coho salmon fry displaying signs of EMS were divided into three lots. Two lots were treated with either a thiamine HCl (500 ppm) bath or a control bath for 1 h. The pH and chloride content of the control bath were adjusted to that of the thiamine bath with HCl and NaCl. The third group was left untreated. Data were analyzed as a completely randomized design using the General Linear Model of SAS for means, variance, and correlation coefficients (SAS 1994). For statistical analysis, fry survival was transformed to the arcsine of the square root of the decimal equivalent of the percentage of fry survival. Differences among means were separated using Duncan's new multiple-range test.

Results

Eggs from the low survival group had less total thiamine, free thiamine, and TP than eggs from the higher survival groups (Figure 1). Egg and tissue concentrations of thiamine from captive broodstock are listed in Table 1. Free egg thiamine in captive broodstock was 27.6 nmol/g, whereas free thiamine in Lake Michigan fish was less than 2 nmol/g (Figure 1). Muscle TPP of captive broodstock was 11.11 nmol/g, whereas TPP in Lake Michigan fish ranged from 7.5 to 9.6 nmol/g (Figure 2). No differences were observed in the muscle concentrations of thiamine among the three treatment groups (Figure 2), although there were decreasing numerical trends in the concentrations of thiamine compounds as survival decreased. A correlation ($r = 0.62$) was observed between egg free thiamine and fry survival (Figure 3). There was also a correlation ($r = 0.52$) between TP and fry survival (Figure 4). Fry treated with 500 ppm of thiamine had 91% survival, whereas eggs treated in a control bath or left untreated displayed 15 and 18% survival, respectively.

Total ascorbic acid concentrations in the coho salmon eggs averaged 114, 128, and 105 μg/g wet weight for the low, medium, and high survival groups (Table 2), respectively, and there was no correlation with fry survival (Figure 5). Most of the ascorbate was in the reduced form (75–90%), which indicates

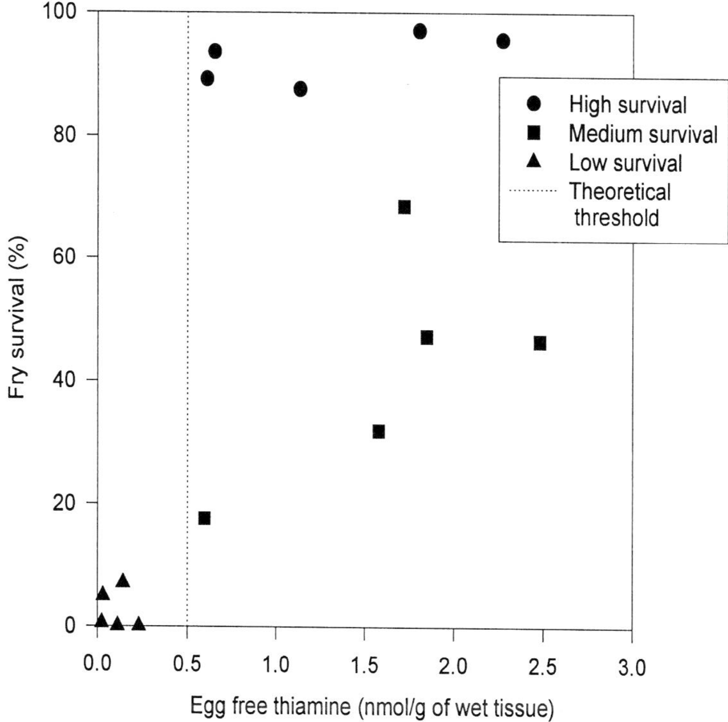

FIGURE 3.—Relationship (r = 0.61, P = 0.01) between egg free thiamine and fry survival in Lake Michigan coho salmon with estimated threshold level of thiamine causing EMS.

that the handling of the samples was appropriate. Also, there were no significant differences in egg mineral concentrations (Table 2).

Mean body fat percentage and concentration of contaminants were not different ($P > 0.10$) among the adults that produced the three egg survival groups (Table 3). The females from the low survival group were longer ($P < 0.06$) and they tended to be heavier than the females of the medium or high survival groups. Fish age was not determined. Aldrin, lindane, terphynl, hexachlorobenzene, octachlorostyrene, heptachlor, mirex, pentachlorostyrene, hexachlorostyrene, heptachlorostyrene, and Firemaster BP-6 were all below the limits of detection. There were no differences among survival groups for mercury and the 15 chlorinated compounds listed in Table 3.

Discussion

Many questions remain about the etiology of EMS. Fry from eggs with low thiamine concentrations have been linked with the syndrome. Field biologists have improved fry survival by using a thiamine solution to water-harden eggs or by immersing fry in a thiamine bath (Bylund and Lerche 1995; Hornung et al. 1998, this volume). However, the underlying cause of low thiamine concentrations in eggs of broodstock whose progeny suffer from EMS is unknown. Furthermore, the time sequence of thiamine deposition into the egg is not known. Data from lake trout show that egg thiamine levels were reduced when amprolium, a thiamine antagonist, was administered 3 months before spawning (Honeyfield et al. 1998, this volume). The deposition process of thiamine into the egg is relevant to the understanding of EMS. If the major portion of thiamine is deposited into the egg at the same time that vitellogenin is deposited, then alterations in the dietary supply of thiamine to the broodfish during this period may affect egg thiamine depositions. On the other hand, if thiamine is passively moved into the egg throughout the year, then factors that affect the supply of thiamine on a long-term basis would be important to identify. Egg concentrations of total thiamine were strikingly different between the Lake Michigan coho (1.5–6.3 nmol/g) and the captive broodstock (29.8 nmol/g) fed a thiamine-replete diet, but differences in concentrations of total thiamine in muscle between the captive broodstock (13.0 nmol/g) and the Lake Michigan coho (8.4–11.2 nmol/g) were not as great. Comparison of these data with data from other wild

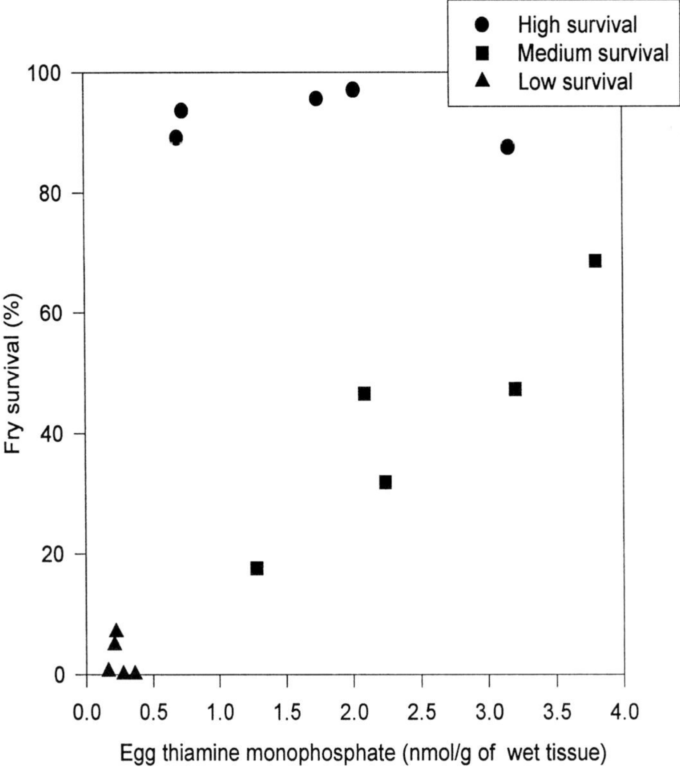

FIGURE 4.—Relationship (r = 0.52, P = 0.04) between egg thiamine monophosphate and fry survival in Lake Michigan coho salmon.

populations indicates that the Lake Michigan egg values were low and the captive broodstock egg values were intermediate to those of Lake Superior coho (65 nmol/g) and Pacific Coast coho (7.7 nmol/g; Marcquenski and Brown 1997).

A thiamine-destroying enzyme (thiaminase) in the forage fishes alewife and rainbow smelt is hypothesized to be the cause of low egg thiamine levels. Information is lacking to determine if there is a difference in thiaminase activity in young versus old alewives, the effect of environmental stress on enzyme activity in forage fish, or whether environmental or other factors alter the sensitivity of the salmonid to the presence of thiaminase.

Careful inspection of the data from the medium and high survival groups (Figure 3) suggests that there are differences in the pattern. If the data from the medium and low survival groups are evaluated together, there appears to be a linear relationship ($r = 0.90$, $P < 0.001$) between survival and egg thiamine (Figure 3). An increase in egg thiamine corresponds to a higher fry survival. In contrast, the relationship observed between the high and low survival groups suggests a threshold effect. In other words, when thiamine is below a threshold concentration, EMS is observed. This threshold for free thiamine in the egg appears to be less than 1 nmol/g. A linear response for an essential vitamin is not the norm; a threshold response would be expected, which suggests that there may be another factor involved in EMS. The relationship between egg TP and fry survival ($r = 0.97$, $P < 0.001$) shown in Figure 4 is similar to that observed in Figure 3 for free thiamine within the low and medium survival groups. The linear response observed may or may not be indicative of an intermediate stage of EMS. Our guess is that there are multiple factors that contribute to the observed signs associated with the syndrome. Also, it remains to be determined if low thiamine is the cause or simply a consequence of EMS, but it is clear that thiamine is involved in this malady.

The body burdens of the fish used in the present study provide little support for the involvement of contaminants in EMS. However, measurement of contaminants in the eggs may be more important. Alternatively, we may need to look for other organic compounds or at the metabolites of contaminants.

TABLE 3.—Mean (SE) muscle concentrations of contaminants from the low (2.5%), medium (42.2%), and high (92.6%) survival groups of Lake Michigan coho salmon broodstock. Means in a row with a similar superscript are not significantly different $P < 0.06$.

	Survival group		
Variable	High	Medium	Low
Length (cm)	23.3[a] (0.290)	23.3[a] (0.695)	25.1[b] (0.556)
Weight (kg)	4.4 (0.197)	4.5 (0.695)	5.6 (0.509)
Fat (%)	2.2 (0.250)	2.3 (0.240)	2.4 (0.254)
Mercury (ppm)	0.174 (0.009)	0.150 (0.008)	0.160 (0.009)
Toxaphene (ppm)	0.390 (0.049)	0.400 (0.038)	0.370 (0.015)
4,4′-DDD (ppm)	0.033 (0.001)	0.038 (0.005)	0.035 (0.002)
4,4′-DDE (ppm)	0.442 (0.035)	0.454 (0.039)	0.460 (0.033)
4,4′-DDT (ppm)	0.032 (0.002)	0.038 (0.004)	0.038 (0.003)
Total DDT (ppm)	0.508 (0.038)	0.530 (0.048)	0.533 (0.037)
Dieldrin (ppm)	0.019 (0.003)	0.022 (0.005)	0.028 (0.003)
PCB A-1254 (ppm)	0.998 (0.055)	1.025 (0.084)	1.051 (0.070)
α-Chlordane (ppm)	0.026 (0.003)	0.033 (0.005)	0.032 (0.004)
γ-Chlordane (ppm)	0.009 (0.001)	0.010 (0.002)	0.011 (0.001)
cis-Nonachlordane (ppm)	0.033 (0.003)	0.089 (0.050)	0.039 (0.003)
trans-Nonachlordane (ppm)	0.091 (0.004)	0.095 (0.007)	0.077 (0.007)
Oxychlordane (ppm)	0.010 (0.001)	0.010 (0.001)	0.010 (0.001)
Total chlordane (ppm)	0.170 (0.009)	0.185 (0.017)	0.168 (0.015)
Heptachlor epoxide (ppm)	0.004 (0.001)	0.005 (0.001)	0.005 (0.001)

Although coho salmon females are not deficient in ascorbate, the level in the eggs is significantly less than the saturation level reported in rainbow trout eggs (Blom and Dabrowski 1995). There was no relationship between ascorbic acid and minerals in the eggs of coho salmon in the present study. Sandnes et al. (1984) reported a high correlation between iron and ascorbic acid, and between zinc and ascorbic acid, in cod *Gadus morhua* ovary. However, samples for this analysis were collected during ovarian development of cod. In the present study, dehydroascorbic acid was numerically higher in the low survival group (Table 2), which suggests that there may have been an increase in oxidative stress. Preliminary research with dioxinlike compounds that were extracted from Lake Michigan lake trout eggs and reinjected into rainbow trout eggs resulted in evidence of oxidative stress, DNA degradation, and increased programmed cell death in the emerging fry (D. Tillitt, Biological Resources Division, U.S. Geological Survey, personal communication). Unfortunately, we did not measure egg or tissue concentrations of dioxins in this study.

Muscle concentrations of contaminants measured in the females (Table 4) did not correlate with fry survival. Miller (1993) and Miller and Amrhein (1995) reported that egg concentrations of selected chlorinated contaminants reflected the body burden of the contaminant of the female. Fry survival was negatively correlated (Table 4) to length ($r = -0.55$) and weight ($r = -0.49$). There also was a negative correlation between length and egg thiamine ($r = -0.54$). Possible reasons for this may include differences in forage selection by large and small fish or differences in total body load of contaminants. Both length and weight are positively correlated to dieldrin, α-chlordane, and γ-chlordane. Furthermore, the low survival group had the highest numerical muscle concentration of dieldrin (Table 3). Not surprisingly, there are

TABLE 4.—Correlation of coefficients.

Variable	TPP	TP	Thiamine	Total thiamine	Length	Weight	Fat	Mercury	Toxaphene	4,4′-DDD	4,4′-DDE	4,4′-DDT	Total DDT
TPP	1.00	0.83	0.67	0.89	−0.24	−0.14	−0.00	−0.31	−0.02	0.10	−0.27	0.04	−0.23
TP		1.00	0.78	0.96	−0.40	−0.21	0.04	−0.17	0.08	0.09	−0.12	−0.07	−0.10
Thiamine			1.00	0.89	−0.54	−0.39	−0.07	−0.25	0.22	−0.03	−0.22	−0.21	−0.21
Total thiamine				1.00	−0.44	−0.27	−0.00	−0.25	0.11	0.06	−0.20	−0.10	−0.18
Length					1.00	0.94	0.49	−0.12	0.22	0.40	0.44	0.47	0.46
Weight						1.00	0.62	−0.21	0.27	0.41	0.47	0.44	0.48
Fat							1.00	−0.36	0.33	0.36	0.43	0.50	0.44
Mercury								1.00	0.17	0.09	0.29	0.13	0.27
Toxaphene									1.00	0.68	0.75	0.69	0.76
4,4′-DDD										1.00	0.75	0.82	0.80
4,4′-DDE											1.00	0.78	0.99
4,4′-DDT												1.00	0.83
Total DDT													1.00
Dieldrin													
PCB A-1254													
α-Chlordane													
γ-Chlordane													
cis-Nonachlordane													
trans-Nonachlordane													
Oxychlordane													
Total chlordane													
Heptachlor-epoxide													
Fry survival													

Variable	Dieldrin	PCB A-1254	α-Chlor-dane	γ-Chlor-dane	*cis*-Nona-chlordane	*trans*-Nona-chlordane	Oxy-chlordane	Total chlordane	Heptachlor epoxide	Fry survival
TPP	0.07	−0.30	0.14	−0.16	0.56	0.05	−0.05	0.02	0.12	0.19
TP	−0.05	−0.19	0.08	−0.09	0.52	0.32	0.15	0.15	0.13	0.54
Thiamine	−0.18	−0.23	−0.07	−0.17	0.20	0.28	0.03	0.06	−0.01	0.64
Total thiamine	−0.07	−0.25	0.05	−0.19	0.46	0.15	0.07	0.10	0.09	0.53
Length	0.76	0.49	0.63	0.49	−0.13	0.01	0.26	0.35	0.47	−0.55
Weight	0.87	0.48	0.68	0.53	−0.17	0.08	0.35	0.41	0.60	−0.49
Fat	0.82	0.52	0.73	0.66	−0.31	0.43	0.55	0.65	0.84	−0.31
Mercury	−0.41	0.14	−0.28	−0.08	−0.13	0.16	−0.19	−0.01	−0.33	0.28
Toxaphene	0.38	0.73	0.61	0.67	−0.24	0.71	0.38	0.77	0.47	0.06
4,4′-DDD	0.53	0.76	0.73	0.74	−0.19	0.65	0.58	0.79	0.66	−0.15
4,4′-DDE	0.48	0.95	0.72	0.70	−0.21	0.72	0.60	0.85	0.61	−0.14
4,4′-DDT	0.61	0.85	0.80	0.84	−0.11	0.58	0.38	0.81	0.60	−0.40
Total DDT	0.51	1.00	0.75	0.74	−0.21	0.73	0.60	0.87	0.63	−1.17
Dieldrin	1.00	0.57	0.84	0.71	−0.21	0.25	0.46	0.60	0.79	−0.46
PCB A-1254		1.00	0.80	0.80	−0.25	0.71	0.60	0.88	0.85	−0.31
α-Chlordane			1.00	0.73	−0.03	0.62	0.66	0.88	0.85	−0.31
γ-Chlordane				1.00	−0.48	0.49	0.32	0.73	0.62	−0.38
cis-Nona-chlordane					1.00	−0.12	−0.07	−0.15	−0.23	0.10
trans-Nona-chlordane						1.00	0.70	0.90	0.59	0.32
Oxy-chlordane							1.00	0.76	0.81	0.04
Total chlordane								1.00	0.81	−0.04
Heptachlor epoxide									1.00	−0.30
Fry survival										1.00

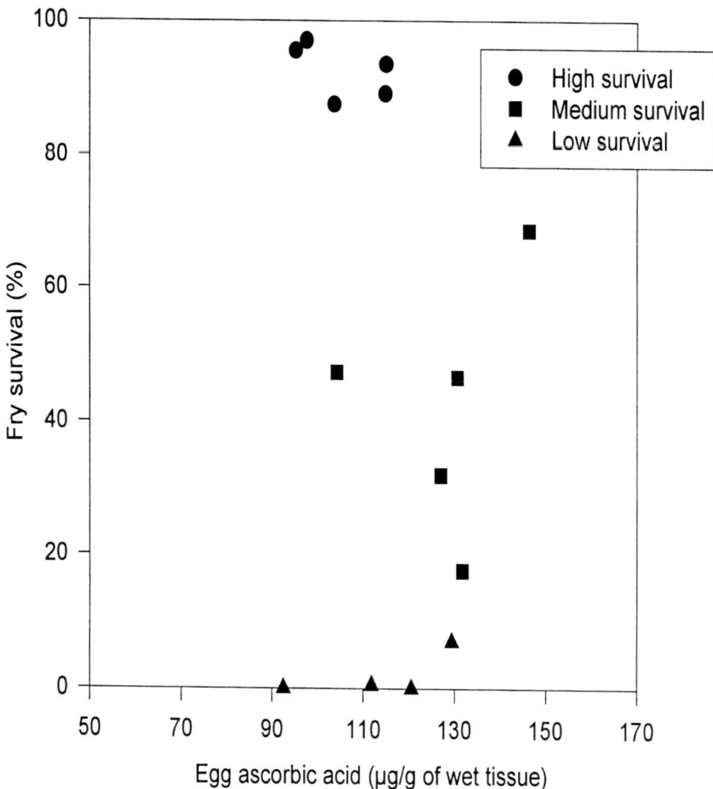

FIGURE 5.—Relationship (r = 0.20, P = 0.40) between egg ascorbic acid concentration and fry survival in Lake Michigan coho salmon.

multiple correlations among the DDT family of compounds, the chlordane family, dieldrin, PCB, and heptachlor epoxide. Mercury was not strongly correlated to most other contaminants.

Although thiamine therapy offers an immediate treatment for EMS, it merely treats the symptom and not the cause of the problem. The recent increase in the incidence of EMS along with bacterial kidney disease in salmonids and reproductive failure observed in yellow perch *Perca flavescens* in Lake Michigan (S. Marcquenski, Wisconsin Department of Natural Resources, personal communication) are indicators of a larger, more insidious ecosystem problem. Determining the underlying cause of EMS would be a step toward understanding and addressing other reproductive dysfunction and disease issues affecting the Great Lakes fishery.

In conclusion, low egg thiamine concentrations were associated with coho salmon fry mortality. Free thiamine concentrations were found to be very low in Lake Michigan coho salmon eggs (1–2 nmol/g) versus captive coho salmon broodstock (28 nmol/g). Finally, there was little or no evidence to support a role of contaminants as a factor in EMS.

References

Bengtsson, B. E., and six coauthors. 1994. Reproductive disturbances in Baltic fish. Swedish Environmental Protection Agency Report 4319, Stockholm.

Bengtsson, B.-E., C. Hill, and S. Nellbring. 1996. Report from the second workshop on reproduction disturbances in fish. Swedish Environmental Protection Agency Report 4534, Stockholm.

Blom, J. H., and K. Dabrowski. 1995. Reproductive success of female rainbow trout (*Oncorhynchus mykiss*) in response to graded dietary ascorbyl monophosphate levels. Biology of Reproduction 52:1073–1080.

Blom, J. H., and K. Dabrowski. 1996. Ascorbic acid metabolism in fish: is there a maternal effect on the progeny? Aquaculture 147:215–224.

Brown, S. B., D. C. Honeyfield, and L. Vandenbyllaardt. 1998. Thiamine analysis in fish tissues. Pages 73–81 *in* G. McDonald, J. D. Fitzsimons, and D. C. Honeyfield, editors. Early life stage mortality syndrome in fishes of the Great Lakes and Baltic Sea. American Fisheries Society, Symposium 21, Bethesda, Maryland.

Bylund, G., and O. Lerche. 1995. Thiamine therapy of M 74 affected fry of Atlantic salmon *Salmo salar*. Bulletin of the European Association of Fish Pathologists 15(3):93–97.

Dabrowski, K. 1991. Ascorbic acid status in high mountain charr, *Salvelinus alpinus*, in relation to reproductive cycle. Environmental Biology of Fishes 31:213–217.

Dabrowski, K., R. E. Ciereszko, J. H. Blom, and J. S. Ottobre. 1995. Relationship between vitamin C and plasma concentrations of testosterone in female rainbow trout, *Oncorhynchus mykiss*. Fish Physiology and Biochemistry 14:409–414.

Dabrowski, K., and S. Hinterleitner. 1989. Applications of a simultaneous assay of ascorbic acid, dehydroascorbic acid, and ascorbic sulfate in biological materials. Analyst (London) 114:83–87.

Fisher, J. P., J. Fitzsimons, G. F. Combs, Jr., and J. M. Spitsbergen. 1996. Naturally occurring thiamine deficiency causing reproductive failure in Finger Lakes Atlantic salmon and Great Lakes trout. Transactions of the American Fisheries Society 125:167–178.

Fisher, J. P., and six coauthors. 1995. Reproductive failure of landlocked Atlantic salmon from New York's Finger Lakes: investigations into the etiology and epidemiology of the "Cayuga syndrome." Journal of Aquatic Animal Health 7:81–94.

Fitzsimons, J. D. 1995. The effect of B-vitamins on a swim-up syndrome in Lake Ontario lake trout. Journal of Great Lakes Research 21(Supplement 1):286–289.

Fitzsimons, J. D., S. Huestis, and B. Williston. 1995. Occurrence of a swim-up syndrome in Lake Ontario lake trout in relation to contaminants and cultural practices. Journal of Great Lakes Research 21(Supplement 1):277–285.

Honeyfield, D. C., K. Fynn-Aikins, J. D. Fitzsimons, and J. A. Mota. 1998. Effect of dietary amprolium on egg and tissue thiamine concentrations in lake trout. Pages 172–177 *in* G. McDonald, J. D. Fitzsimons, and D. C. Honeyfield, editors. Early life stage mortality syndrome in fishes of the Great Lakes and Baltic Sea. American Fisheries Society, Symposium 21, Bethesda, Maryland.

Hornung, M. W., L. Miller, R. E. Peterson, S. Marcquenski, and S. B. Brown. 1998. Efficacy of thiamine, astaxanthin, β-carotene, and thyroxine treatments in reducing early mortality syndrome in Lake Michigan salmonid embryos. Pages 124–134 *in* G. McDonald, J. D. Fitzsimons, and D. C. Honeyfield, editors. Early life stage mortality syndrome in fishes of the Great Lakes and Baltic Sea. American Fisheries Society, Symposium 21, Bethesda, Maryland.

Johansson, N., P. Jonsson, O. Svanberg, A. Södergren, and J. Thulin. 1995. Reproduction disorders in Baltic fish. Swedish Environmental Protection Agency Report 4347, Solna.

Marcquenski, S. V. 1996. Characterization of early mortality syndrome (EMS) in salmonids from the Great Lakes. Pages 73–75 *in* Bengtsson et al. (1996).

Marcquenski, S. V., and S. B. Brown. 1997. Early mortality syndrome in the Great Lakes. Pages 135–152 *in* R. M. Rolland, M. Gilbertson, and R. E. Peterson, editors. Chemically induced alterations in functional development and reproduction in fishes. SETAC (Society of Environmental Toxicology and Chemistry), Pensacola, Florida.

Miller, M. A. 1993. Maternal transfer of organochlorine compounds in salmonines to their eggs. Canadian Journal of Fisheries and Aquatic Sciences 50:1405–1413.

Miller, M. A. 1994. Organochlorine concentration dynamics in Lake Michigan chinook salmon (*Oncorhynchus tshawytscha*). Archives of Environmental Contamination and Toxicology 27:367–374.

Miller, M. A., and J. F. Amrhein. 1995. Maternal transfer of organochlorine compounds in Lake Superior siscowet (*Salvelinus namaycush siscowet*) to their eggs. Bulletin of Environmental Contamination and Toxicology 55:96–103.

Norrgren, L., editor. 1994. Report from the Uppsala workshop on reproduction disturbances in fish. Swedish Environmental Protection Agency Report 4346, Uppsala.

Price, H. A., R. L. Welch, R. H. Scheel, and L. A. Warren. 1986. Modified multi-residue method for chlordane, toxaphene, and polychlorinated biphenyls in fish. Bulletin of Environmental Contamination and Toxicology 37:1–9.

Sandnes, K., K. Julshamn, and O. R. Braekkan. 1984. Interrelationship between ascorbic acid and trace elements in ovarian development in fish. Pages 213–217 *in* I. Wegger, F. J. Tagwerker, and J. Moustgaard, editors. Proceedings of workshop on ascorbic acid in domestic animals. Royal Danish Agricultural Society, Copenhagen.

SAS (Statistical Analysis System). 1994. SAS/STAT guide for personal computers, version 6.10. SAS Institute Inc., Cary, North Carolina.

Simonin, H., J. Skea, H. Dean, and J. Symula. 1990. Summary of reproductive studies of Lake Ontario salmonids. Pages 15–16 *in* M. Mac and M. Gilbertson, editors. Proceedings of the roundtable on contaminant-caused reproductive problems in salmonids. Great Lakes Science Advisory Board, Biological Effects Subcommittee, Windsor, Ontario.

American Fisheries Society Symposium 21:146–153, 1998

Relationship between Induction of the Phase I Enzyme System and Oxidative Stress: Relevance for Lake Trout from Lake Ontario and Early Mortality Syndrome of their Offspring

VINCE P. PALACE
Department of Zoology, University of Manitoba, Winnipeg, Manitoba R3T 2N6, Canada

SCOTT B. BROWN
Environment Canada, National Water Research Institute Burlington, Ontario L7R 4A6, Canada

CHRIS L. BARON
Department of Fisheries and Oceans, Freshwater Institute, Central and Arctic Region Winnipeg, Manitoba R3T 2N6, Canada

JOHN D. FITZSIMONS
Environment Canada, National Water Research Institute

JACK F. KLAVERKAMP
Department of Zoology, University of Manitoba, and Department of Fisheries and Oceans, Freshwater Institute

Abstract.—By exposing lake trout *Salvelinus namaycush* and lake sturgeon *Acipenser fulvescens* to planar organochlorines in the laboratory, we have revealed a relationship between induction of the Phase I or mixed function oxidase enzyme system and oxidative stress. Indices of oxidative stress in fish exposed to organochlorines include depleted tissue stores of antioxidant vitamins and elevated concentrations of membrane breakdown products. Given the historically different organochlorine contaminant concentrations in lake trout from Lakes Ontario and Superior, an examination of Phase I induction and oxidative stress in these populations was warranted. Lake trout from Lake Ontario had greater hepatic and renal Phase I activity and lower concentrations of the antioxidant vitamin tocopherol than lake trout from Lake Superior. Lipid hydroperoxide concentrations, a measure of oxidative membrane breakdown and general oxidative stress, were also significantly higher in liver of lake trout from Lake Ontario. The relationship between oxidative stress in adult lake trout from Lake Ontario and early mortality syndrome (EMS) of their offspring was also examined. The elevated oxidative stress indices found in adult female lake trout from Lake Ontario were not correlated with the appearance of EMS in their offspring. Concentrations of antioxidant vitamins in embryos and depletion of these vitamins throughout development also did not differ between embryos with EMS and those without EMS. Eggs that later developed EMS were initially lighter in color and had lower total carotenoid concentrations. Additional work concerning the relationships of the various proretinoid forms with EMS is required. Although lake trout from Lake Ontario exhibit some oxidative stress responses, EMS among their offspring does not appear to be directly related to oxidative stress or the depletion of antioxidant vitamins.

Because they are easily and sensitively measured, Phase I or mixed function oxidase enzyme activities have become an important tool for determining environmental exposures of fish to chlorinated hydrocarbons (Hodson et al. 1991). Despite considerable research concerning Phase I enzymes in fish, the relationship between enzyme induction and cellular mechanisms of toxicity has not been clearly established. However, results from some of the available studies indicate that induction of the Phase I enzyme system can increase the proliferation of oxygen radicals (Lehtinen 1990), resulting in damage to cellular components (i.e., oxidative stress) including lipid membranes, proteins, and DNA (Stohs et al. 1990).

Phase I biotransformation of some substrates, including the reproductive hormone estrogen and some organochlorine contaminants, can produce metabolites that cyclically remove hydrogen atoms from cellular molecules and surrender them to other weak oxidants present in the cell (Liehr and Roy 1990; Winston and Di Giulio 1991). This is known as redox cycling. Redox cycling by transformed metabolites increases oxygen radical production and oxidative stress (Winston and Di Giulio 1991). In addition, metabolites of exogenous contaminant molecules, including PCBs, can mobilize ferrous iron from low molecular weight fractions. These liberated ferrous iron ions can increase oxygen radical proliferation, especially that of the highly reactive hydroxyl radical ($OH^{\cdot}$), by reacting with peroxides in Fenton-type reactions (Smith and De Matteis 1990):

$$H_2O_2 + Fe^{2+} \rightarrow Fe^{3+} + OH^- + OH^{\cdot}$$
(Fenton reaction).

Thus, organisms exposed to compounds that induce Phase I enzymes can have greater biotransformation of endogenous molecules and xenobiotics, both of which result in greater oxidative stress (Lehtinen 1990). Although this process has been widely studied in mammals (Al-Bayati et al. 1987; Shara and Stohs 1987), it has only recently been considered in fish.

These recent studies in fish have found that depletion of antioxidant vitamins and production of oxidative stress may also be related to the elevated mortality of salmonid embryos from Baltic waters (Pettersson 1996). This high mortality in salmon from the Baltic region is referred to as M74 and resembles the early mortality syndrome (EMS) of lake trout *Salvelinus namaycush* from the lower North American Great Lakes (Bengtsson and Hill 1996). Both M74 and EMS occur when yolk resorption is almost completed, when contaminants that were maternally deposited in the yolk have reached their maximal concentration in the developing embryo (Giesy et al. 1986).

We have examined the linkage between Phase I enzyme induction and oxidative stress in fish exposed to planar organochlorines in the laboratory and in lake trout collected from contaminated sites within the Great Lakes (Palace 1996; Palace et al. 1996a, 1996b). Additionally, the relationship between high oxidative stress in adult female lake trout from Lake Ontario and the prevalence of EMS among their offspring has been evaluated. The objectives of these laboratory and field studies on adult and early life history stages were threefold:

1. To examine the hypothesis that Phase I induction is related to oxidative stress, by exposing fish to inducing contaminants in controlled laboratory experiments.
2. To extend the examination of this hypothesis to include lake trout from different locations within the Great Lakes. The locations were chosen based on their different organochlorine contaminant concentrations, which have historically resulted in different Phase I activities of their resident fish populations (Luxon et al. 1987). Specifically, lake trout from Lake Ontario and from the less contaminated Lake Superior were compared.
3. To investigate whether oxidative stress and the accompanying depletion of antioxidant vitamins are related to the appearance of EMS in lake trout from Lake Ontario.

A review of several studies is presented to provide an overview of the accumulated evidence that links Phase I enzyme induction to oxidative stress and EMS. The appropriate publications should be referred to for detailed experimental descriptions.

Laboratory Exposures

Two separate laboratory exposures, using different fish test species, different Phase I inducing contaminants, and different methods of dose administration, aided in our evaluation of the relationship between Phase I induction and induced oxidative stress. In the first experiment, juvenile lake trout were intraperitoneally injected with 3,3′,4,4′,5-pentachlorobiphenyl (PCB 126) suspended in corn oil to achieve nominal doses of 0 (control), 0.6, 6.3, or 25 μg PCB 126/kg body weight ($N = 30$ for each dose group; Palace et al. 1996a). Each of the dose groups was subsampled ($N = 5$) at 1, 3, 6, 13, 20, and 30 weeks after the single dose was administered. After 30 weeks, only lake trout from the two highest dose groups had elevated hepatic Phase I enzyme activity, measured as ethoxyresorufin-*O*-deethylase (EROD), compared with the control group (Table 1). The two highest dose groups also had elevated hepatic concentrations of thiobarbituric acid reactive substances (TBARS; Table 1), a measure of oxidative membrane breakdown, 30 weeks after exposure. Statistical analysis using stepwise linear regression revealed that Phase I activity was a strong predictor of TBARS ($P < 0.001$). The antioxidant vitamins tocopherol and retinol were also depleted in fish with elevated Phase I activity (data not shown). Depletion of these vitamins has previously been shown to occur in oxidatively stressed organisms (Ribera et al. 1991; Liebler 1993).

TABLE 1.—Phase I enzyme activity and TBARS concentrations in liver of lake trout 30 weeks after exposure to pentachlorobiphenyl 126 (PCB). Data are expressed as mean ± SE (N = 5). Means labeled with different letters are statistically different from each other based on results from a randomized one way analysis of variance (ANOVA) followed by Duncan's multiple-range test ($P < 0.05$).

PCB dose group (μg/kg)	Phase I enzyme activity[a] (nmol · min^{-1} · mg protein^{-1})	TBARS[b] (nmol/g)
0	0.035 ± 0.009 z	31.94 ± 8.14 z
0.6	0.0696 ± 0.014 z	33.26 ± 3.46 z
6.3	1.539 ± 0.56 y	0.05 ± 10.62 y
25	3.906 ± 0.26 x	78.55 ± 7.75 y

[a] Phase I enzyme activity was measured as ethoxyresorufin-O-deethylase and is expressed as quantity of resorufin produced per unit time and weight of microsomal protein.

[b] Oxidative membrane breakdown is expressed as quantity of TBARS produced per unit weight of wet liver.

TABLE 2.—Phase I enzyme activity and lipid peroxide concentrations in liver of lake sturgeon 27 d after exposure to 2,3,7,8-tetrachlorodibenzofuran (TCDF). Data are expressed as mean ± SE (N = 5). Means labeled with different letters are statistically different from each other based on results of a randomized one way ANOVA followed by Duncan's multiple-range test ($P < 0.05$).

TCDF dose group (ng/kg)	Phase I enzyme activity[a] (pmol · min^{-1} · mg protein^{-1})	Lipid peroxides[b] (nmol/g)
0	1.06 ± 0.03 z	5.81 ± 3.85 z
0.16	1.28 ± 0.02 y	35.58 ± 13.72 y
1.6	1.89 ± 0.19 x	49.72 ± 8.06 x

[a] Phase I enzyme activity was measured as ethoxyresorufin-O-deethylase and is expressed as quantity of resorufin produced per unit time and weight of microsomal protein.

[b] Oxidative membrane breakdown is expressed as quantity of lipid peroxides produced per unit weight of wet liver.

In the second laboratory experiment, lake sturgeon *Acipenser fulvescens* were orally dosed with gelatin containing 2,3,7,8-tetrachlorodibenzofuran (TCDF) to achieve nominal doses of 0 (control), 0.16, or 1.6 ng TCDF/kg body weight (N = 10 for each dose group; Palace et al. 1996b). Each of the groups was subsampled (N = 5) 10 and 27 d after the single dose was administered. Shorter exposure times were used in this experiment than in the first experiment because TCDF is more readily metabolized than PCB 126 (Muir et al. 1992). Analyses similar to those in the first experiment were performed except that the level of TBARS as a measure of oxidative stress was replaced by a more specific and less variable assay for lipid hydroperoxides (Ohishi et al. 1985).

Despite the use of a different test fish species, method of dose administration, and inducing contaminant, the results obtained from this experiment were consistent with those from the first experiment. Sturgeon exposed to TCDF had induced hepatic Phase I enzyme activity and elevated concentrations of lipid hydroperoxides (Table 2). Furthermore, hepatic Phase I enzyme activity was positively correlated with lipid hydroperoxide concentrations in the liver ($R^2 = 0.52$, $P < 0.001$). Tocopherol concentrations were also depleted in the livers of sturgeon exposed to TCDF (data not shown), further confirming that greater oxidative stress resulted from exposure to the contaminant (Packer 1991).

Results from these two laboratory studies directly addressed the first hypothesis. Fish exposed to organochlorine contaminants that induce the Phase I enzyme system had elevated oxidative stress and depleted stores of antioxidant vitamins. Furthermore, these effects appeared with different inducing contaminants and test fish species.

Great Lakes Studies

Having established a relationship between induction of the Phase I enzyme system and oxidative stress in fish exposed to organochlorine contaminants in the laboratory, we evaluated this relationship, and the second hypothesis, in lake trout from the Great Lakes. Adult female lake trout captured during the fall of 1994 at Port Weller, Lake Ontario (N = 30), had greater Phase I activity and higher oxidative stress than lake trout captured from the less contaminated site of Black Bay on Lake Superior (N = 7; Palace 1996). The lake trout from Lake Ontario had 3.3 times greater Phase I activity in liver (Table 3) and 15 times greater Phase I activity in kidney (data not shown) than lake trout from Lake Superior.

In addition to higher hepatic and renal Phase I enzyme activities, the lake trout from Lake Ontario also were subject to greater oxidative stress, as shown by elevated hepatic lipid peroxide concentrations (Table 3). However, unlike the results from our laboratory experiments, there was no statistically significant relationship between Phase I activity and lipid hydroperoxide concentrations in lake trout from the

TABLE 3.—Phase I enzyme activity and concentrations of lipid peroxides and tocopherol in liver of adult female lake trout from Lakes Ontario and Superior. Data are expressed as mean ± SE (N = 30 for Port Weller and N = 7 for Black Bay). Means labeled with different letters are statistically different from each other based on comparisons using Dunnett's one-tailed test ($P < 0.05$).

Location	Phase I enzyme activity[a] (nmol · min^{-1} · mg protein^{-1})	Lipid peroxides[b] (nmol/g)	Tocopherol[c] (μg/g)
Port Weller, Lake Ontario	0.46±0.09 z	44.18±3.89 z	462±103 z
Black Bay, Lake Superior	0.14±0.03 y	16.23±4.03 y	2897±995 y

[a] Phase I enzyme activity was measured as ethoxyresorufin-*O*-deethylase and is expressed as quantity of resorufin produced per unit time and weight of microsomal protein.

[b] Oxidative membrane breakdown is expressed as quantity of lipid peroxides extracted per unit weight of wet liver.

[c] Tocopherol concentrations are expressed as quantity per unit weight of wet liver.

Great Lakes. It should be emphasized that Phase I enzyme activities were induced 150- to 200-fold in fish exposed to contaminants in the laboratory but only 3.3 to 15-fold in lake trout from Lake Ontario versus those from Lake Superior. Therefore, although oxygen radicals resulting from Phase I activity may contribute to oxidative stress, the level of Phase I activity in lake trout from Lake Ontario is probably not sufficient to be solely responsible for this condition. Moreover, lake trout from Lake Ontario contain higher concentrations of other potential oxidants, including redox active metals (J. F. Klaverkamp, Department of Fisheries and Oceans, and K. Wautier, Biotech West, unpublished data), than lake trout from Lake Superior. These metals may contribute to the elevated membrane oxidation in lake trout from Lake Ontario by a mechanism that is separate from the induction of Phase I enzymes (Winston and Di Giulio 1991).

The lake trout captured from Lake Superior in 1994 had tocopherol concentrations that were 6.3 times greater in liver (Table 3) and 35 times greater in kidney (data not shown) than lake trout from Lake Ontario (Palace 1996). Long-term exposures of lake trout and other aquatic organisms to inducing contaminants have consistently resulted in depleted stores of tocopherol (Ribera et al. 1991; Palace et al. 1996a, 1996b; Brown et al., in press). Although greater antioxidant consumption of tocopherol may be responsible for lower tocopherol concentrations in trout from Lake Ontario (Burton and Traber 1990), dietary differences between the Lake Ontario and Lake Superior populations could also influence tissue concentrations of the vitamin (Packer 1991). Regardless of the factors involved, greater concentrations of tocopherol in lake trout from Lake Superior would afford them greater protection against oxidant-mediated cell injury (Maellaro et al. 1990).

Oxidative Stress, Antioxidants, and EMS

Adult Lake Trout

Higher Phase I activity, greater tissue concentrations of redox active metals, and lower concentrations of antioxidant vitamins could all contribute to the higher oxidative stress in lake trout from Lake Ontario compared with lake trout from Lake Superior. Because other studies have shown that antioxidant vitamin depletion and oxidative stress may be related to greater mortality of embryonic salmonids (Pettersson 1996), this relationship was examined in offspring of lake trout from Lake Ontario and from a reference site.

In addition to the 1994 collections from Lake Ontario described above, adult female lake trout were also captured from a less contaminated reference site on Lake Manitou during the fall of 1994 (N = 6; Palace 1996). Phase I enzyme activity, oxidative stress indices, and concentrations of antioxidant vitamins were assessed in liver tissue collected from adult females at both of these locations.

To allow comparisons based on the prevalence of EMS in their offspring, the adult lake trout from Lake Ontario were divided into two subpopulations: a high EMS group, the offspring of which exhibited more than 10% mortality from EMS (N = 13); and a low EMS group, the offspring of which exhibited less than 10% mortality from EMS (N = 14). The two subpopulations of adult lake trout from Lake Ontario had 2.5–3 times greater hepatic Phase I enzyme activities, measured as EROD, than adult female lake trout from the

TABLE 4.—Phase I enzyme activity and concentrations of lipid peroxides and tocopherol in liver of adult female lake trout from Lakes Ontario and Manitou. Data are expressed as mean ± SE (N = 13 for females whose offspring had >10% EMS, N = 14 for females whose offspring had <10% EMS, and N = 6 for Lake Manitou). Means labeled with different letters are statistically different from each other based on results from a randomized one way ANOVA followed by Duncan's multiple-range test ($P < 0.05$).

Location	Phase I enzyme activity[a] (nmol · min^{-1} · mg protein^{-1})	Lipid peroxides[b] (nmol/g)	Tocopherol[c] (μg/g)
Lake Ontario >10% EMS in offspring	0.61 ± 0.15 z	43.1 ± 3.9 z	419 ± 106 z
Lake Ontario <10% EMS in offspring	0.51 ± 0.09 z	41.7 ± 4.7 z	889 ± 191 y
Lake Manitou (EMS not present)	0.22 ± 0.03 y	26.5 ± 3.4 y	414 ± 75 z

[a] Phase I enzyme activity was measured as ethoxyresorufin-*O*-deethylase activity and is expressed as quantity of resorufin produced per unit time and weight of microsomal protein.

[b] Oxidative membrane breakdown is expressed as quantity of lipid peroxides extracted per unit weight of wet liver.

[c] Tocopherol concentrations are expressed as quantity per unit weight of wet liver.

control site at Lake Manitou (Table 4). However, there were no significant differences in the levels of Phase I activity of the adult lake trout between the high and low EMS groups from Lake Ontario. Similarly, both subpopulations of lake trout from Lake Ontario had 1.5–2 times greater concentrations of hepatic lipid peroxides than the reference lake trout from Lake Manitou (Table 4), but no differences related to the prevalence of EMS in the offspring were apparent. Of the oxidative stress variables measured in adults, only hepatic vitamin E concentrations were different between the high and low EMS groups from Lake Ontario. Lake trout from the low EMS group had hepatic vitamin E concentrations that were approximately 2 times greater than those found in lake trout from the high EMS group from Lake Ontario and in lake trout from Lake Manitou (Table 4). However, statistical analysis revealed no significant correlation between the lower hepatic vitamin E concentrations of adult lake trout and mortality related to EMS within the offspring.

Embryonic Lake Trout

Eggs stripped from the adult females from Lake Ontario and Lake Manitou were fertilized and reared separately in the laboratory. Each female's embryos were monitored throughout their development to the post-swim-up stage for survival and the appearance of EMS. Additionally, the concentrations of antioxidant vitamins were determined in subsamples of the embryos (N = 4) taken at six developmental stages: green eggs (0 degree-days), eyed (247 degree-days), prehatch (524 degree-days), posthatch (686 degree-days), pre-swim-up (836 degree-days), and post-swim-up (964 degree-days). Egg color was recorded only at the green egg stage. The potential for generating oxygen radicals by induced Phase I enzymes was assessed in the embryos at the post-swim-up stage using an immunohistochemical method to detect the Cyp1A protein (Smolowitz et al. 1991).

The capacity for Phase I activity to be induced increases in salmonid embryos near the time of hatching (Binder and Stegeman 1983). However, immunohistochemical staining analysis for Cyp1A protein content, which has previously been shown to correlate well with Phase I activity, showed no significant differences between the high and low EMS embryos from Lake Ontario and embryos from the reference site on Lake Manitou at the post-swim-up stage (data not shown; Palace 1996). These results are surprising given the higher Phase I activity of Lake Ontario adults compared with Lake Manitou adults. Furthermore, embryos from Lake Ontario would be expected to contain higher concentrations of maternally deposited organochlorine contaminants in their lipid-rich yolks (Walker and Peterson 1991).

Because of the high content of unsaturated fatty acids in eggs and the increasing aerobic metabolism that generates oxidative radicals in developing embryos, and because antioxidant enzymes are not synthesized until late in embryonic development, early antioxidant protection by vitamins is essential (Cowey et al. 1985). Tissue stores of vitamins A, C, and E can be depleted by their increased use as anti-

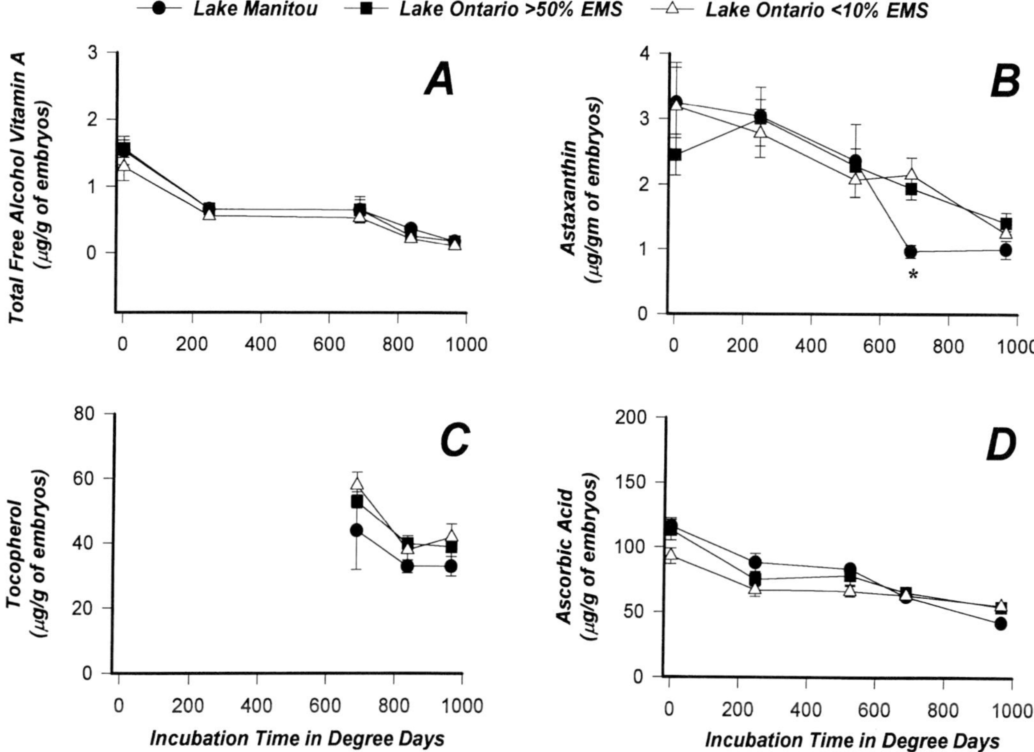

FIGURE 1.—Concentrations (microgram per gram of embryos) of total free alcohol vitamin A (e.g., retinol + didehydroretinol) (**A**), the provitamin A compound astaxanthin (**B**), tocopherol (**C**), and ascorbic acid (**D**) in lake trout embryos. Data are expressed as mean ± SE (N = 13, 14, and 6 for >10% EMS population from Lake Ontario, <10% EMS population from Lake Ontario, and Lake Manitou population, respectively). The asterisk in (**B**) indicates a mean that is significantly different from the other two means for the same sample period based on results from Duncan's multiple-range test ($P < 0.05$).

oxidants (Chatterjee and Nandi 1991; Ribera et al. 1991; Liebler 1993). However, we found similar concentrations of vitamin A, measured as the free alcohol forms (e.g., retinol + didehydroretinol; Figure 1A) and as the predominant provitamin form, astaxanthin (Figure 1B), in the embryos of the high and low EMS groups from Lake Ontario and the reference lake at all of the developmental stages that were analyzed. Eggs produced by females whose offspring later developed EMS were lighter in color than those produced by females whose offspring did not develop EMS (data not shown). Carotenoids other than astaxanthin, including canthaxanthin, could contribute to this difference in color. In fact, eggs subsampled from batches that developed EMS had lower total carotenoid stores, but this difference was not evident at any of the other developmental stages that were analyzed (data not shown). Clearly, additional work concerning the relationships of the various proretinoid forms with EMS is required.

Tocopherol (Figure 1C) and ascorbic acid (Figure 1D) concentrations were not consistently different between these populations at any of the developmental stages that were considered. This lack of accelerated vitamin depletion in embryos from Lake Ontario with EMS compared with unaffected and reference embryos indicates that EMS may not be related to greater oxidative stress in lake trout embryos. However, whole body antioxidant concentrations may not be representative of the concentrations found in specific tissues, which could be more predictive of EMS mortality.

The lack of consistent correlations between oxidative stress and EMS in lake trout embryos from this study is significant in light of other recent information. Specifically, strong correlations between M74 and oxidative stress, measured as malonaldehyde concentrations, have been reported for salmon from Swedish waters (Pettersson 1996). These studies have also shown significant depletions of vitamin A compounds in salmon embryos with M74 compared with unaffected embryos (Pettersson 1996). However, fortification of North American salmonid embryos with vitamin A compounds was shown to have no significant effect on EMS in steelhead trout *Oncorhynchus mykiss* from Lake Michigan (Hornung et al. 1996).

Biological differences between Baltic salmon and lake trout from the Great Lakes may partially explain the contrasting results for the two species. For example, spawning activity in salmon is accompanied by a significant period of fasting, which alone has been shown to increase indices of oxidative stress in mammals (Pohjanvirta et al. 1990). Because lake trout do not restrict feeding to the same extent during spawning, oxidative stress variables would be less affected.

Summary and Conclusions

Two laboratory studies using different Phase I enzyme-inducing contaminants and test fish species enabled us to establish a correlation between Phase I enzyme induction and oxidative stress with its accompanying antioxidant vitamin depletion. However, a comparison of lake trout from traditionally more contaminated Lake Ontario with those from Lake Superior showed that although oxidative stress was higher and antioxidant concentrations were lower in Lake Ontario fish, these differences were not correlated with Phase I enzyme activity. Lower Phase I enzyme inductions in Great Lakes fish compared with fish from the laboratory experiments may be the root of this fundamental difference between the laboratory and field results. Additionally, in contrast to recent reports concerning Baltic salmon with M74, a detailed examination of oxidative stress and antioxidant concentrations in lake trout from Lake Ontario revealed few significant relationships with EMS. Only egg color and the concentration of total carotenoids in green eggs were different between the EMS and non-EMS populations. The discrepancy between the results from the Great Lakes and the Baltic region may arise from biological differences between lake trout and Baltic salmon.

References

Al-Bayati, Z. A. F., W. J. Murray, and S. J. Stohs. 1987. 2,3,7,8-tetrachlorodibenzo-p-dioxin induced lipid peroxidation in hepatic and extrahepatic tissues of male and female rats. Archives of Environmental Contamination and Toxicology 16:159–166.

Bengtsson, B.-E., and C. Hill. 1996. Summary of the second workshop on reproduction disturbances in fish. Pages 9–10 *in* B.-E. Bengtsson, C. Hill, and S. Nellbring, editors. Report from the second workshop on reproduction disturbances in fish. Swedish Environmental Protection Agency Report 4534, Stockholm.

Binder, R. L., and J. J. Stegeman. 1983. Basal levels and induction of hepatic aryl hydrocarbon hydroxylase activity during the embryonic period of development in brook trout. Biochemical Pharmacology 32:1324–1327.

Brown, S. B., and five coauthors. In press. Biochemical and histological responses in broodstock rainbow trout (*Oncorhynchus mykiss*) exposed to 2,3,4,7,8-pentachloro-dibenzofuran. Environmental Toxicology and Chemistry.

Burton, G. W., and M. G. Traber. 1990. Vitamin E: antioxidant activity, biokinetics and bioavailability. Annual Review of Nutrition 10:357–382.

Chatterjee, I. B., and A. Nandi. 1991. Ascorbic acid: a scavenger of oxyradicals. Indian Journal of Biochemistry and Biophysics 28:233–236.

Cowey, C. B., J. G. Bell, D. Knox, A. Fraser, and A. Youngson. 1985. Lipids and antioxidant systems in developing eggs of salmon (*Salmo salar*). Lipids 20:567–572.

Giesy, J. P., J. Newsted, and D. L. Garling. 1986. Relationships between chlorinated hydrocarbon concentrations and rearing mortality of chinook salmon (*Oncorhynchus tshawytscha*) eggs from Lake Michigan. Journal of Great Lakes Research 12:82–98.

Hodson, P. V., and nine coauthors. 1991. Protocols for measuring mixed function oxygenases of fish liver. Canadian Technical Report of Fisheries and Aquatic Sciences 1829.

Hornung, M. W., L. Miller, R. Peterson, S. Marcquenski, and S. B. Brown. 1996. Evaluation of nutritional and pathogenic factors in early mortality syndrome in Lake Michigan salmonids. Pages 82–83 *in* B.-E. Bengtsson, C. Hill, and S. Nellbring, editors. Report from the second workshop on reproduction disturbances in fish. Swedish Environmental Protection Agency Report 4534, Stockholm.

Lehtinen, K. J. 1990. Mixed function oxygenase enzyme responses and physiological disorders in fish exposed to kraft pulp mill effluents: a hypothetical model. Ambio 19:259–265.

Liebler, D. C. 1993. The role of metabolism in the antioxidant function of vitamin E. Critical Reviews in Toxicology 23:147–169.

Liehr, J. G., and D. Roy. 1990. Free radical generation by redox cycling of estrogens. Free Radical Biology & Medicine 8:415–423.

Luxon, P. L., P. V. Hodson, and U. Borgmann. 1987. Hepatic aryl hydrocarbon hydroxylase activity of lake trout (*Salvelinus namaycush*) as an indicator of organic pollution. Environmental Toxicology and Chemistry 6:649–657.

Maellaro, E., A. F. Casini, B. Del-Bello, and M. Comporti. 1990. Lipid peroxidation and antioxidant systems in the liver injury produced by glutathione depleting agents. Biochemical Pharmacology 39:1513–1521.

Muir, D. C. G., A. L. Yarechewski, D. A. Metner, and W. L. Lockhart. 1992. Dietary 2,3,7,8-tetrachlorodibenzofuran in rainbow trout: accumulation, disposition and hepatic mixed-function oxidase enzyme induction. Toxicology and Applied Pharmacology 117:65–74.

Ohishi, N., H. Ohkawa, A. Miike, T. Tatano, and K. Yagi. 1985. A new assay for lipid peroxides using a methylene blue derivative. Biochemistry International 10:205–211.

Packer, L. 1991. Protective role of vitamin E in biological systems. American Journal of Clinical Nutrition 53:1050s–1055s.

Palace, V. P., and five coauthors. 1996a. Oxidative stress in lake trout (*Salvelinus namaycush*) exposed to 3,3',4,4',5-pentachlorobiphenyl (PCB 126). Environmental Toxicology and Chemistry 15:955–960.

Palace, V. P., T. A. Dick, S. B. Brown, C. L. Baron, and J. F. Klaverkamp. 1996b. Oxidative stress in lake sturgeon (*Acipenser fulvescens*) orally exposed to 2,3,7,8-tetrachlorodibenzofuran. Aquatic Toxicology 35:79–92.

Palace, V. P. 1996. Oxidative stress in lake trout (*Salvelinus namaycush*) exposed to organochlorine contaminants that induce the phase I biotransformation enzyme system. Doctoral dissertation. University of Manitoba, Winnipeg.

Pettersson, A. 1996. Decreased astaxanthin levels in the Baltic salmon and the M74 syndrome. Pages 28–29 *in* B.-E. Bengtsson, C. Hill, and S. Nellbring, editors. Report from the second workshop on reproduction disturbances in fish. Swedish Environmental Protection Agency Report 4534, Stockholm.

Pohjanvirta, R., and five coauthors. 1990. Studies on the role of lipid peroxidation in the acute toxicity of TCDD in rats. Pharmacology & Toxicology 66:399–408.

Ribera, D., J. F. Narbonne, X. Michel, D. R. Livingstone, and S. O'Hara. 1991. Responses of antioxidants and lipid peroxidation in mussels to oxidative damage exposure. Comparative Biochemistry and Physiology 100C:177–181.

Shara, M. A., and S. J. Stohs. 1987. Biochemical and toxicological effects of 2,3,7,8-tetrachlorodibenzo-p-dioxin (TCDD) congeners in female rats. Archives of Environmental Contamination and Toxicology 16:599–605.

Smith, A. G., and F. De Matteis. 1990. Oxidative injury mediated by the hepatic cytochrome P-450 system in conjunction with cellular iron. Effects on the pathway of haem biosynthesis. Xenobiotica 20:865–877.

Smolowitz, R. M., M. E. Hahn, and J. J. Stegeman. 1991. Immunohistochemical localization of cytochrome P4501A1 induced by 3,3',4,4'-tetrachlorobiphenyl and by 2,3,7,8-tetrachlorodibenzofuran in liver and extrahepatic tissues of the teleost *Stenotomus chrysops* (scup). Drug Metabolism and Disposition 19:113–123.

Stohs, S. J., M. A. Shara, N. Z. Alsharif, Z. Z. Wahba, and Z. A. Al-Bayati. 1990. 2,3,7,8-tetrachlorodibenzo-p-dioxin induced oxidative stress in female rats. Toxicology and Applied Pharmacology 106:126–135.

Walker, M. K., and R. E. Peterson. 1991. Potencies of polychlorinated dibenzo-p-dioxin, dibenzofuran, and biphenyl congeners, relative to 2,3,7,8-tetrachlorodibenzo-*p*-dioxin, for producing early life stage mortality in rainbow trout (*Oncorhynchus mykiss*). Aquatic Toxicology 21:219–238.

Winston, G. W., and R. T. Di Giulio. 1991. Prooxidant and antioxidant mechanisms in aquatic organisms. Aquatic Toxicology 19:137–161.

American Fisheries Society Symposium 21:154–159, 1998

Thiaminase Activity in Alewives and Smelt in Lakes Huron, Michigan, and Superior

YING Q. JI[1] AND IRA R. ADELMAN[2]
Department of Fisheries and Wildlife, University of Minnesota
1980 Folwell Avenue, St. Paul, Minnesota 55108-6124, USA

Abstract.—Smelt *Osmerus mordax* and alewives *Alosa pseudoharengus* were collected from Lakes Huron and Michigan in spring and fall and from Lake Superior in spring to determine the activity of thiaminase, a thiamine-destroying enzyme, in those species. Greater thiaminase activity was found in the viscera (1,902 pmol · g^{-1} · min^{-1} for smelt and 1,705 pmol · g^{-1} · min^{-1} for alewives) than in the eviscerated body (180 pmol · g^{-1} · min^{-1} for smelt and 235 pmol · g^{-1} · min^{-1} for alewives). The average whole body thiaminase activity when all of the samples were pooled was 362 pmol · g^{-1} · min^{-1} for smelt and 357 pmol · g^{-1} · min^{-1} for alewives. Large differences were found in thiaminase activities between smelt and alewives from different locations in the Great Lakes region and at different sampling times. These differences may be species-, location-, or season-specific.

Smelt *Osmerus mordax* and alewives *Alosa pseudoharengus* are major items in the diet of lake trout *Salvelinus namaycush* in the Great Lakes (Jude et al. 1987; Diana 1990; Miller and Holey 1992; Conner et al. 1993). Both of these species contain thiaminase, an enzyme that destroys thiamine (Deutsch and Hasler 1943; Gnaedinger and Krzeczkowski 1966). Consumption of thiaminase causes rapid thiamine deficiency in humans and other mammals (Murata 1965) and may cause a thiamine deficiency in fish (Coble 1965; Ishihara et al. 1978; Ji et al. 1998, this volume).

Recent studies have suggested that thiamine deficiency may be the cause of early mortality syndrome (EMS) in lake trout larvae, the symptoms of which include anorexia, loss of equilibrium, hyperexcitability, and eventual death (Fitzsimons 1995; Fisher et al. 1996). This deficiency could result from consumption of forage species containing thiaminase, particularly smelt and alewives. A resultant thiamine deficiency could then be responsible, at least in part, for the poor reproductive success of lake trout in the Great Lakes.

The destruction of thiamine by thiaminase was first characterized as Chastek's paralysis when raw carp, which are high in thiaminase, were fed to foxes (Green and Evans 1940). Symptoms included anorexia, weakness, convulsions, and paralysis. Thiaminase has since been found in many species of both marine and freshwater fish (Deutsch and Hasler 1943; Neilands 1947; Hilker and Peter 1966; Grieg and Gnaedinger 1971; Ishihara et al. 1973).

The purpose of this study was to determine the levels of thiaminase activity in smelt and alewives in Lakes Huron, Michigan, and Superior and to determine the differences in these levels among the species, lakes, locations within lakes, and fish caught at different times of the year. Because of the uncertainty regarding whether thiaminase is present in the viscera, musculature, or both (Neilands 1947; Grieg and Gnaedinger 1971), separate analyses were conducted on viscera and the remaining eviscerated fish.

Methods

Sample Collection and Preparation

Alewives and smelt were collected from the Harbor Beach, Oscoda, Alpena, and Cheboygan areas of Lake Huron; the Saugatuck area of Lake Michigan; and the Apostle Islands area of Lake Superior (smelt only) from late April to early June 1987 (Figure 1). Alewives and smelt were also collected from the Frankfort, Benton Harbor, Waukegon, Manistique, Sturgeon Bay, and Saugatuck areas of Lake Michigan from late August to late October 1987. Smelt weight averaged 27 g (range, 7–62 g) and alewife weight averaged 14 g (range, 3–33 g). All of the samples were collected by U.S. Fish and Wildlife Service research vessels trawling at about 10–70 m, 8–25 km off shore. Once the fish were out of the water, they were frozen within 10–30 min.

The samples were transported to the laboratory on dry ice and stored in a −20°C freezer until they were analyzed. For analysis, frozen fish were

[1] Present address: Minnesota Department of Agriculture, 90 West Plato Boulevard, St. Paul, Minnesota 55107, USA.
[2] To whom reprint requests should be addressed.

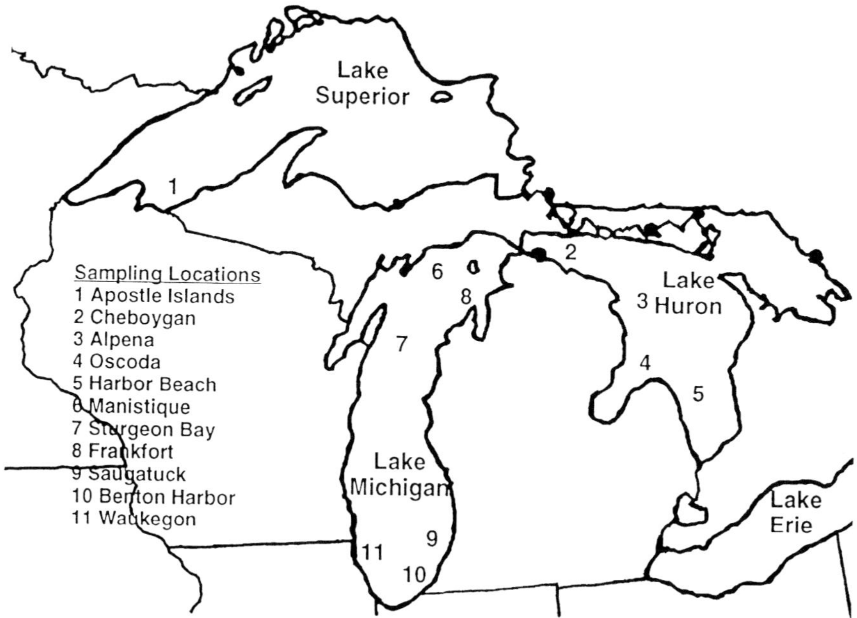

FIGURE 1.—Locations in Lakes Huron, Michigan, and Superior from which smelt and alewives were collected.

thawed, body weight was measured, and viscera and body samples were prepared separately. All contents of the gastrointestinal tract were removed before thiaminase analysis. Because viscera were not weighed separately, a viscera to body weight relationship for each species was used to calculate whole body thiaminase activity. Data for calculating the relationship for both smelt and alewives were provided by G. H. Ketola (Biological Resources Division, U.S. Geological Survey, unpublished data). To calculate whole body thiaminase activity, the activity of the eviscerated body was multiplied by the proportion of the whole body comprising the eviscerated fish (89% for smelt and 92% for alewives) and added to the activity of the viscera multiplied by the proportion of the whole body comprising the viscera (11% for smelt and 8% for alewives).

Thiaminase Assay

The thiaminase assay of Edwin and Jackman (1974) was used with minor modifications. Thiazole-2-^{14}C-labeled thiamine (Amersham Corp., Arlington Heights, Illinois) was dissolved in 0.1 N HCl to give a solution of 10 mCi/mL as stock solution. A working solution was prepared by mixing 0.2 mL of stock solution with 100 mL of citrate phosphate buffer (0.1 M, pH = 6.4) containing nonradioactive thiamine at a concentration of 14.97 nmol/mL, resulting in a specific activity of 2,821 disintegrations per minute per nanomole (dpm/nmol) of thiamine.

A 1-g sample of body tissue or viscera was placed in a round bottom tube, ground and homogenized in 2 mL of citrate phosphate buffer, and centrifuged for 10 min at 3,000 g at room temperature. One-half milliliter of supernatant was pipetted into a centrifuge tube, mixed with 0.5 mL of thiamine solution, and incubated for 10 min at 37°C. After incubation, 2 mL of ethyl acetate was added to the tube, which was spun vigorously to induce absorption of thiazole by ethyl acetate. The extraction was done only once because preassay testing indicated that the extraction efficiency was 93% or better. The tube was then centrifuged for 10 min at 3,000 g to separate ethyl acetate from the aqueous portion of the sample. The 0.5-mL upper layer was pipetted into a scintillation vial containing 5 mL of Ecocint O, a liquid scintillation cocktail (National Diagnostics, Manville, New Jersey).

Radioactivity was measured with a Beckman Instruments (Fullerton, California) LS-1000 Liquid Scintillation Spectrometer. For each batch of samples, a blank of 0.5 mL of citrate phosphate buffer was analyzed in place of the 0.5-mL sample to correct for background radioactivity. A standard of 0.5

mL of ethyl acetate containing 7 mL of [^{14}C]toluene (400,000 dpm/mL) was used to measure the counting efficiency.

The thiaminase activity, expressed as picomoles of thiamine destroyed per minute per gram of sample, was calculated according to the following formula:

thiaminase activity =
[(sample CPM − blank) × DF]/ CF × SA × AT × SW,

where CPM is counts per minute, DF is dilution factors, CE is counting efficiency (0.914), SA is specific activity, AT is assay time (10 min), and SW is sample weight.

During preassay testing of the procedures, a known amount of radioactive thiamine was incubated with carp intestine, a tissue high in thiaminase activity, for 30 min to degrade all of the thiamine into thiazole. After the procedures described above, 85% of the radioactivity was recovered.

Multiple regression was used to analyze overall differences in thiaminase activity between species, differences within and between species in different regions of the lakes, differences between sampling times, and the relationship between fish size and thiaminase activity. Statistical comparisons were conducted for five different regions (Lake Superior, Apostle Islands region; north and south Lake Michigan; and north and south Lake Huron) because these locations might represent ecologically distinct areas. The north Lake Michigan region included Manistique, Sturgeon Bay, and Frankfort; the south Lake Michigan region included Saugatuck, Benton Harbor, and Waukegon; the north Lake Huron region included Cheboygan and Alpena; and the south Lake Huron region included Oscoda and Harbor Beach (Figure 1). Samples collected from 25 April to 4 June 1987 were designated spring samples and those collected from 27 August to 31 October 1987 were designated fall samples.

Analysis of variance was used to compare thiaminase activities where the experimental design was balanced, that is, where samples were available from all compared locations and times. *F*-tests and *t*-tests were used in conjunction with multiple regression analysis, analysis of variance, and for multiple group comparisons. A *t*-test was also used to compare thiaminase activities between viscera and eviscerated bodies and between smelt and alewives when all of the samples were pooled.

TABLE 1.—Thiaminase activity (pmol · g^{-1} · min^{-1}) in viscera, eviscerated body, and whole body of all smelt and alewives assayed. Standard errors are shown in parentheses.

Tissue	Smelt	Alewife
Whole body	362 (18)	357 (18)
Eviscerated body	180 (17)	235 (17)
Viscera	1,902 (61)	1,705 (57)

Results

By far, the greatest activity of thiaminase occurred in the viscera of both alewives and smelt, but thiaminase was also present in the eviscerated bodies of both species (Table 1). Smelt had significantly greater thiaminase activity in the viscera than alewives ($P < 0.05$), and alewives had significantly greater activity in the eviscerated body than smelt ($P < 0.05$). Because these differences were opposite for the two tissue groups, whole body thiaminase activity was not significantly different between smelt and alewives when samples from all locations and seasons were combined ($P > 0.05$).

Multiple regression analysis indicated that considerable variation in thiaminase activity occurred between smelt and alewives among regions in the Great Lakes and during different sampling seasons (Table 2). This variation included highly significant interactions between species and region and between species and season ($P < 0.0001$). Because of an imbalance in the availability of data from all locations and times, interactions between region and season, although potentially significant, could not be computed. There was no relationship between fish size and thiaminase activity for either smelt or alewives ($P > 0.05$).

Thiaminase activities of smelt from Lakes Huron, Michigan, and Superior during the spring sampling were not significantly different ($P > 0.05$; Table 2). Thiaminase activities of spring-sampled alewives from Lake Michigan were significantly higher than those from Lake Huron, both regions combined, but they were not different from those from the southern region of Lake Huron when locations were considered separately. Spring samples for both species from both lakes indicated significant differences between lakes ($P < 0.05$) and between species ($P < 0.0001$), whereas the interaction between lakes and species was not significant ($P > 0.05$).

Among the fall samples within Lake Michigan, there were significant differences between species, regions, and their interaction ($P < 0.01$; Table 2). Smelt

TABLE 2.—Mean thiaminase activity (pmol · g^{-1} · min^{-1}) in alewives and smelt in different regions of the Great Lakes and in different seasons. Standard errors are shown in parentheses.

	Alewife				Smelt			
Lake and region	*N*	Spring	*N*	Fall	*N*	Spring	*N*	Fall
Superior					28	249 (20)		
Michigan								
North			44	242 (23)			36	313 (18)
South	18	576 (57)	24	240 (19)	12	341 (37)	59	517 (50)
Combined			68	241 (22)			95	440 (39)
Huron								
North	24	514 (43)			24	183 (16)		
South	24	362 (19)			24	476 (50)		
Combined	48	438 (26)			48	330 (34)		

had higher thiaminase activities in both the northern and southern regions than alewives. Smelt thiaminase activity was significantly higher in the south than in the north ($P < 0.0001$), whereas alewife thiaminase activity was about the same in the two regions.

Thiaminase activities of spring-sampled smelt and alewives were significantly different between the northern and southern regions of Lake Huron (Table 2). Smelt thiaminase activity was significantly higher in the south than in the north ($P < 0.05$). Smelt also had higher thiaminase activity in the south than alewives, but alewife thiaminase activity was significantly higher than that of smelt in the north ($P < 0.05$), which resulted in a significant interaction between species and region ($P < 0.0001$).

The only region for which we had both spring and fall samples was southern Lake Michigan (Table 2). The analysis of these samples indicated that although species were not significantly different ($P > 0.05$), both season and interaction between season and species were significant ($P < 0.02$ and 0.0001, respectively). The results of the analysis ($P < 0.05$) were: smelt had higher thiaminase activity than alewives in fall; alewife thiaminase activity was higher in spring than in fall; and alewives had higher thiaminase activity than smelt in spring.

Discussion

Thiaminase was present in all smelt and alewives, but the level of thiaminase activity was highly variable. Large differences occurred among locations, species at a given location, and time of year. Lack of samples from all locations during both seasons made it impossible to statistically determine in an integrated manner the differences in thiaminase activity among species, lakes, and seasons. The highly significant interactions allow us to conclude only that thiaminase activities are significantly different between alewives and smelt at different locations and possibly during different seasons. These differences may be species-, location-, and time-specific. Sampling would need to be repeated at several locations for several years to determine if the differences that we detected are repeatable at different times.

The level of thiaminase found in smelt and alewives in this study was consistent with that found in most previous reports. Fujita (1954), Gnaedinger and Krzeczkowski (1966), Hilker and Peter (1966), Hirn and Pekkanen (1975), and Anglesea and Jackson (1986) reported thiaminase activity in smelt and alewives or other fish species ranging from about 10 to 1,500 pmol · g^{-1} · min^{-1} (converted from originally reported units), which was similar to the levels found in individual fish in the present study: 76–1,282 pmol · g^{-1} · min^{-1} for alewives and 69–1,478 pmol · g^{-1} · min^{-1} for smelt.

Recent studies have linked EMS in salmonids to thiaminase activities in their forage species. Fitzsimons (1995) suggested that the presence of EMS in different Great Lakes regions might be the result of higher thiaminase activities in alewives than in smelt, as reported by Gnaedinger and Krzeczkowski (1966). However, Gnaedinger and Krzeczkowski (1966) analyzed only one smelt and three alewives; moreover, their smelt was from Lake Erie and their alewives were from Lake Michigan. Our results indicate that single samples are poor predictors of overall thiaminase levels in a species and that thiaminase levels in both species are highly variable. The presence of EMS in some regions of the Great Lakes but not in others is more likely caused by a combination of the percentage of thiaminase-containing species in the diet and the level of thiaminase activity in individual species at the time and location of consumption by lake trout.

Although thiaminase has been purified (Murata 1965) and a bacterial thiaminase gene has been cloned and expressed in *Escherichia coli* (Abe et al. 1987), its physiological significance is not clear. It is probably not active as a thiamine-destroying enzyme in living cells. In species containing the enzyme, it may be used for thiamine synthesis (Fujita 1954). Any attempt to explain the wide variation of thiaminase activities found in this study would be premature because we do not know what would cause thiaminase activity to change.

Various attempts have been made to feed thiaminase-containing species to other fish, with inconsistent results; sometimes the fish show overt symptoms of thiamine deficiency and sometimes they do not (Wolf 1942; Harrington 1954; Coble 1965; Ji et al. 1998). The variable results may be attributable to a variety of circumstances. The thiaminase acts on dietary thiamine; therefore, a period of storage of the dietary fish may be necessary to destroy the thiamine. However, almost complete destruction of large quantities of naturally occurring thiamine, as well as supplementary thiamine, can occur within 30 min, as demonstrated in our preliminary experiment with carp intestine (see "Methods") and in studies by Krampitz and Woolley (1944) and Melnick et al. (1945). In live fish in a natural environment, thiamine destruction would have to occur in the gastrointestinal tract, but considering the rapid rate of the reaction, this certainly seems plausible. Melnick et al. (1945) found that about 50% of ingested thiamine was destroyed in the gastrointestinal tract of human subjects after ingestion of raw clams containing thiaminase. Thiamine destruction might be less severe in the coldwater salmonids, but the reaction rate in vitro is not greatly affected by temperature. Krampitz and Woolley (1944) found only a 50% difference in the amount of thiamine destroyed in a given time at temperatures of 0 and 37°C.

Because smelt and alewives are predominant forage species for Great Lakes salmonids (Diana 1990; Miller and Holey 1992; Conner et al. 1993) and high thiaminase activities have been confirmed in these species in this study, thiamine deficiency as a result of the presence of high levels of thiaminase seems a plausible cause of early mortality syndrome in salmonids.

Acknowledgments

This work is the result of research sponsored by the Minnesota Sea Grant Program, which is supported by the National Oceanic and Atmospheric Administration Office of Sea Grant, United States Department of Commerce, under grant R/F-23. This paper is journal reprint number JR 433 of the Minnesota Sea Grant College Program. We thank the staff of the U.S. Fish and Wildlife Service for collecting fish samples, George H. Ketola (U.S. Geological Survey) for providing data on body and visceral weights of smelt and alewives, George R. Spangler for providing suggestions for conducting this research, and Ronald W. Hardy and an anonymous reviewer for suggestions for revision of the original manuscript.

References

Abe, M., S. Ito, M. Kimoto, R. Hayashi, and T. Nishimune. 1987. Molecular studies on thiaminase I. Biochimica et Biophysica Acta 909:213–221.

Anglesea, J. D., and A. J. Jackson. 1986. Thiaminase activity in fish silage and moist fish feed. Animal Feed Science and Technology 13:39–46.

Coble, D. D. 1965. Effect of raw smelt on lake trout. Canadian Fish Culturist 36:27–34.

Conner, D. J., C. R. Bronte, J. H. Selgeby, and H. L. Collins. 1993. Food of salmonine predators in Lake Superior, 1981–87. Great Lakes Fishery Commission Technical Report 59.

Deutsch, H. F., and A. D. Hasler. 1943. Distribution of a vitamin B-1 destructive enzyme in fish. Proceedings of the Society for Experimental Biology and Medicine 53:63–65.

Diana, J. S. 1990. Food habits of angler-caught salmonines in western Lake Huron. Journal of Great Lakes Research 16:271–278.

Edwin, E. E., and R. Jackman. 1974. A rapid radioactive method for determination of thiaminase activity and its use in the diagnosis of cerebrocortical necrosis in sheep and cattle. Journal of the Science of Food and Agriculture 25:357–368.

Fisher, J. P., J. D. Fitzsimons, G. F. Combs, Jr., and J. M. Spitsbergen. 1996. Naturally occurring thiamine deficiency causing reproductive failure in Finger Lakes Atlantic salmon and Great Lakes lake trout. Transactions of the American Fisheries Society 125:167–178.

Fitzsimons, J. D. 1995. The effect of B-vitamins on a swim-up syndrome in Lake Ontario lake trout. Journal of Great Lakes Research 21 (Supplement 1):286–289.

Fujita, A. 1954. Thiaminase. Pages 389–421 *in* F. F. Nord, editor. Advances in enzymology and related subjects of biochemistry. Volume XV. Interscience Publishers, Inc., New York.

Gnaedinger, R. H. and R. A. Krzeczkowski. 1966. Heat inactivation of thiaminase in whole fish. Commercial Fisheries Review 28:11–14.

Green, R. G., and C. A. Evans. 1940. A deficiency disease of foxes. Science 92:154–155.

Grieg, R. A., and R. H. Gnaedinger. 1971. Occurrence of thiaminase in some common aquatic animals of the United States and Canada. NOAA (National Oceanic and Atmospheric Administration) NMFS (National Marine Fisheries Service) SSRF (Special Scientific Report-Fisheries) 631.

Harrington, R., Jr., 1954. Contrasting susceptibilities of two fish species to a diet destructive to vitamin B-1. Journal of the Fisheries Research Board of Canada 11:529–534.

Hilker, D. M., and O. F. Peter. 1966. Anti-thiamin activity in Hawaii fish. Journal of Nutrition 89:419–421.

Hirn, J., and T. J. Pekkanen. 1975. Quantitative analysis of thiaminase activity in certain fish species. Nordisk Veterinaermedicin 27:646–648.

Ishihara, T., K. Hara, M. Yagi, and M. Yasuda. 1978. Studies on thiaminase I in marine fish–VIII. Thiaminase requirement of yellowtail fed anchovy. Bulletin of the Japanese Society of Scientific Fisheries 44:659–664.

Ishihara, T., H. Kinari, and M. Yasuda. 1973. Studies on thiaminase I in marine fish–II. Distribution of thiaminase in marine fish. Bulletin of the Japanese Society of Scientific Fisheries 39:55–59.

Ji, Y. Q., J. J. Warthesen, and I. R. Adelman. 1998. Thiamine nutrition, synthesis, and retention in relation to lake trout reproduction in the Great Lakes. Pages 99–111 *in* G. McDonald, J. D. Fitzsimons, and D. C. Honeyfield, editors. Early life stage mortality syndrome in fishes of the Great Lakes and Baltic Sea. American Fisheries Society, Symposium 21, Bethesda, Maryland.

Jude, D. J., F. J. Tesar, S. F. Deboe, and T. J. Miller. 1987. Diet and selection of major prey species by Lake Michigan salmonines 1973–1982. Transactions of the American Fisheries Society 116:677–691.

Krampitz, L. O., and D. W. Woolley. 1944. The manner of inactivation of thiamine by fish tissue. Journal of Biological Chemistry 152:9–17.

Melnick, D., M. Hochberg, and B. L. Oser. 1945. Physiological availability of the vitamins. II. The effect of dietary thiaminase in fish products. Journal of Nutrition 30:81–88.

Miller, M. A., and M. E. Holey. 1992. Diets of lake trout inhabiting nearshore and offshore Lake Michigan environments. Journal of Great Lakes Research 18:51–60.

Murata, K. 1965. Thiaminase. Pages 220–254 *in* N. Shimozono and E. Katsura, editors. Review of Japanese literature on beriberi and thiamine. Kyoto University, Japan.

Neilands, J. B. 1947. Thiaminase in aquatic animals of Nova Scotia. Journal of the Fisheries Research Board of Canada 7:94–99

Wolf, L. E. 1942. Fish diet disease of trout. Fisheries Research Bulletin 2, New York State Conservation Department, Albany.

American Fisheries Society Symposium 21:160–171, 1998

Reduced Egg Thiamine Levels in Inland and Great Lakes Lake Trout and Their Relationship with Diet[1]

JOHN D. FITZSIMONS
Bayfield Institute, Department of Fisheries and Oceans
Burlington, Ontario L7R 5R9, Canada

SCOTT B. BROWN[2]
Freshwater Institute, Department of Fisheries and Oceans
Winnipeg, Manitoba R3T 2N6, Canada

Abstract.—Lake trout *Salvelinus namaycush* eggs were collected from 18 separate locations in the Great Lakes and inland lakes to evaluate the relationship between diet and egg thiamine content. Thiamine concentrations in the eggs of lake trout whose diet consisted primarily of rainbow smelt *Osmerus mordax* and alewife *Alosa pseudoharengus* were one-ninth to one-seventeenth those of eggs of lake trout whose diet lacked either of these two species and was composed of lake herring *Coregonus artedi*, yellow perch *Perca flavescens*, cyprinids, or invertebrates. Within the Great Lakes, concentrations of thiamine in the eggs of lake trout increased in the order Ontario, Erie, Michigan, Huron < Superior and reflected the proportion of smelt, alewives, or both in the diet. Of the three forms of thiamine found in eggs, free thiamine was the most important and the form most affected by a diet of alewives or smelt. Collections from inland lakes were similar in terms of thiamine content and its relationship to diet composition. Average free thiamine concentrations in lake trout from Lakes Ontario, Erie, Michigan, and Huron were 1.5 to 4 times a threshold of 0.8 nmol/g that has been associated with the development of a thiamine-responsive early mortality syndrome. In contrast, the concentration of free thiamine in Lake Superior lake trout eggs was 26 times the threshold. We concluded that the reduction in egg thiamine concentrations in lake trout whose diet was primarily smelt or alewives was the result of their high thiaminase content, because published thiamine contents could not explain the patterns observed. Egg thiamine concentrations in lake trout were unaffected by maternal age.

Fisher et al. (1996) reported that levels of thiamine in the eggs of lake trout *Salvelinus namaycush* from Lakes Ontario and Erie were much lower than those found in hatchery fish. These low thiamine levels are of concern because they have been associated with a swim-up mortality syndrome in lake trout (Fitzsimons 1995; Fitzsimons et al. 1995; Fisher et al. 1996; Fitzsimons and Brown 1996; Brown et al. 1998b, this volume) for which thiamine has a therapeutic effect (Fitzsimons 1995). This syndrome, which is associated with anorexia, ataxia, hyperexcitability, and loss of equilibrium, affects larval lake trout around the swim-up stage. The clinical signs and timing of the syndrome are consistent with a deficiency of thiamine, an essential vitamin that is important, particularly in its phosphorylated forms, for normal carbohydrate metabolism and nerve function (Combs 1992). Thiamine concentrations decline by approximately 50% between fertilization and swim-up (Sato et al. 1987; Brown et al. 1998b).

Lake trout in Lakes Ontario and Erie feed almost exclusively on alewives *Alosa pseudoharengus* and rainbow smelt *Osmerus mordax* (Rand and Stewart, in press; F. Cornelius, New York Department of Environmental Conservation [NYDEC], personal communication). Because these species have high thiaminase levels (Nielands 1947; Gnaedinger 1964; Ji and Adelman 1998, this volume), Fisher et al. (1996) speculated that the low egg thiamine concentrations measured in lake trout from Lakes Ontario and Erie might reflect thiamine degradation by thiaminase in the gut, with the result that less thiamine was available for deposition into the eggs. Alewives and smelt also constitute an important part of the diet of lake trout in Lake Michigan (Miller and Holey 1992; Madenjian et al. 1998) and Lake Huron (Diana 1990; J. Johnson, Michigan Department of Natural Resources [MDNR], personal communication) but a smaller proportion in Lake Superior (Fisher and Swanson 1996; M. Gallinat, Red Cliff Band of Lake Superior Chippewa Indians, personal communication). Consequently, egg thiamine levels in lake trout from these lakes may also be affected. Other

[1] Portions of this publication were presented at the Second Workshop on Reproductive Disturbances in Fish, Stockholm, Sweden (1995).

[2] Current address: Environment Canada, Canada Center for Inland Waters, 867 Lakeshore Road, Box 5050, Burlington, Ontario L7R 4A6, Canada.

TABLE 1.— Summary of diet information for lake trout from the Great Lakes and inland lakes where eggs were collected for thiamine analysis, based on the percentage composition by weight in summer diets of adults. Abbreviations for species or groups: LH, lake herring; WF, lake whitefish; BC, bloater chub; CY, cyprinids; INV, invertebrates (includes *Mysis*, *Hyallela*, or zooplankton); YP, yellow perch; AW, alewife; RS, rainbow smelt. The presence of a species in unknown proportions is indicated with x.

				Species or group						
Lake	Site abbreviation	Region	Period	LH (WF)	BC (CY)	INV	YP	AW	RS	Source
				Great Lakes						
Ontario	LO	Southern	1993					90	5	Rand and Stewart, in press
Erie	LE	Eastern	1990–1993						95	F. Cornelius, NYDEC, personal communication
Huron	LH	Western	1994					44	46	J. Johnson, MDNR, personal communication
	LH	Eastern	1992		x			29	67	R. Payne, OMNR, personal communication
Michigan	LM	Southwestern	1994–1995		3			95		Madenjian et al. 1998
	LM	Offshore	1994–1995		19			80		Madenjian et al. 1998
Superior	LSP	Southwest	1994	58					24	M. Gallinat, Red Cliff Band of Lake Superior Chippewa Indians, personal communication
	LSP	Southwest[a]	1993	70–95						Fisher and Swanson 1996
				Inland lakes						
382	382				(x)	x				S. B. Brown, DOE, personal communication
Roddy	RL			(x)	(x)		x			S. B. Brown, DOE, personal communication
Opeongo	OL			80			20			Matuszek et al. 1990
Manitou	LU								x	D. Anderson, OMNR, personal communication
Simcoe	LS		1983	64					14	M. McMurtry, OMNR, personal communication
Seneca	SL							80–90		D. Kosowski, NYDEC, personal communication
Big Rideau	BR			x				80–90		J. Hoyle, OMNR, personal communication
Charleston	CL		1983					67–75		B. Kryshka, OMNR, personal communication

[a] Siscowet lake trout.

factors may be involved as well, such as contaminant effects on either the use or storage of thiamine (Yagi 1979), differences in the thiamine content of prey species (Fitzsimons et al. 1998, this volume), or changes in biological productivity, because thiamine is obtained through the diet from bacterial and algal production (Carlucci and Bowes 1972; Nishijima and Hata 1977).

Our objective was to collate information to assess the possible relationship between the diet of adult lake trout and egg thiamine concentrations. We were specifically interested in comparing egg thiamine levels of lake trout whose diets were composed of smelt or alewives, two marine invaders that are the major component of contemporary diets of lake trout in Lakes Michigan, Huron, Erie, and Ontario (Miller and Holey 1992; Madenjian et al. 1998; Rand and Stewart, in press; J. Johnson, personal communication; F. Cornelius, personal communication), with those of lake trout whose diets lacked these two species. The native coregonids, particularly lake herring *Coregonus artedi*, were historically important in the diet of lake trout throughout the Great Lakes and in some inland lakes (Scott and Crossman 1973). Of all the native coregonids in the Great Lakes, the lake herring is now the only significant dietary component of lake trout, and that only in Lake Superior (Fisher and Swanson 1996; M. Gallinat, personal communication). Bloater chub *Coregonus hoyi* are present in the diet of lake trout from parts of Lake Michigan (Madenjian et al. 1998). Samples were also collected from inland lakes, where lake trout also feed on smelt and alewives but where alternative diet items include lake herring, yellow perch *Perca flavescens*, cyprinids, and invertebrates.

Methods

Fish Collections

Fish were collected from 18 locations (Figure 1, Table 1) in 1994 and 1995 using gill nets and trap nets. All lake trout were of the lean variety (see Krueger and Ihssen 1995) with the exception of those from Isle Royale in Lake Superior, where siscowets, a fat variety, were collected. At the time of collection, the length of all females was determined, but only some of the fish were weighed. Age determinations based on coded wire tag data (1994 western Lake Ontario), fin clips (1994 Lake Simcoe), or otoliths (1995 Isle Royale) were used to assess the potential relationship between maternal age and egg thiamine content. Samples of ripe or ovulated eggs, which were collected from live females that had been killed by a blow to the head, were frozen (−20°C) until the time of analysis.

Thiamine Analysis

Thiamine was analyzed according to the methods of Brown et al. (1998a, this volume). All data were corrected for recoveries of each of the three forms: thiamine pyrophosphate, thiamine monophosphate, and free thiamine. Concentrations of the three forms were summed on a molar basis and expressed as nanomoles per gram wet weight. Thiamine data were included from Fisher et al. (1996) for Lake Erie lake trout to facilitate a broader comparison of thiamine levels and dietary linkages in the Great Lakes. Analysis of total thiamine for the Lake Erie samples was by the thiochrome method (AOAC International 1990).

Adult Lake Trout Diets

Information on diet obtained from published and unpublished sources was used to establish the major dietary items for lake trout at each of the collection locations (Table 1). Only the most recent data were used, and this information was verified by local fisheries personnel to ensure that it reflected current conditions. The presence or absence of smelt or alewives in a lake was also verified by local fisheries personnel. Where annual data were available, only information from the summer was used, because this is the period (e.g., July–October) when the greatest change in egg weight occurs (Martin 1970) and the greatest thiamine transfer to the egg occurs (J. Fitzsimons, Department of Fisheries and Oceans, unpublished observations), so it likely represents the period of greatest thiamine requirement by the parent. Moreover, Ji et al. (1998, this volume) estimated a thiamine turnover rate of 40 d for lake trout muscle, the largest repository of thiamine in the body of this species (estimated at 70%; S. Brown, Department of the Environment [DOE], unpublished observations). As a consequence, thiamine deposition during oogenesis, a process that lasts about 180 d, would presumably be strongly dependent on dietary intake.

Statistical Analysis

The linear relationship between adult age and egg thiamine concentration was evaluated using regression analysis. Differences within lakes were tested by means of *t*-tests, and differences between years and between group means of fish collected in each lake were tested by analysis of variance (ANOVA) computed using the Systat statistical package (Wilkinson 1992).

The analysis represents a lakewide overview of egg thiamine levels and combines like data from both inland and Great Lakes. Because of the variation in known diets from each of the lakes sampled (see Table 1), the data for each lake were placed in one of four general categories: (1) >50% alewives in the diet; (2) <50% of alewives in the diet, with the remainder composed mainly of smelt; (3) a low proportion of smelt in the diet, along with other items that did not include alewives; and (4) no smelt or alewives in the diet.

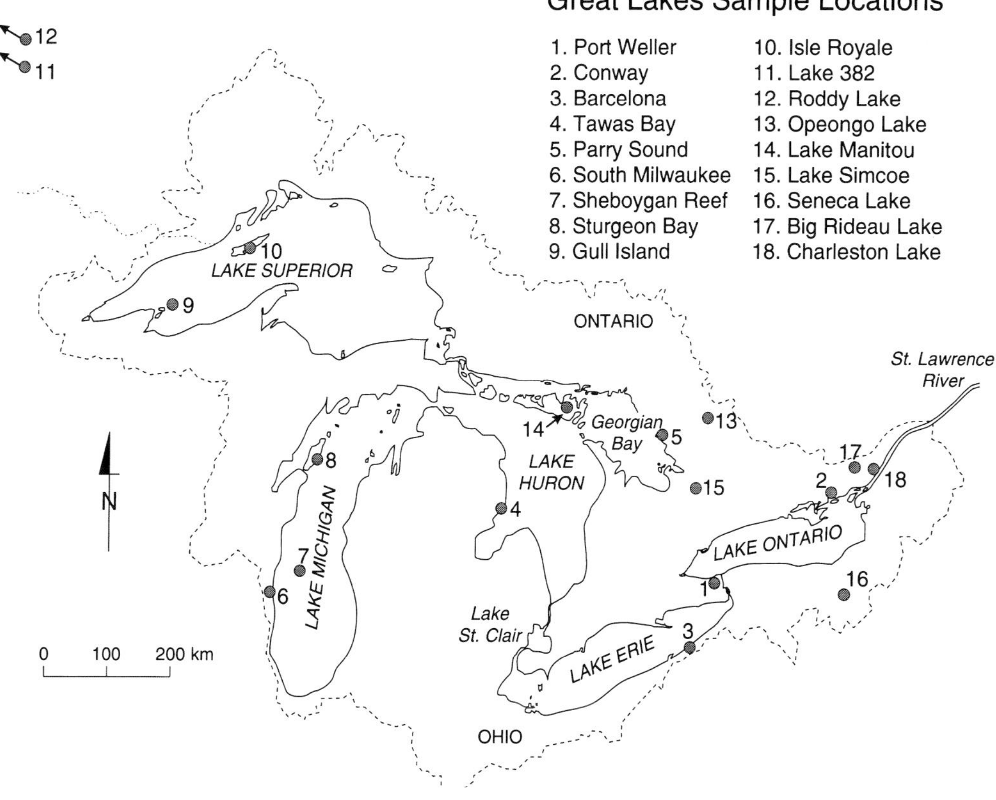

FIGURE 1.—Map showing sampling locations in the Great Lakes and inland lakes where lake trout eggs were collected from 1992 to 1995. The dotted line shows the limit of the Great Lakes drainage basin.

Independent variables used in each category were the mean parameter values calculated for each lake. The Bartlett or the Hartley test was used to test for homogeneity of variance, and, where necessary, data were log-transformed to obtain more uniform variances. Pairwise comparisons were conducted by applying the least-significant-difference test to the least-squares means produced by the ANOVAs. A P-value ≤ 0.05 was considered significant. For clarity of presentation, arithmetic means with standard errors were used in the figures.

Results

General Observations

Data for the 21 collections from 18 locations (Figure 1) shown in Table 2 indicate a variability of greater than 40 times in mean total thiamine concentrations. On the basis of the individual forms (thiamine pyrophosphate, thiamine monophosphate, and free thiamine) in lean lake trout, the variability in concentration was 6, 9, and 291 times, respectively, indicating that most of the between site difference was attributable to free thiamine, the major form of thiamine in eggs at spawning time. This was true for the Great Lakes and inland lakes (Figure 2). Because thiamine can be converted from one form to another (Gubler 1991) and all of the forms may be involved in the expression of early mortality syndrome, we have chosen to limit all further comparisons to total thiamine, the sum of all three forms.

Age Effect

Maternal age had no effect on egg thiamine levels for stocks exhibiting low (Lake Ontario, Port Weller), intermediate (Lake Simcoe), or high (Lake Superior, Isle Royale) average levels of thiamine. There was no relationship between maternal age and total thiamine content in egg samples from western Lake Ontario (Port Weller) during 1994 and 1995 (Figure 3; F = 1.83, r^2 = 0.05, P =

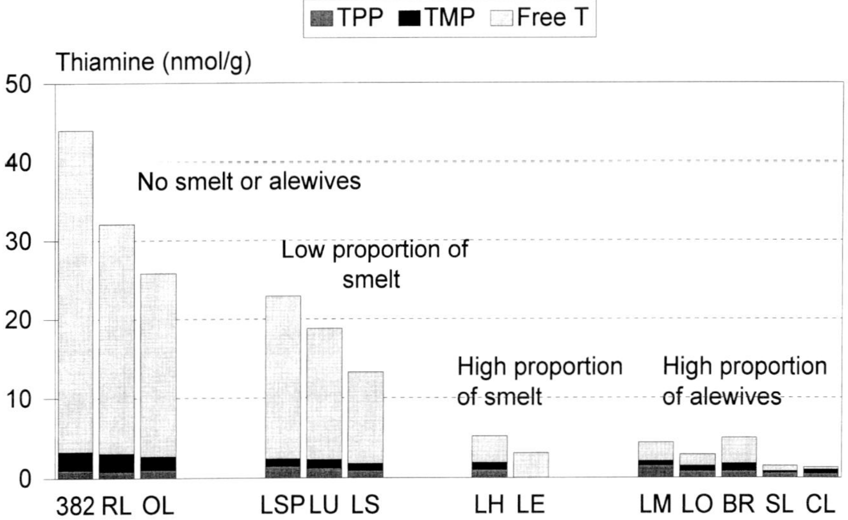

FIGURE 2.—Mean concentrations of thiamine pyrophosphate (TPP), thiamine monophosphate (TMP), and free thiamine (Free T) in lake trout eggs from the Great Lakes and inland lakes combined. Means represent whole lake means. Labels above bars indicate relative proportions of smelt or alewives in the diet. Definitions of site abbreviations are given in Table 1. Data for Lake Erie are from Fisher et al. (1996) and represent total thiamine.

0.19; age range, 5–14 years; mean age, 8.6 years; $N = 42$). This was also the case in Lake Simcoe ($F = 0.23$, $r^2 = 0.02$, $P = 0.64$; age range, 6–15 years; mean age, 9.6 years; $N = 12$) and at Isle Royale ($F = 2.09$, $r^2 = 0.23$, $P = 0.19$; age range, 13–18 years; mean age, 15.3 years; $N = 9$). Given the lack of an age effect, all further comparisons were based on mean thiamine concentration without consideration of age.

Year to Year Variation

Using a two-way analysis of variance on three lakes sampled in 1994 and 1995 (Lake Ontario [Port Weller], Charleston Lake, and Lake Manitou), no significant ($F = 1.5$, $P = 0.217$) year to year variation was evident. As a result, data were pooled across the 2 years for each of the three lakes to derive the mean values used in between lake comparisons.

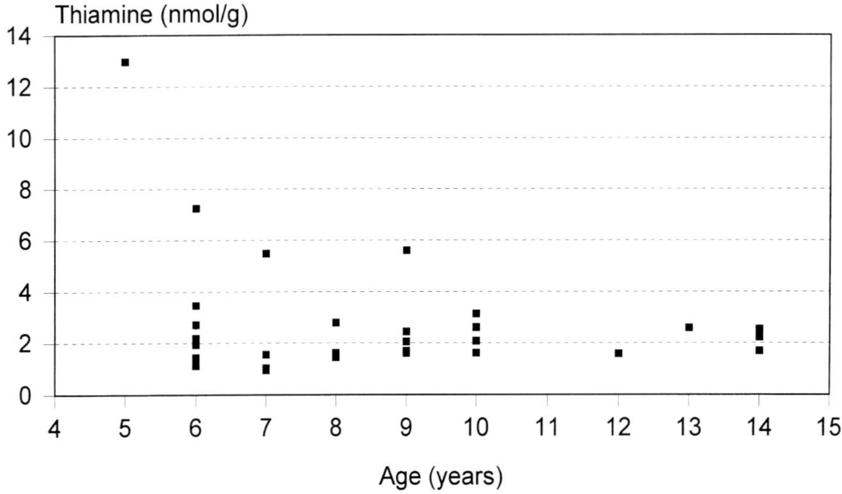

FIGURE 3.—Relationship between the total egg thiamine concentration and maternal age for lake trout collected at Port Weller during the fall of 1994 and 1995.

TABLE 2.—Summary of concentrations (nmol/g) of thiamine pyrophosphate (TPP), thiamine monophosphate (TMP), free thiamine (FT), and total thiamine in lake trout eggs from various Great Lakes and inland lakes. Values shown are means ± SE (*N*).

Lake	Location	Date	TPP	TMP	FT	Total thiamine
			Great Lakes			
Ontario	Port Weller	25 October–14 November 1994	0.9 ± 0.0 (30)	0.5 ± 0.1 (30)	1.2 ± 0.4 (30)	2.6 ± 0.4 (30)
	Port Weller	2 November 1995	0.8 ± 0.0 (12)	0.4 ± 0.0 (12)	1.5 ± 0.5 (12)	2.7 ± 0.5 (12)
	Conway	2 November 1995	0.4 ± 0.1 (11)	1.4 ± 0.2 (11)	2.2 ± 1.0 (11)	4.0 ± 1.1 (11)
Erie[a]	Barcelona	10 November 1992				3.1 ± 0.3 (5)
Huron	Tawas Bay	October 1994	1.0 ± 0.2 (11)	0.8 ± 0.1 (11)	3.4 ± 1.1 (11)	5.2 ± 1.3 (11)
	Parry Sound	October 1994	0.8 ± 0.2 (6)	1.0 ± 0.1 (6)	3.2 ± 0.7 (6)	4.9 ± 0.9 (6)
Michigan	South Milwaukee	18 October 1994	1.3 ± 0.3 (8)	0.6 ± 0.2 (8)	3.0 ± 1.7 (6)	4.9 ± 2.1 (8)
	Sheboygan Reef	17 October 1994	2.0 ± 0.2 (12)	0.8 ± 0.1 (12)	2.1 ± 0.7 (12)	5.0 ± 0.9 (12)
	Sturgeon Bay	26 October 1994	0.9 ± 0.1 (10)	0.4 ± 0.1 (10)	2.0 ± 0.8 (10)	3.3 ± 0.9 (10)
Superior	Gull Island	14 October 1994	1.4 ± 0.1 (8)	1.0 ± 0.1 (8)	20.5 ± 3.2 (8)	22.9 ± 3.2 (8)
	Isle Royale[b]	20–26 June 1995	0.1 ± 0.0 (9)	1.6 ± 0.3 (9)	24.1 ± 2.1 (9)	25.8 ± 2.1 (9)
			Inland lakes			
382		21–24 September 1994	1.0 ± 0.1 (3)	2.3 ± 0.2 (3)	40.7 ± 4.5 (3)	43.9 ± 4.7 (3)
Roddy		25–27 September 1994	0.8 ± 0.2 (5)	2.3 ± 0.2 (5)	29.0 ± 2.6 (5)	32.1 ± 2.6 (5)
Opeongo		13–23 October 1995	1.0 ± 0.2 (6)	1.7 ± 0.3 (6)	23.1 ± 2.0 (6)	25.8 ± 2.2 (6)
Manitou		17–18 October 1994	1.2 ± 0.1 (18)	1.2 ± 0.2 (18)	17.0 ± 1.0 (18)	19.4 ± 1.1 (18)
Manitou		23 October 1995	1.3 ± 0.1 (6)	1.0 ± 0.1 (6)	14.9 ± 2.1 (6)	17.2 ± 2.3 (6)
Simcoe	North Georgina Island	25–31 October 1994	0.9 ± 0.1 (12)	0.9 ± 0.1 (12)	11.5 ± 1.2 (12)	13.4 ± 1.3 (12)
Seneca		17–18 October 1995	0.6 ± 0.1 (11)	0.2 ± 0.0 (11)	0.7 ± 0.1 (11)	1.5 ± 0.1 (11)
Big Rideau		1995	0.4 ± 0.1 (10)	0.9 ± 0.1 (10)	0.9 ± 0.3 (10)	2.1 ± 0.4 (10)
Charleston		1994	0.3 ± 0.0 (13)	0.8 ± 0.1 (13)	0.4 ± 0.1 (13)	1.5 ± 0.1 (13)
Charleston		8–10 November 1995	0.7 ± 0.1 (11)	0.2 ± 0.0 (11)	0.1 ± 0.0 (11)	1.0 ± 0.1 (11)

[a] From Fisher et al. 1996.

[b] Siscowet lake trout.

Within Lake Variation

Samples collected from locations within Lakes Superior, Michigan, Huron, and Ontario did not indicate any significant within lake variation despite some variation in the relative proportions of smelt and alewives in the diet. In southwestern Lake Superior, the mean thiamine concentration in eggs of lean lake trout from Gull Island (22.9 ± 3.2 nmol/g) did not differ ($t = -0.78$, $P = 0.45$) from that of eggs of siscowet lake trout from offshore at Isle Royale (25.8 ± 2.1 nmol/g). The diet of lake trout from southwestern Lake Superior was composed of 24% smelt during the summer months (M. Gallinat, personal communication), whereas the proportion of smelt was negligible for the offshore siscowet lake trout (Fisher and Swanson 1996). Similarly, no site to site variation was evident among three sites evaluated in western Lake Michigan ($F = 0.04$, $P = 0.97$). The mean thiamine concentration in Lake Michigan at Sheboygan reef (5.0 ± 0.9 nmol/g), where 80% of the adult lake trout diet consisted of alewives, did not differ from concentrations in either South Milwaukee (4.9 ± 2.1 nmol/g) or Sturgeon Bay (3.3 ± 0.9 nmol/g), where 95% of the diet was composed of alewives (Madenjian et al. 1998). The mean thiamine level in lake trout eggs from Tawas Bay (5.2 ± 1.3 nmol/g) on western Lake Huron did not differ from that in lake trout from Parry Sound (4.9 ± 0.9 nmol/g) on eastern Lake Huron, despite some variation in the relative proportions of smelt and alewives in the diet of lake trout from western (44:46%; J.

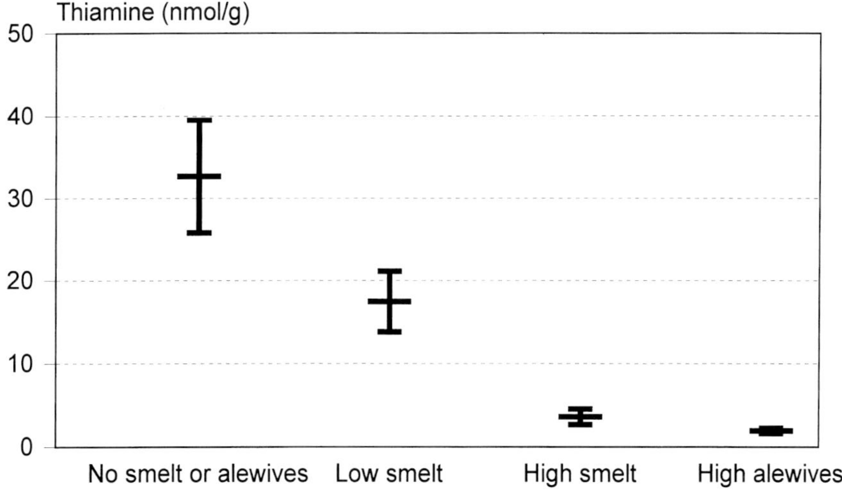

FIGURE 4.—Mean concentrations (±SE) of total thiamine for groups of lakes where lake trout diets had no smelt or alewives, a low proportion of smelt, a high proportion of smelt and some alewives, or a high proportion of alewives.

Johnson, personal communication) and eastern (67:29%; R. Payne, Ontario Ministry of Natural Resources [OMNR], personal communication) Lake Huron. The mean thiamine concentration in eggs of lake trout collected at Port Weller in western Lake Ontario in 1995 (2.7 ± 0.5 nmol/g) did not differ from that in lake trout eggs collected at Conway in eastern Lake Ontario (4.0 ± 1.1 nmol/g). The proportion of alewives in the diet of lake trout in Lake Ontario was 90% (Rand and Stewart, in press).

Lake to Lake Variation

When lakes were grouped according to the relative proportion of smelt and alewives in lake trout diets for each lake and compared, diet had a significant effect (F = 58.17, $P < 0.001$, $r^2 = 0.95$) on between lake variation in egg thiamine concentrations (Figure 4). For Lake 382, Opeongo Lake, and Roddy Lake, where neither smelt nor alewives are present in lake trout diets, the average egg thiamine level was highest overall (32.7 nmol/g). Where smelt composed a small percentage of the diet and there were no alewives in the diet, as in Lakes Superior, Manitou, and Simcoe, the mean egg thiamine concentration (17.2 nmol/g) exhibited a significant ($P = 0.05$) decline of almost 50% compared with that in lakes where both smelt and alewives were absent from the diet. Where smelt was a major component of the diet and alewives constituted a small proportion of the diet, as in Lakes Erie and Huron, there was a further significant ($P = 0.001$) decline in mean egg thiamine concentration (3.6 nmol/g) of almost fivefold from that in lakes where alewives were absent and smelt composed a small percentage of the diet. Moreover, compared with those lakes where both smelt and alewives were absent from the diet, this level represented an almost 10 times decline in the mean egg thiamine concentration. Finally, in those lakes where alewives composed a major portion of the diet, as in Big Rideau, Seneca, and Charleston lakes and Lakes Ontario and Michigan, the mean egg thiamine concentration (1.9 nmol/g) was lowest overall and exhibited a further significant ($P = 0.044$) decline of almost 50% from that in lakes where alewives were a minor component of the diet. Overall, this represented a 17 times decline in average egg thiamine concentration from that in lakes where both smelt and alewives were absent from the diet.

Discussion

This synopsis supports the hypotheses of Fitzsimons (1995) and Fisher et al. (1996) that salmonid diets containing either smelt or alewives are associated with low egg thiamine concentrations, although the exact relationship between the actual proportion of these two species in the diet and reductions in egg thiamine levels remains unclear. Stocks with a high proportion of alewives in the diet were found to have the lowest egg thiamine concentrations relative to those whose diet contained neither smelt nor alewives, whose mean egg thiamine concentrations were much higher.

For those stocks in which smelt composed the highest proportion of the diet but with alewives also present, egg thiamine concentrations were still depressed, but not to the same extent as for those stocks in which alewives dominated the diet. Moreover, as the diet became more diverse and other species such as herring were included in higher proportions, the mean egg thiamine concentration showed the smallest difference relative to stocks in which smelt and alewives were absent from the diet.

The variation in mean egg thiamine levels for stocks eating either mostly smelt or mostly alewives may be related to the ecological characteristics of these two schooling pelagic species. With a temperature preferenda of 17°C, alewives would tend to occur above the thermocline during the summer months, whereas smelt, which have a thermal preferenda of 7°C, would occur below the thermocline, where they could co-occur with lake herring, which have a thermal preferenda of 12°C (Wismer and Christie 1987). As a result, lake trout may alternate between the two species, leading to considerable variation in thiamine levels depending on the actual amount of smelt consumed. Compensation of body stores of thiamine may also occur during the consumption of lake herring, particularly at low levels of smelt consumption.

It is only in Lakes Ontario and Erie (Fisher et al. 1996) and Seneca and Charleston lakes (Fitzsimons, unpublished observations) that thiamine levels have been associated with a swim-up mortality syndrome and thus represent a deficiency. Nevertheless, thiamine concentrations in lake trout eggs from Lakes Michigan and Huron were also low relative to those in eggs from Lake Superior by a factor of fivefold and were just above a tentative egg thiamine threshold concentration for early mortality syndrome that lies between 1.4 and 3.0 nmol/g total thiamine, based on Lake Ontario lake trout eggs (Brown et al. 1998b). Early mortality syndrome is the only effect of the thiamine deficiency identified so far. Its absence in Lakes Michigan and Huron in recent years (C. Edsall, U.S. Geological Survey, personal communication) is consistent with the thiamine levels measured in this study that were above the threshold concentration. The threshold for sublethal effects may be higher, however; mortality is a relatively crude indicator of a thiamine deficiency (Halver 1989), and for other end points lake trout from lakes other than Lakes Erie and Ontario may also be thiamine deficient. For example, Fisher et al. (1996) reported decreased yolk conversion efficiency and bradycardia in thiamine-deficient larval Atlantic salmon *Salmo salar*, Halver (1957) reported poor appetite and muscle atrophy in thiamine-deficient larval chinook salmon *Oncorhynchus tshawytscha*, and Spannhof et al. (1978) noted reduced hemoglobin and hematocrit in thiamine-deficient juvenile rainbow trout *O. mykiss*.

The low thiamine concentrations in the eggs of lake trout that feed predominantly on either smelt or alewives are consistent with the high thiaminase contents of these two species (Ji and Adelman 1998a) and the hypothesis that elevated thiaminase in the diet results in the destruction of thiamine in the gut of the lake trout. Thiaminase activity in the gut of a predator such as lake trout is consistent with reported activities (Krampitz and Wooley 1944; Melnick et al. 1945) and the temperature (Krampitz and Wooley 1944) and pH requirements (Deolalkar and Sohonie 1954) for thiaminase. Ji and Adelman (1998) reported similar levels of thiaminase in smelt and alewives from the Great Lakes. These data are in contrast to data from an earlier report by Gnaedinger (1964) that indicated far higher levels of thiaminase in alewives, a difference Ji and Adelman (1998) attributed to interlake variation. In contrast to the similar thiaminase contents of smelt and alewives, Fitzsimons et al. (1998), working with samples from Lakes Michigan and Ontario, found that alewives had approximately six times more thiamine in their muscle than smelt. Based on the average thiaminase activity reported by Ji and Adelman (1998) of 360 pmol of thiamine destroyed per gram of tissue per minute and a thiamine concentration of 10,000 pmol/g in alewives (Fitzsimons et al. 1998), it would take 27 min to completely destroy the thiamine in an alewife under these conditions. Similarly, for smelt with the same thiaminase activity as alewives but lower thiamine content (1,700 pmol/g; Fitzsimons et al. 1998), it would take only 5 min to completely destroy the thiamine. Although it is not known how well the conditions of the assay used by Ji and Adelman (1998) actually reflect conditions in the gut of a predator, these intervals are well within the reported 3- to 6-d digestion times for fish meals (Vonk 1929; Karpevitch and Bokoff 1937), which suggests that the potential for destruction of thiamine within the gut of a predator is high. Other results also support the proposed relevance of thiaminase activity in prey, rather than their thiamine content, in the determination of lake trout egg thiamine concentrations. Fitzsimons et al. (1998) reported that the thiamine content of alewives was 1.5 times higher than that of the coregonids bloater chub and lake herring, yet the mean egg thiamine concentration of Lake

Superior lake trout that fed predominantly on lake herring was 5–8 times higher than that of lake trout eggs from Lakes Michigan and Ontario.

The two to ninefold variation in egg thiamine concentrations noted between lake trout consuming smelt and those consuming alewives was similar to the results reported for thiamine-deficient Atlantic salmon from the Finger Lakes of New York State (Fisher et al. 1996). These authors found that the mean egg thiamine concentration of Atlantic salmon from Cayuga Lake that fed on alewives was approximately one-fifth that of Atlantic salmon from Little Clear Pond, a control lake where resident Atlantic salmon fed on smelt. These authors attributed the differences to an earlier reported difference in the thiaminase content of smelt and alewives (Gnaedinger 1964; Gnaedinger and Krzeczkowski 1966). However, based on the pattern of thiamine levels and diet in this study and the findings of Ji and Adelman (1998) that indicated a similar thiaminase content of smelt and alewives, the observations of Fisher et al. (1996) likely represent differences in the proportions of the two species in the diets of Atlantic salmon from the two locations. Differences in the thiamine content of the two prey species may also be involved (Fitzsimons et al. 1998). Fisher et al. (1996) had also speculated that the lack of significant reproductive problems in lake trout from Seneca Lake, in contrast to Atlantic salmon from this same lake, was the result of a more diverse diet that presumably contained some prey items lacking thiaminase. Based on the present study, however, the eggs of lake trout from Seneca Lake had thiamine concentrations that were one-third to one-half those of lake trout from Lakes Michigan and Ontario. Because lake trout in Lakes Michigan and Ontario feed predominantly on alewives, it seems reasonable to conclude, based on the low egg thiamine concentrations in lake trout from Seneca Lake, that they, like Atlantic salmon, are also feeding heavily on alewives.

The pattern of free thiamine representing the major form of thiamine in the eggs of lake trout with no thiaminase in the diet and being the form most affected by a diet high in thiaminase is consistent with findings in hatchery fish fed a thiamine antagonist, amprolium, in their food. Honeyfield et al. (1998a, this volume) reported that free thiamine accounted for more than 98% of the thiamine found in eggs of lake trout reared on a thiamine-replete diet. When amprolium was added to the diet at the rate of 0.05%, however, these authors observed a 93% decrease in free thiamine but no significant change in either thiamine monophosphate or thiamine pyrophosphate. Free thiamine was also the predominant form in lake trout plasma (Brown et al. 1998a), although thiamine pyrophosphate, the biologically active form, predominated in the red blood cells, liver, muscle, and kidney of this species. Thiamine pyrophosphate does not become an important constituent of the total thiamine concentration of lake trout eggs until hatch, when most of the free thiamine appears to be converted to thiamine pyrophosphate (Brown et al. 1998b).

The declines in egg thiamine concentrations noted in this study appear to represent a unique sensitivity of the ovary, relative to other tissues, to the effects of decreased thiamine uptake by the parent. Honeyfield et al. (1998a) observed a 31 and 53% decline in liver and muscle thiamine pyrophosphate, the major form in these tissues, when the diet of hatchery fish contained 0.05% amprolium relative to an amprolium-free control diet. In contrast, these same authors noted a 93% decline in the free thiamine concentration in the ovaries of the group fed amprolium. Similarly, Brown et al. (1998a) compared the amount of thiamine in the bodies of non-thiamine-deficient and thiamine-deficient lake trout and noted a 94% decline in the egg free thiamine concentration in the thiamine-deficient group yet only 40 and 63% declines in the thiamine pyrophosphate concentrations in the livers and kidneys of the thiamine-deficient group.

For the ranges in age and thiamine concentration that we evaluated, age differences cannot account for the observed variation in thiamine egg content among lakes. For lake trout from Lakes Ontario, Simcoe, and Superior, where relative egg thiamine concentrations were low, intermediate, and high, respectively, no significant relationships were evident between egg thiamine content and maternal age. Age-related differences in egg thiamine concentration, however, may occur in younger fish. Size-dependent changes in the diet of juvenile lake trout have been reported for Lakes Superior (Dryer et al. 1965; Fisher and Swanson 1996), Michigan (Jude et al. 1987), and Ontario (Elrod and O'Gorman 1991), where they were related to a transition from either an invertebrate to a piscine diet or from a benthic to a pelagic piscine diet. Both of these changes could potentially affect egg thiamine concentrations. Invertebrates have thiamine concentrations that are intermediate to those of prey fish (Fitzsimons et al. 1998), whereas benthic fish such as sculpin appear to lack thiaminase (Nielands 1947) and have high thiamine concentrations in their muscle (Fitzsimons et al. 1998).

Some of the lakes sampled, such as Lakes Michigan and Ontario, have high burdens of organic contaminants (Baumann and Whittle 1988), which have been associated with reduced thiamine levels in rats (Yagi 1979). It seems unlikely, however, that such contaminants played a major role in the observed lake to lake differences in egg thiamine concentrations. Lake trout from Charleston, Seneca, and Big Rideau lakes, which feed on alewives and are relatively uncontaminated with organic compounds (Fisher et al. 1996; W. Scheider, Ministry of Environment and Energy, unpublished data), all had lower egg thiamine concentrations than lake trout from Lake Ontario, which also feed on alewives but in contrast are heavily contaminated with chlorinated hydrocarbons (Ontario 1995; Heustis et al. 1996).

Our findings indicate a strong association between a diet high in thiaminase, dominated by the two marine invaders smelt and alewives, and reduced egg thiamine concentrations in lake trout to the extent that concentrations in some locations are deficient (Fisher et al. 1996; Brown et al. 1998b). Such a diet has been speculated to contribute to reduced egg thiamine concentrations and associated thiamine-responsive early mortality syndromes in the eggs of Lake Michigan coho salmon *Oncorhynchus kisutch* and chinook salmon (Honeyfield et al. 1998b, this volume) as well as Baltic salmon (Amcoff et al. 1998, this volume). All of these species are salmonids, which tend to have higher dietary requirements for thiamine (Halver 1989), and so may be especially sensitive. Nevertheless, other nonsalmonid species in the Great Lakes may also be affected. Smelt and alewives are also important in the diets of walleye *Stizostedion vitreum*, burbot *Lota lota*, yellow perch, American eel *Anguilla rostrata*, and northern pike *Esox lucius* (Scott and Crossman 1973).

The documentation of the negative effects of smelt and alewives on salmonid nutriture, which in turn can affect reproduction, is but one more negative effect associated with these two species. Their effects on thiamine can be added to predation on the larval stages of several fish species, including lake whitefish *Coregonus clupeaformis*, lake trout, emerald shiner *Notropis atherinoides*, yellow perch, deepwater cisco *Coregonus johannae*, and deepwater sculpin *Myoxocephalus thompsoni* (Smith 1970; Crowder 1980; Jude and Tesar 1985; Eck and Wells 1987; Evans and Loftus 1987; Krueger et al. 1995). If our hypothesis regarding the effect of a smelt or alewife diet on egg thiamine concentrations is correct, it is unlikely that full restoration of lake trout can occur if smelt or alewives are a major part of their diet. Moreover, restoration of Atlantic salmon, another species whose thiamine levels are affected by diet (Fisher et al. 1996; Fynn-Aikins et al., in press), may be similarly affected if smelt or alewives are a major part of their diet.

Acknowledgments

We are greatly indebted to L. Vandenbyllaardt, who did all of the thiamine analyses. We also thank R. Allan, C. Bronte, G. Cholwek, F. Cornelius, C. Edsall, B. Henderson, B. Kryshka, M. Keir, M. Keniry, S. Marcquenski, E. McIntyre, P. Mettner, K. Osika, V. Palace, J. Radford, S. Schram, B. Timmins, M. Toneys, D. Walsh, and B. Williston, whose assistance with the collection of these samples contributed enormously to the scope of this study. We also thank Victor Cairns, Arthur Niimi, Michael Hornung, and an anonymous reviewer, who provided valuable comments on an earlier draft.

References

Amcoff, P., H. Börjeson, J. Lindeberg, and L. Norrgren. 1998. Thiamine concentrations in feral Baltic salmon exhibiting the M74 syndrome. Pages 82–89 *in* McDonald et al. (1998).

AOAC (Association of Official Analytical Chemists) International. 1990. Official methods of analysis, 15th edition, volume 2. AOAC International, Arlington, Virginia.

Baumann, P. C., and D. M. Whittle. 1988. The status of selected organics in the Laurentian Great Lakes: an overview of DDT, PCBs, dioxins, furans, and aromatic hydrocarbons. Journal of Aquatic Toxicology 11:241–257.

Brown, S. B., D. C. Honeyfield, and L. Vandenbyllaardt. 1998a. Thiamine analysis in fish tissues. Pages 73–81 *in* McDonald et al. (1998).

Brown, S. B., J. D. Fitzsimons, V. P. Palace, and L. Vandenbyllaardt. 1998b. Thiamine and early mortality syndrome in lake trout. Pages 18–25 *in* McDonald et al. (1998).

Carlucci, A. F., and P. M. Bowes. 1972. Determination of vitamin B12, thiamine, and biotin in Lake Tahoe waters using modified marine bioassay techniques. Limnology and Oceanography 17:774–776.

Combs, G. F. 1992. The vitamins. Academic Press, San Diego, California.

Crowder, L. B. 1980. Alewife, rainbow smelt and native fishes in Lake Michigan: competition or predation? Environmental Biology of Fishes 5:225–233.

Deolalkar, S. T., and K. Sohonie. 1954. Thiaminase from fresh-water, brackish-water and salt-water fish. Nature 4402:489–490.

Diana, J. S. 1990. Food habits of angler-caught salmonines in western Lake Huron. Journal of Great Lakes Research 16:271–278.

Dryer, W. R., L. F. Erkkila, and C. L. Tetzloff. 1965. Food of lake trout in Lake Superior. Transactions of the American Fisheries Society 94:169–176.

Eck, G. W., and L. Wells. 1987. Recent changes in Lake Michigan's fish community and their probable causes, with emphasis on the role of alewife (*Alosa pseudoharengus*). Canadian Journal of Fisheries and Aquatic Sciences 44(Supplement 2):53–60.

Elrod, J. H., and R. O'Gorman. 1991. Diet of juvenile lake trout in southern Lake Ontario in relation to abundance and size of prey fishes, 1979–1987. Transactions of the American Fisheries Society 120:290–302.

Evans, D. O., and D. H. Loftus. 1987. Colonization of inland lakes in the Great Lakes region by rainbow smelt, *Osmerus mordax*: their freshwater niche and effects on indigenous fishes. Canadian Journal of Fisheries and Aquatic Sciences 44(Supplement 2):249–266.

Fisher, J. P., J. D. Fitzsimons, G. F. Combs, Jr., and J. M. Spitsbergen. 1996. Naturally occurring thiamine deficiency causing reproductive failure in Finger Lakes Atlantic salmon and Great Lakes lake trout. Transactions of the American Fisheries Society 125:167–178.

Fisher, S. J., and B. L. Swanson. 1996. Diets of siscowet lake trout from the Apostle Islands region of Lake Superior, 1993. Journal of Great Lakes Research 22 (Supplement 2):463–468.

Fitzsimons, J. D. 1995. The effect of B-vitamins on a swim-up syndrome in Lake Ontario lake trout. Journal of Great Lakes Research 21(Supplement 1):286–289.

Fitzsimons, J. D., and S. B. Brown. 1996. Effect of diet on thiamine levels in Great Lakes lake trout and relationship with early mortality syndrome. Pages 76–78 *in* B.-E. Bengtsson, C. Hill, and S. Nellbring, editors. Report from the second workshop on reproduction disturbances in fish. Swedish Environmental Protection Agency Report 4534, Stockholm.

Fitzsimons, J. D., S. B. Brown, and L. Vandenbyllaardt. 1998. Thiamine levels in food chains of the Great Lakes. Pages 90–98 *in* McDonald et al. (1998).

Fitzsimons, J. D., S. Huestis, and B. Williston. 1995. Occurrence of a swim-up syndrome in Lake Ontario lake trout in relation to contaminants and cultural practices. Journal of Great Lakes Research 21(Supplement 1):277–285.

Fynn-Aikins, K., D. C. Honeyfield, P. Bowser, and J. D. Fitzsimons. In press. Early mortality syndrome in Atlantic salmon fry from fish fed dietary amprolium. Transactions of the American Fisheries Society.

Gnaedinger, R. H. 1964. Thiaminase activity in fish: an improved assay method. Fishery Industrial Research 2:55–59.

Gnaedinger, R. H., and R. A. Krzeczkowski. 1966. Heat inactivation of thiaminase in whole fish. Commercial Fisheries Review 28(8):11–14.

Gubler, C. J. 1991. Thiamin. Pages 234–281 *in* L. J. Machlin, editor. Handbook of vitamins, second edition. Marcel Dekker, New York.

Halver, J. E. 1957. Nutrition of salmonid fishes. III. Water-soluble vitamin requirements of chinook salmon. Journal of Nutrition 62:225–243.

Halver, J. E. 1989. Fish nutrition, second edition. Academic Press, New York.

Heustis, S. Y., M. R. Servos, D. M. Whittle, and D. G. Dixon. 1996. Temporal and age-related trends in levels of polychlorinated biphenyl congeners and organochlorine contaminants in Lake Ontario lake trout (*Salvelinus namaycush*). Journal of Great Lakes Research 22:310–330.

Honeyfield, D. C., K. Fynn-Aikins, J. D. Fitzsimons, and J. A. Mota. 1998a. Effect of dietary amprolium on egg and tissue thiamine concentrations in lake trout. Pages 172–177 *in* McDonald et al. (1998).

Honeyfield, D. C., J. G. Hnath, J. Copeland, K. Dabrowski, and J. H. Blom. 1998b. Correlation of nutrients and environmental contaminants in Lake Michigan coho salmon with incidence of early mortality syndrome. Pages 135–145 *in* McDonald et al. (1998).

Ji, Y. Q., and I. R. Adelman. 1998. Thiaminase activity in alewives and smelt in Lakes Huron, Michigan, and Superior. Pages 154–159 *in* McDonald et al. (1998).

Ji, Y. Q., J. J. Warthesen, and I. R. Adelman. 1998. Thiamine nutrition, synthesis, and retention in relation to lake trout reproduction in the Great Lakes. Pages 99–111 *in* McDonald et al. (1998).

Jude, D. J., and F. J. Tesar. 1985. Recent changes in the inshore forage fish of Lake Michigan. Canadian Journal of Fisheries and Aquatic Sciences 42:1154–1157.

Jude, D. J., F. J. Tesar, S. F. Deboe, and T. J. Miller. 1987. Diet and selection of major prey species by Lake Michigan salmonines, 1973–1982. Transactions of the American Fisheries Society 116:677–691.

Karpevitch, A., and E. Bokoff. 1937. The rate of digestion in marine fishes. Zoologicheskii Zhurnal 16:28–44. (Russian; English summary.)

Krampitz, L. O., and D. W. Wooley. 1944. The manner of inactivation of thiamine by fish tissue. Journal of Biological Chemistry 152:9–17.

Krueger, C. C., and P. E. Ihssen. 1995. Review of genetics of lake trout in the Great Lakes: history, molecular genetics, physiology, strain comparisons, and restoration management. Journal of Great Lakes Research 21(Supplement 1):348–363.

Krueger, C. C., D. L. Perkins, E. L. Mills, and J. E. Marsden. 1995. Predation by alewives on lake trout fry in Lake Ontario: role of an exotic species in preventing restoration of a native species. Journal of Great Lakes Research 21(Supplement 1):458–469.

Madenjian, C. P., T. J. DeSourcie, and R. M. Stedman. 1998. Ontogenetic and spatial patterns in diet and growth of lake trout in Lake Michigan. Transactions of the American Fisheries Society 127:236–252.

Martin, N. V. 1970. Long-term effects of diet on the biology of the lake trout and the fishery in Lake Opeongo, Ontario. Journal of the Fisheries Research Board of Canada 27:125–146.

Matuszek, J. E., B. J. Shuter, and J. M. Casselman. 1990. Changes in lake trout growth and abundance after introduction of cisco into Lake Opeongo, Ontario. Transactions of the American Fisheries Society 119:718–729.

McDonald, G., J. D. Fitzsimons, and D. C. Honeyfield, editors. 1998. Early life stage mortality syndrome in fishes of the Great Lakes and Baltic Sea. American Fisheries Society, Symposium 21, Bethesda, Maryland.

Melnick, D., M. Hochberg, and B. L. Oser. 1945. Physiological availability of the vitamins. II. The effect of dietary thiaminase in fish products. Journal of Nutrition 30:81–88.

Miller, M. A., and M. E. Holey. 1992. Diets of lake trout inhabiting nearshore and offshore Lake Michigan environments. Journal of Great Lakes Research 18(Supplement 1):51–60.

Nielands, J. B. 1947. Thiaminase in aquatic animals of Nova Scotia. Journal of the Fisheries Research Board of Canada 7:94–99.

Nishijima, T., and Y. Hata. 1977. Distribution of thiamine, biotin, and vitamin B12 in Lake Kojima. I. Distribution in lake water. Bulletin of the Japanese Society of Scientific Fisheries 44:815–818.

Ontario. 1995. Guide to eating Ontario sport fish. 1995–1996. Queen's Printer for Ontario, Toronto.

Rand, P. S., and D. S. Stewart. In press. Dynamics of salmonine diets and foraging in Lake Ontario 1983–1993: a test of a bioenergetic model prediction. Canadian Journal of Fisheries and Aquatic Sciences.

Sato, M., R. Yoshinaka, R. Kuroshima, H. Morimoto, and S. Ikeda. 1987. Changes in water soluble vitamin contents and transaminase activity of rainbow trout egg during development. Nippon Suisan Gakkiaishi 53:795–799.

Scott, W. B., and E. J. Crossman. 1973. Freshwater fishes of Canada. Bulletin of the Fisheries Research Board of Canada 184.

Smith, S. H. 1970. Species interactions of the alewife in the Great Lakes. Transactions of the American Fisheries Society 99:754–765.

Spannhof, S. L., K. P. Hase, M. Mehl, and A. Plantikow. 1978. Wirkung gleichzeitigen thiamine- und sauerstoffmangels auf den physiologichen zustand von forellensetzlingen. Fischerei-Forschung Wissenschaftliche Schriftenreihe 16:21–24.

Vonk, H. J. 1929. Das pepsin verschiedener vertebraten. Zeitschrift fur Vergleichende Physiologie 5:685–702.

Wilkinson, L. 1992. Systat: the system for statistics. Systat, Inc., Evanston, Illinois.

Wismer, D. A., and A. E. Christie. 1987. Temperature relationships of Great Lakes fishes: a data compilation. Great Lakes Fishery Commission Special Publication 87-3, Ann Arbor, Michigan.

Yagi, N. 1979. Effects of PCB, DDT and other organochloride compounds on thiamine metabolism in rat. Journal of the Japanese Society of Food and Nutrition 32:55–60.

American Fisheries Society Symposium 21:172–177, 1998

Effect of Dietary Amprolium on Egg and Tissue Thiamine Concentrations in Lake Trout

DALE C. HONEYFIELD
Biological Resources Division, U.S. Geological Survey
Research and Development Laboratory
Wellsboro, Pennsylvania 16901, USA

KOFI FYNN-AIKINS
Biological Resources Division, U.S. Geological Survey,
Tunison Laboratory of Aquatic Sciences
Cortland, New York 13045, USA

JOHN D. FITZSIMONS
Great Lakes Laboratory of Fisheries, Aquatic Sciences, Bayfield Institute
Burlington, Ontario L7R 4A6, Canada

JENNIFER A. MOTA
Biological Resources Division, U.S. Geological Survey
Research and Development Laboratory

Abstract.—Dietary amprolium, a thiamine antagonist, was fed to lake trout *Salvelinus namaycush* broodstock from April to October before spawning to determine its effect on egg and tissue concentrations of thiamine, thiamine monophosphate, and thiamine pyrophosphate. The thiamine concentration of eggs from fish fed no amprolium was 61.8 nmol/g, whereas the concentration of thiamine in fish fed 0.05 and 0.10% amprolium was 4.02 and 1.71 nmol/g ($P < 0.01$), respectively. In lake trout fed 0.10% amprolium beginning in August, egg free thiamine concentration was reduced to 11.6 nmol/g. No sign of early mortality syndrome was observed in sac fry from eggs in this study, which suggests that thiamine concentrations in the egg were not low enough to be below a critical threshold or that factors other than thiamine are involved in early mortality syndrome.

The reproductive success of Great Lakes lake trout *Salvelinus namaycush*, coho salmon *Oncorhynchus kisutch*, chinook salmon *O. tshawytscha*, and some strains of steelhead trout *O. mykiss*, as well as Atlantic salmon *Salmo salar* in the New York Finger Lakes (Cayuga Lake) and the Baltic Sea, has markedly declined since 1992 because of an increase in a particular type of larval mortality. This larval mortality, which occurs between hatch and swim-up, has been called swim-up syndrome in Great Lakes lake trout (Fitzsimons et al. 1995), Cayuga syndrome in Finger Lakes Atlantic salmon (Fisher et al. 1995, 1996), and M74 in Baltic Sea Atlantic salmon (Bengtsson et al. 1994; Norrgren 1994; Johansson et al. 1995). The clinical signs of affected species include erratic swimming, hyperexcitability, dark coloration, lethargy, anemia, emaciation, and anorexia before death. Recent data reported for Lake Michigan (Marcquenski and Brown 1997) indicate fry mortality of 70% for coho salmon, 60% for chinook salmon, 35% for steelhead trout, and 80% for lake trout; these rates have increased from less than 30% before 1990 (Simonin et al. 1990). Many questions remain about the etiology of early mortality syndrome (EMS), but low egg thiamine concentrations have been linked with the various mortality syndromes.

Total thiamine concentration in lake trout eggs collected from lakes with early life stage mortality (Fitzsimons and Brown 1995) were 1.28 nmol/g for Charleston Lake, 2.25 nmol/g for Lake Ontario, 3.2 nmol/g for Lake Erie, and 3.4 nmol/g for Lake Michigan. In the same report, egg thiamine concentrations were higher in lakes where EMS was absent: 9.0 nmol/g for Lake Simcoe, 14.7 nmol/g for Lake Superior, 15.1 nmol/g for Lake Manitou, 25.3 nmol/g for Lake 375, and 32.1 nmol/g for Lake 442. Similarly, in Lake Michigan coho salmon, three studies have reported low egg thiamine concentrations in groups exhibiting high incidence of EMS (1.2–1.9 nmol/g, Marcquenski and Brown 1997; less than 0.9 nmol/g, Hornung et al. 1995; and 1.1–1.8 nmol/g, Honeyfield et al. 1998, this volume). Fry loss was absent or minimal in coho eggs from Lake Michigan with total thiamine concentrations greater than 0.9 nmol/g (Hornung et al. 1995) and 2.1–6.3 nmol/g (Honeyfield et al. 1998) and in coho eggs from Lake Superior with concentrations of 65 nmol/g (Marcquenski and Brown 1997). Finally, studies with Baltic Sea salmon (Amcoff et al. 1995) and Atlantic salmon (Fisher et al. 1996) reported high incidences of fry loss when total egg thiamine was less than 1.0 nmol/g. These data suggest that there is a critical threshold concentration for the onset of EMS.

Fry survival can be improved by water hardening eggs or immersing sac fry in a thiamine solution (Bylund and Lerche 1995; Koski et al. 1995; Fisher et al. 1996). Although these results do not constitute evidence of a cause and effect relationship, they do indicate that thiamine likely plays an important role in the development of EMS.

In related research, other water-soluble vitamins and thyroxine gave variable results, but they were generally less effective than thiamine in the treatment of EMS. Fitzsimons (1995) found that riboflavin, folic acid, nicotinic acid, and pyridoxine had no beneficial effect. In contrast, Hornung et al. (1995) found that treatment of fry with 2 mg/L thyroxine reduced EMS-related mortality from 40 to 17%. J. Hnath (Michigan Department of Natural Resources, personal communication) found a 40% improvement in fry survival of Lake Michigan chinook salmon by treating fry in an immersion bath of vitamin C (100–1,000 mg/L). The metabolic functions of thyroxine and ascorbic acid are different from that of thiamine. Therefore, it remains to be determined if the beneficial effects of thyroxine and ascorbic acid can be substantiated by others and shown to be directly related to EMS. One hypothesis for the cause of low concentrations of thiamine in eggs concerns a thiamine-destroying enzyme, thiaminase, in forage fish. Rainbow smelt *Osmerus mordax* and alewife *Alosa pseudoharengus* are forage fishes of salmonids and are known to contain high levels of thiaminase (Neilands 1947; Gnaedinger and Krzeczkowski 1966). Among the Great Lakes, the occurrence of EMS is high in Lakes Michigan and Ontario, low in Lake Erie (Fitzsimons et al. 1995), and nonexistent in Lakes Superior and Huron (Mac et al. 1985). In the New York Finger Lakes, the syndrome afflicts Atlantic salmon from Cayuga, Keuka, and Seneca lakes, all of which have alewife and smelt populations (Fisher et al. 1996).

TABLE 1.—Composition of experimental diets.

Ingredient	Composition (%) Diet 1	Diet 2	Diet 3
Herring meal (70%)	32.0	32.0	32.0
Corn gluten meal	18.0	18.0	18.0
Blood flour	8.6	8.6	8.6
Herring oil	8.0	8.0	8.0
Dextrin	30.0	29.95	29.9
Choline chloride	0.5	0.5	0.5
Vitamin premix[a]	0.5	0.5	0.5
Mineral premix[b]	0.2	0.2	0.2
Ascorbic acid	0.2	0.2	0.2
Ameribond, pellet binder	2.0	2.0	2.0
Amprolium chloride	0.0	0.05	0.1

[a] Vitamin premix supplied per kilogram of diet: vitamin A, 3,297 IU; vitamin D, 220 IU; vitamin E, 175 IU; vitamin K, 5.5 mg; ascorbic acid, 330 mg; biotin, 180 mg; vitamin B_{12}, 10 mg; folic acid, 4.4 mg; niacin, 110 mg; pantothenate, 50 mg; pyridoxine, 15.5 mg; riboflavin, 30 mg; thiamine, 17.6 mg (diet 1 only).

[b] Mineral premix (Bernhart-Tomarelli, ICN Nutritional Biochemical, Cleveland, Ohio) supplied per kilogram of diet: calcium carbonate, 630 mg; calcium phosphate, 22,050 mg; citric acid, 68.1 mg; cupric citrate-2½ H_2O, 13.8 mg; ferric citrate-5H_2O, 1,674 mg; magnesium oxide, 750 mg; manganese citrate, 250.5 mg; potassium iodide, 0.3 mg; potassium phosphate dibasic, 2,430 mg; potassium sulfate, 2,040 mg; sodium chloride, 918 mg; sodium phosphate, 64.2 mg; zinc citrate-2H_2O, 39.9 mg.

In contrast, fish from Skaneateles Lake, which has neither smelt nor alewife, are not afflicted with EMS. Thus, Fisher et al. (1996) have proposed that EMS is a result of fishes consuming alewives and smelt.

Mac et al. (1985) suggested that EMS in lake trout is caused by contaminants; however, no direct cause and effect connection has been demonstrated (Fitzsimons et al. 1995). Furthermore, the incidence of EMS has increased while levels of organochlorine and heavy metal toxicants that are widely measured in fish flesh have decreased (Leatherland 1993). Lesser known contaminants or their metabolites have not been ruled out; of particular concern are those compounds that act on the endocrine system. Exposure of fishes to endocrine-disrupting compounds has been associated with a decrease in fertility (Moccia et al. 1986; Leatherland 1993, 1994; Hontela et al. 1995). One conclusion that may be drawn is that

TABLE 2.—Mean levels of thiamine pyrophosphate (TPP), thiamine monophosphate (TP), and free thiamine (T) in eggs of lake trout fed three levels of amprolium. Means with the same letters in the same column are not significantly different ($P > 0.01$).

	Mean egg concentration			
Diet	TPP	TP	T	*N*
Diet 1, 0% amprolium	0.29 z	0.35 z	61.78 z	12
Diet 2, 0.05% amprolium	0.25 yz	0.34 z	4.02 y	9
Diet 3, 0.10% amprolium	0.15 y	0.20 z	1.71 y	6
Diet 3, 0.10% amprolium (Aug)	0.13 y	0.27 z	11.59 y	9
Pooled SE	0.02	0.04	4.49	

if contaminants are involved in the etiology of EMS, and given the fact that there is an absence of typical signs and pathology of acute or chronic toxicity, then the role of contaminants is through an unidentified mechanism.

Early mortality syndrome has not previously been experimentally induced in broodstock under laboratory conditions. Experimental injection of healthy lake trout fry with pyrithiamine, a thiamine antagonist, has resulted in fry mortality resembling that of EMS (J. D. Fitzsimons, Bayfield Institute, personal communication). Thiamine deficiency has been reported in carp *Cyprinus carpio* and rainbow trout (nonanadromous *Oncorhynchus mykiss*) fed diets containing amprolium, a thiamine antagonist (Aoe et al. 1969). A means of reproducing EMS in the laboratory would facilitate the search for the cause of EMS. Therefore, the objectives of this study were to evaluate the ability of amprolium to reduce egg thiamine concentrations in lake trout and to determine if EMS symptoms could be produced in fry hatched from eggs of lake trout fed amprolium.

Materials and Methods

Diets were formulated with 29–30% dextrin to be high in carbohydrates (Table 1) to increase the metabolic demand for thiamine. Amprolium was supplemented at three concentrations (0, 0.05, and 0.10%). Dietary ingredients were chosen to produce a low-thiamine feed. First time spawning 4-year-old lake trout were allocated to one of four dietary treatments. Fish on three of the four treatments were fed the basic test diet with 0, 0.05, or 0.10% amprolium added, beginning 1 April 1995 through spawning in October and November 1995. Fish in the fourth treatment group were fed a commercial broodstock feed (Zeigler Brothers, Inc., Gardners, Pennsylvania) from April through July followed by diet 3 containing 0.10% amprolium from 1 August through spawning. The delay in administration of amprolium to the fourth group was to correspond with an expected surge in vitellogenesis. Therefore the fourth treatment was to determine the effect of amprolium on egg thiamine concentrations when amprolium was given only during the latter stages of egg maturation.

Adult lake trout (Seneca strain) were maintained in 2.74-m circular tanks adjacent to large windows inside the fish culture laboratory. All aspects of physical behavior, number of fish spawning, and number of eggs per female in the experimental fish were the same as in fish maintained in outside facilities. Standard hatchery practices for salmonids (Piper et al. 1982) were used for spawning, fertilization, and egg incubation. Eggs were incubated in Heath trays. Well water with a constant temperature of 9°C was used throughout the study.

Tissue, red blood cell, and egg concentrations of free thiamine, thiamine monophosphate, and thiamine pyrophosphate were determined using the high-pressure liquid chromatography method of Brown et al. (1998, this volume). Blood samples were collected on 15 June, 28 July, and at spawning (October–November). Fish were sedated with tricaine methanesulfonate (MS-222) and blood was collected from the tail vein in heparinized syringes. Blood was centrifuged to remove the plasma. Red blood cells were resuspended in normal saline and centrifuged twice. Washed cells were stored frozen (−80°C). At spawning, four fish per treatment group were killed using an overdose of MS-222. Tissue was immediately collected and stored frozen (−80°C) for analysis of thiamine concentrations. Eggs from 6 to 12 fishes were collected from each treatment group and an aliquot of their eggs was incubated. The incidence of EMS in the fry was monitored from hatching through swim-up by visual observation for symptoms. The remaining unfertilized eggs were stored frozen for thiamine analysis. Data were analyzed as a completely randomized design using the General

TABLE 3.—Mean levels of thiamine pyrophosphate (TPP), thiamine monophosphate (TP), and free thiamine (T) in tissues of lake trout fed three levels of amprolium. Means with the same letter in the same column are not significantly different ($P > 0.01$).

	Mean tissue concentration (nmol/g of wet tissue)											
	Liver			Muscle			Kidney			Heart		
Diet	TPP	TP	T	TPP	TP	T	TPP	TP	T	TPP	TP	T
Diet 1[a]	5.32 z	2.59 yz	1.80 z	4.10 z	0.80 z	0.35 yz	2.15	1.51	1.07	41.20 z	11.01 z	4.37 z
Diet 2[b]	3.68 yz	2.88 yz	1.02 y	1.93 y	0.44 y	0.35 yz	2.40	1.69	2.14	15.20 x	3.57 y	0.92 y
Diet 3[c]	3.33 y	1.83 y	1.51 yz	1.01 y	0.23 y	0.31 y	1.57	1.09	0.50	9.45 x	3.14 y	1.59 y
Diet 3[c] (Aug)	4.50 yz	3.59 z	1.70 yz	3.90 z	0.83 z	0.38 z	1.50	1.11	1.04	24.38 y	5.24 y	1.01 y
Pooled SE	0.32	0.24	0.15	0.37	0.07	0.01	0.25	0.16	0.27	3.51	0.96	0.41

[a] Diet 1, 0% amprolium.
[b] Diet 2, 0.05% amprolium.
[c] Diet 3, 0.10% amprolium.

Linear Model of SAS for means and analysis of variance (SAS 1994). Differences among means were separated using Duncan's new multiple-range test (SAS 1994).

Results and Discussion

This study with lake trout and an associated study with Atlantic salmon (Fynn-Aikins et al., in press) constitute steps toward developing a laboratory model for the study of EMS. The data show that dietary amprolium is an effective thiamine antagonist that reduces the deposition of thiamine into the egg.

Free thiamine is the predominant form of thiamine found in lake trout eggs (Table 2). Fish fed no amprolium had higher levels of free thiamine in eggs than fish fed either 0.05 or 0.10% amprolium. Lake trout fed 0.10% amprolium beginning in August (versus April) also had significantly lower thiamine levels than the controls. In August there is a significant increase in estrogen-stimulated vitellogenesis in salmonids (Crim and Idler 1978). In addition, estrogen stimulates the synthesis of a thiamine carrier protein in avian and amphibian species, and it has been postulated that this estrogen-stimulated thiamine carrier protein is specific for the transport of thiamine into the eggs of fish as well (Adiga and Murty 1983). The results from fish fed amprolium starting in August are consistent with the hypothesis that a carrier protein exists. Thiamine values for the group fed amprolium beginning in August were more variable than those observed in the other treatment groups. Free thiamine values ranged from 1.36 to 46.52 nmol/g of egg in the August group, and if the highest two values are removed from the data, the mean changes from 11.59 to 5.56 nmol/g. This latter mean is numerically similar to that found with diet 2, which suggests that feeding lake trout broodstock a thiamine antagonist during the latter phase of egg development will result in lower, but highly variable, egg thiamine levels among individual fishes.

In contrast to the egg data, the predominant form of thiamine found in liver, muscle, kidney, and heart (Table 3) was thiamine pyrophosphate (TPP), which is the active form or the cofactor in thiamine-containing enzymes (Gubler 1991). Heart tissue from fish fed no amprolium contained the highest level of TPP, followed by liver and muscle. There was a decrease in TPP concentration in these three tissues when fish were fed diets containing 0.10% amprolium from April through spawning. Muscle TPP was similar between the groups fed no amprolium and those fed 0.10% amprolium beginning in August. Lake Michigan coho salmon with high, medium, and low incidences of EMS showed no differences in muscle TPP concentrations (Honeyfield et al. 1998). When Atlantic salmon were fed three dietary levels of amprolium, as in the present lake trout study (April through spawning), no differences were observed in muscle TPP (Fynn-Aikins et al., in press). In contrast, lake trout fed a thiamine antagonist beginning in April had lower muscle concentrations of thiamine. It appears that lake trout stores of thiamine are more labile than those of Atlantic salmon and possibly coho salmon muscle.

The effect of amprolium on red blood cell (RBC) concentration of thiamine (Table 4) was measurable at first sampling (15 June). Total thiamine and TPP in RBC were reduced as dietary levels of amprolium increased ($P < 0.05$). Free thiamine and thiamine monophosphate levels in RBC from fish fed 0.10% amprolium were lower than those from fish fed no amprolium. Total thiamine concentration in RBCs decreased from June through spawning with all three

TABLE 4.—Mean concentrations of thiamine pyrophosphate (TPP), thiamine monophosphate (TP), and free thiamine (T) in red blood cells of lake trout fed three levels of amprolium. Means with the same letters in the same column within a sampling period are not significantly different ($P > 0.05$).

Diet	Red blood cell concentration (nmol/g of wet tissue)			Total
	TPP	TP	T	thiamine
		15 June		
Diet 1[a]	1.34 z	0.87 z	0.33 z	2.54 z
Diet 2[b]	0.66 y	0.22 y	0.12 yz	0.99 y
Diet 3[c]	0.39 x	0.16 y	0.03 y	0.58 x
Pooled SE	0.150	0.085	0.130	0.191
		28 July		
Diet 1[a]	0.14 z	0.91 z	0.35 z	1.39 z
Diet 2[b]	0.08 y	0.29 y	0.42 y	0.78 y
Diet 3[c]	0.08 y	0.19 y	0.45 x	0.72 y
Pooled SE	0.020	0.223	0.015	0.225
		Spawning (Oct–Nov)		
Diet 1[a]	0.22 z	0.24 z	0.17 z	0.63 z
Diet 2[b]	0.15 yz	0.11 y	0.15 zy	0.40 y
Diet 3[c]	0.08 y	0.08 y	0.14 y	0.30 y
Pooled SE	0.069	0.046	0.015	0.117

[a] Diet 1, 0% amprolium.
[b] Diet 2, 0.05% amprolium.
[c] Diet 3, 0.10% amprolium.

dietary treatments. We surmise that the lowest levels observed at spawning were related to the fasting state of the fish. Feed was offered daily up to 2 weeks before spawning, although feed intake decreased in early September and all feeding ceased by mid to late October, or approximately 1 month before spawning. From this we concluded that RBC thiamine concentrations are affected by amprolium and are a function of time. However, in nonreproductive fish, RBC TPP concentrations of young rainbow trout did not decrease during a 30-week study (Masumoto et al. 1987). Thus, the use of a single RBC thiamine measurement cannot reliably determine thiamine status in reproductive lake trout.

No EMS deaths were observed in fry of lake trout in the present study. The lack of signs of EMS is in contrast to our Atlantic salmon study, in which EMS was observed (Fynn-Aikins et al., in press). In both studies, egg concentration of thiamine was reduced with amprolium, demonstrating that amprolium is an effective experimental tool for reducing egg thiamine levels. The presence of fry mortality in Atlantic salmon and not in lake trout suggests that species differences exist or that multiple factors interact to cause EMS.

General observations about the adult lake trout fed amprolium are unremarkable. Spawning, health, and physical appearance were similar to those of lake trout not fed experimental diets. The only observation that can be made about fry from fish fed experimental diets with or without amprolium is that the fry tended to be slower to swim-up by 3–5 d compared with fry from fish fed commercial feed. This did not appear to be related to EMS. Otherwise, no signs or symptoms of EMS were observed.

References

Adiga, P. R., and C. V. R. Murty. 1983. Vitamin carrier proteins during embryonic development in birds and mammals. Pages 111–136 *in* R. Porter and J. Whelan, editors. Molecular biology of egg maturation. Pitman Books, London.

Amcoff, P., L. Norrgren, H. Borjeson, and J. Lindeberg. 1995. Lowered concentrations of thiamine (vitamin B_1) in M74-affected feral Baltic salmon (*Salmo salar*). Pages 38–39 *in* Bengtsson et al. (1995).

Aoe, H., and five coauthors. 1969. Water-soluble vitamin requirements of carp - VI. Requirement for thiamine and effects of antihistamines. Bulletin of the Japanese Society of Scientific Fisheries 35:459–465.

Bengtsson, B.-E., C. Hill, and S. Nellbring, editors. 1995. Report from the second workshop on reproduction disturbances in fish. Swedish Environmental Protection Agency Report 4534, Stockholm.

Bengtsson, B. E., and six coauthors. 1994. Reproductive disturbances in Baltic fish. Swedish Environmental Protection Agency Report 4319, Stockholm.

Brown, S. B., D. C. Honeyfield, and L. Vandenbyllaardt. 1998. Thiamine analysis in fish tissues. Pages 73–81 *in* G. McDonald, J. D. Fitzsimons, and D. C. Honeyfield, editors. Early life stage mortality syndrome in fishes of the Great Lakes and Baltic Sea. American Fisheries Society, Symposium 21, Bethesda, Maryland.

Bylund, G., and O. Lerche. 1995. Thiamine therapy of M74 affected fry of Atlantic salmon, *Salmo salar*. Bulletin of the European Association of Fish Pathologists 15(3):93–97.

Crim, L. W., and D. R. Idler. 1978. Plasma gonadotropin, estradiol and vitellogenin and gonad phosvitin levels in relation to the seasonal reproductive cycles of female brown trout. Annales de Biologie Animale Biochimie Biophysique 18:1001–1005.

Fisher, J. P., J. D. Fitzsimons, G. F. Combs, Jr., and J. M. Spitzbergan. 1996. Naturally occurring thiamine deficiency causing reproductive failure in Finger Lakes Atlantic salmon and Great Lakes trout. Transactions of the American Fisheries Society 125:167–178.

Fisher, J. P., and six coauthors. 1995. Reproductive failure in landlocked Atlantic salmon from New York's Finger Lakes: investigations into the etiology and epidemiology of the "Cayuga syndrome." Journal of Aquatic Animal Health 7:81–94.

Fitzsimons, J. D. 1995. The effect of B-vitamins on a swim-up syndrome in Lake Ontario lake trout. Journal of Great Lakes Research 21(Supplement 1):286–289.

Fitzsimons, J., and S. Brown. 1995. Effect of diet on thiamine levels in Great Lakes Lake trout and relationship with early mortality syndrome. Pages 76–78 *in* Bengtsson et al. (1995).

Fitzsimons, J. D., S. Huestis, and B. Williston. 1995. Occurrence of a swim-up syndrome in Lake Ontario lake trout in relation to contaminants and cultural practices. Journal of Great Lakes Research 21(Supplement 1):277–285.

Fynn-Aikins, K., P. R. Bowser, D. C. Honeyfield, J. D. Fitzsimons, and H. G. Ketola. In press. Effect of dietary amprolium on tissue thiamin and Cayuga syndrome in Atlantic salmon. Transactions of the American Fisheries Society.

Gubler, C. J. 1991. Thiamin. Pages 233–280 *in* L. J. Machlin, editor. Handbook of vitamins, second edition. Marcel Dekker, New York.

Gnaedinger, R. H., and R. A. Krzeczkowski. 1966. Heat inactivation of thiaminase in whole fish. Commercial Fisheries Review 28(8):11–14.

Honeyfield, D. C., J. G. Hnath, J. Copeland, K. Dabrowski, and J. H. Blom. 1998. Correlation of nutrients and environmental contaminants in Lake Michigan coho salmon with incidence of early mortality syndrome. Pages 135–145 *in* G. McDonald, J. D. Fitzsimons, and D.C. Honeyfield, editors. Early life stage mortality syndrome in fishes of the Great Lakes and Baltic Sea. American Fisheries Society, Symposium 21, Bethesda, Maryland.

Hontela, A., P. Dumont, D. Duclos, and R. Fortin. 1995. Endocrine and metabolic dysfunction in yellow perch, *Perca flavescens*, exposed to organic contaminants and heavy metals in the St. Lawrence River. Environmental Toxicology and Chemistry 14:725–731.

Hornung, M. W., L. Miller, R. E. Peterson, S. V. Marcquenski, and S. Brown. 1995. Evaluation of nutritional and pathogenic factors in early mortality syndrome in Lake Michigan salmonids. Pages 82–83 *in* Bengtsson et al. (1995).

Johansson, N., P. Jonsson, O. Svanberg, A. Sodergren, and J. Thulin. 1995. Reproduction disorders in Baltic fish. Swedish Environmental Protection Agency Report 4347, Solna.

Koski, P., M. Pakarinen, and A. Soivio. 1995. A dose-response study of thiamine hydrochloride bathing for the prevention of yolk-sac mortality in Baltic salmon fry (M74 syndrome). Page 46 *in* Bengtsson et al. (1995).

Leatherland, J. F. 1993. Field observations on reproductive and developmental dysfunction of introduced and native salmonids from the Great Lakes. Journal of Great Lakes Research 19:737–751.

Leatherland, J. F. 1994. Reflections on the thyroidology of fishes: from molecules to humankind. Guelph Ichthyology Review 2:1–67.

Mac, M. J., C. C. Edsall, and J. G. Seelye. 1985. Survival of lake trout eggs and fry reared in water from the upper Great Lakes. Journal of Great Lakes Research 11:520–529.

Marcquenski, S. V., and S. B. Brown. 1997. Early mortality syndrome in the Great Lakes. Pages 135–153 *in* R. M. Rolland, M. Gilbertson, and R. E. Peterson, editors. Chemically induced alterations in functional development and reproduction in fishes. SETAC (Society of Environmental Toxicology and Chemistry), Pensacola, Florida.

Masumoto, T., R. W. Hardy, and E. Casillas. 1987. Comparison of transketolase activity and thiamine pyrophosphate levels in erythrocytes and liver of rainbow trout (*Salmo gairdneri*) as indications of thiamin status. Journal of Nutrition 117:1422–1426.

Moccia, R., G. Fox, and A. J. Britton. 1986. A quantitative assessment of thyroid histopathology of herring gull (*Larus argentatus*) from the Great Lakes and a hypothesis on the causal role of environmental contaminants. Journal of Wildlife Diseases 22:60–70.

Neilands, J. B. 1947. Thiaminase in aquatic animals of Nova Scotia. Journal of the Fisheries Research Board of Canada 7:94–99.

Norrgren, L., editor. 1994. Report from the Uppsala workshop on reproduction disturbances in fish. Swedish Environmental Protection Agency Report 4346, Uppsala.

Piper, R. G., and five coauthors. 1982. Fish hatchery management. U.S. Fish and Wildlife Service, Washington, DC.

SAS (Statistical Analysis System). 1994. SAS/STAT guide for personal computers, version 6.10. SAS Institute Inc., Cary, North Carolina.

Simonin, H., J. Skea, H. Dean, and J. Symula. 1990. Summary of reproductive studies of Lake Ontario salmonids. Pages 15–16 *in* M. Mac and M. Gilbertson, editors. Proceedings of the roundtable on contaminant-caused reproductive problems in salmonids. Great Lakes Science Advisory Board, Biological Effects Subcommittee, Windsor, Ontario.